MW00835562

Advancing Nursing Practice

Exploring Roles and Opportunities for Clinicians, Educators, and Leaders

Advancing Nursing Practice

Exploring Roles and Opportunities for Clinicians, Educators, and Leaders

Carolyn Hart, PhD, RN, CNE

Dean of Nursing and Associate Professor
Coker University
Hartsville, South Carolina

Pegge L. Bell, PhD, RN, WHNP

Dean, College of Nursing & Health Sciences (retired)
Barry University
Miami Shores, Florida

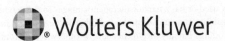 Wolters Kluwer

Philadelphia • Baltimore • New York • London
Buenos Aires • Hong Kong • Sydney • Tokyo

Vice President and Publisher: Julie K. Stegman
Manager, Nursing Education and Practice Content: Jamie Blum
Acquisitions Editor: Michael Kerns
Senior Development Editor: Julie Vitale
Editorial Coordinator: Vinoth Ezhumalai
Editorial Assistant: Molly Kennedy
Marketing Manager: Brittany Clements
Senior Production Project Manager: Alicia Jackson
Manager, Graphic Arts & Design: Steve Druding
Art Director: Jennifer Clements
Manufacturing Coordinator: Karin Duffield
Prepress Vendor: TNQ Technologies

Copyright © 2022 Wolters Kluwer.

All rights reserved. This book is protected by copyright. No part of this book may be reproduced or transmitted in any form or by any means, including as photocopies or scanned-in or other electronic copies, or utilized by any information storage and retrieval system without written permission from the copyright owner, except for brief quotations embodied in critical articles and reviews. Materials appearing in this book prepared by individuals as part of their official duties as U.S. government employees are not covered by the above-mentioned copyright. To request permission, please contact Wolters Kluwer at Two Commerce Square, 2001 Market Street, Philadelphia, PA 19103, via email at permissions@lww.com, or via our website at shop.lww.com (products and services). 12/2020

9 8 7 6 5 4 3 2 1

Printed in China

Library of Congress Cataloging-in-Publication Data

ISBN-13: 978-1-975111-72-4

Cataloging in Publication data available on request from publisher.

This work is provided "as is," and the publisher disclaims any and all warranties, express or implied, including any warranties as to accuracy, comprehensiveness, or currency of the content of this work.

This work is no substitute for individual patient assessment based upon healthcare professionals' examination of each patient and consideration of, among other things, age, weight, gender, current or prior medical conditions, medication history, laboratory data and other factors unique to the patient. The publisher does not provide medical advice or guidance and this work is merely a reference tool. Healthcare professionals, and not the publisher, are solely responsible for the use of this work including all medical judgments and for any resulting diagnosis and treatments.

Given continuous, rapid advances in medical science and health information, independent professional verification of medical diagnoses, indications, appropriate pharmaceutical selections and dosages, and treatment options should be made and healthcare professionals should consult a variety of sources. When prescribing medication, healthcare professionals are advised to consult the product information sheet (the manufacturer's package insert) accompanying each drug to verify, among other things, conditions of use, warnings and side effects and identify any changes in dosage schedule or contraindications, particularly if the medication to be administered is new, infrequently used or has a narrow therapeutic range. To the maximum extent permitted under applicable law, no responsibility is assumed by the publisher for any injury and/or damage to persons or property, as a matter of products liability, negligence law or otherwise, or from any reference to or use by any person of this work.

shop.lww.com

DEDICATION

I would not be here without acknowledging the sage advice and encouragement from my mentors Diane Billings, Laura Dzurec, and Pegge L. Bell. I will forever be grateful to you for showing me how nursing leaders can truly help and inspire others. To Michelle, Sara, Matt, and Philip—you are my best inspiration. To Matt, Chris, Alex, Amina, and Aria—you bring such happiness to my life!

Carolyn Hart

This venture represents Carolyn's goal of writing a book that inspires career advancement for nurses. I am honored to share in her vision for the book and admire her unwavering commitment despite challenges and a pandemic. I hope this book impresses my daughter, Brooke, who is a natural at writing and a walking thesaurus.

Pegge L. Bell

IN MEMORIAM

We also wish to honor the memory of our colleague, Dr. Anne Thomas. She did not hesitate to support and encourage the work of all nurses and made significant contributions that advanced the profession. Her *In Their Own Words* in Chapter 7 offers only a glimpse into her remarkable accomplishments. Dr. Thomas held leadership roles with the National Organization of Nurse Practitioner Faculties (NONPF), the American Nurses Credentialing Center (ANCC), the American Association of Critical-Care Nurses (AACN), and the Commission on Collegiate Nursing Education (CCNE). As an adult/gerontological nurse practitioner, Dr. Thomas worked in rural, long-term care, occupational, and mental health-care settings. Additionally, she was the director for Research Nursing within the Medical Oncology Research Clinical Unit at the National Cancer Institute and the Director of the Health Promotion Laboratory at the National Institute for Nursing Research. Dr. Thomas served as a mentor and faculty member for Sigma Theta Tau's "Emerging Educational Administrator Institute" where she generously shared her knowledge with future nurse educator leaders across the country. In recognition of her leadership and sustained commitment to NP education and practice, she was named a Fellow in AANP in 2012. We hope that through this text, we can inspire other nurses to continue in her footsteps.

Carolyn Hart and Pegge L. Bell

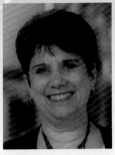

Carolyn Hart, PhD, RN, CNE

Dr. Hart received her diploma in nursing from the Lancaster General School of Nursing in Lancaster, Pennsylvania. Most of her bedside experience in nursing was in the Trauma-Neuro ICU at Lancaster General where she credits her nursing expertise to the mentorship of senior nurses in that unit. In 2002, she received the Weidman Award in Nursing Excellence.

Dr. Hart continued her studies and obtained a BSN from Chamberlain College of Nursing in 2008 and an MSN in Nursing Education from South University in 2009. In 2012, she graduated from the University of Missouri in Kansas City with a PhD in Nursing. Her dissertation topic was development of the Persistence Scale for Online Education in Nursing. Dr. Hart is the only nurse to have attended all three Sigma Theta Tau International Leadership Academies. As a result of these experiences, she specializes in developing new nursing programs that are innovative in meeting the needs of students and communities.

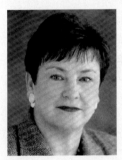

Pegge L. Bell, PhD, RN, WHNP

Dr. Bell began her nursing career after completing an ADN in 1973 from what is now Columbus State University in Georgia. Her clinical experience has since focused on maternal-child services. She completed her BSN in 1976 at Georgia Southwestern University and the MSN from the University of Alabama in Birmingham in 1979. After years of teaching maternal-child nursing, she then assumed academic leadership positions. She completed her PhD at the University of Virginia where she chose the Complex Organizations in Nursing specialization. Returning to an academic position she took the opportunity to complete the women's health nurse practitioner post-MSN certificate. This allowed her to have a faculty practice, opening a new family planning clinic at a local high school, a collaboration with the Arkansas Department of Health. Dr. Bell held several academic administrative positions and used that knowledge to lead the development of Sigma's Emerging Educational Administrator Institute, while also serving as consultant for Sigma's Maternal Child Health Academy sponsored by Johnson and Johnson. She values her legacy of developing nursing leaders and continues to be available for her past mentees.

Contributors

Valerie A. Adelson, MHA, BSN, RN
Senior Consultant
Federal Compliance Consulting
Washington, DC

Nagia Ali, PhD, RN
Professor of Nursing
Ball State University
Muncie, Indiana

Omar Ali, MSN, RN-BC
Staff Nurse II
Eskenazi Health
Indianapolis, Indiana

Kim Amsley-Camp, CNM, MS
Certified Midwife
Keystone Health
Chambersburg, Pennsylvania

Pegge L. Bell, PhD, RN, WHNP
Dean, College of Nursing & Health
    Sciences (retired)
Barry University
Miami Shores, Florida

Grace Buttriss, DNP, RN, CNL
Clinical Nurse Leader Coordinator
Presbyterian School of Nursing
Queens University of Charlotte
Charlotte, North Carolina

Jennifer L. Embree, DNP, RN, NE-BC,
CCNS
Clinical Associate Professor
IU School of Nursing
MSN Leadership in Health Systems
    Coordinator
Magnet Coordinator Eskenazi Health
Indianapolis, Indiana

Carolyn Hart, PhD, RN, CNE
Dean of Nursing and Associate
    Professor
Coker University
Hartsville, South Carolina

Carol Huston, MSN, DPA, FAAN
Professor Emerita
School of Nursing, Trinity Hall
California State University
Chico, California

Anna Jarrett, PhD, ACNS-BC,
ACNP-BC, FNP-BC
Assistant Professor
Eleanor Mann School of Nursing
University of Arkansas
Fayetteville, Arkansas

Kelly Vowell Johnson, EdD, RN
Assistant Professor
Eleanor Mann School of Nursing
University of Arkansas
Fayetteville, Arkansas

John McFadden, PhD, CRNA
Dean and Professor
College of Nursing & Health
    Sciences
Barry University
Miami Shores, Florida

Annie Moore-Cox, PhD, RN
ATI Nursing Education
Strategic Account Executive

Karen Morin, PhD, RN, ANEF, FAAN
Professor Emerita
Associate Editor, *Journal of Clinical
    Nursing*
University of Wisconsin-Milwaukee
Milwaukee, Wisconsin

Margaret Norton-Rosko, DNP, RN,
NEA-BC
Regional Chief Nursing Officer
Loyola Medicine
Chicago, Illinois

Allison L. Scott, DNP, PPCNP-BC, IBCLC
Assistant Professor
Eleanor Mann School of Nursing
University of Arkansas
Fayetteville, Arkansas

Marilou Shreve, DNP, CPNP-BC
Assistant Professor
Eleanor Mann School of Nursing
University of Arkansas
Fayetteville, Arkansas

Tony Umadhay, PhD, CRNA
Associate Professor of
    Anesthesiology & Associate Dean
    for Academic Affairs
College of Nursing & Health
    Sciences
Barry University
Miami Shores, Florida

Cindy Weston, DNP, RN, CCRN,
CNS-CC, FNP-BC
Associate Dean for Clinical and
    Outreach Affairs and Associate
    Professor
College of Nursing
Texas A&M University
Bryan, Texas

In Their Own Words Contributors

Melissa Abreu, MSN-Ed, RN
Scholar's Faculty, Scholars Program
Baptist Health Center for the
 Advancement of Learning
Miami, Florida

Kim Amsley-Camp, CNM, MS
Certified Midwife
Keystone Health
Chambersburg, Pennsylvania

Victoria L. Asturrizaga, MSN, CNM
Jefferson Health
Rowan SOM Department of
 Obstetrics and Gynecology
Sewell, New Jersey

Julia Burke, MSN, RNC-OB, C-EFM
Clinical Educator-Women's and
 Children's Department
Clinical Education & Professional
 Development
Thomas Jefferson University
 Hospitals
Jefferson Health
Turnersville, New Jersey

Cathy Catrambone, PhD, RN, FAAN
Past President, Sigma Theta Tau
 International
Associate Professor
Department of Adult Health and
 Gerontological Nursing
College of Nursing
Rush University
Chicago, Illinois

Joanne Cochran, PhD, CNS, RN
President and CEO
Keystone Health
Chambersburg, Pennsylvania

Cathy Collins-Fulea, DNP, CNM, FACNM
President, American College of
 Nurse-Midwives
Assistant Professor
DNP Clinical Faculty
Frontier Nursing University Hyden,
 Kentucky

Loretta Ford, EdD, NP, FAAN
Co-Founder of the first nurse
 practitioner program
National Women's Hall of Fame
Living Legend of the American
 Academy of Nursing

Jodie C. Gary, PhD, RN
Assistant Professor
College of Nursing
Texas A&M University
Bryan, Texas

Judith Halstead, PhD, RN, FAAN, ANEF
Executive Director
NLN Commission for Nursing
    Education
Accreditation (CNEA)
Past President, National League for
    Nursing

Shakira Henderson, PhD, DNP, MS,
MPH, RNC-NIC, IBCLC
Sr. Administrator, Center for
    Research and Grants
Vidant Health
Greenville, North Carolina

Kathleen E. Hubner, MSN, APRN,
ACNS-BC, ANVP, CNRN
Acute Neurovascular Clinical Nurse
    Specialist and Stroke Coordinator
St. Vincent Neuroscience Institute
Indianapolis, Indiana

Martha Johnson
Deputy CEO/Chief Development
    Officer
Rosemount Center
Washington, DC

Michele Kilmer, DNP, APRN, CPNP-PC
Assistant Professor
The University of Arkansas
Eleanor Mann School of Nursing
Fayetteville, Arkansas

Carol Klingbeil, NDP, RN, CPNP-PC
DNP Program Director
University of Milwaukee
Milwaukee, Wisconsin

Francesca C. Levitt, MSN, RN-BC,
ACNS-BC
Hendricks Regional Health
Danville, Indiana

Kim Litwack, PhD, RN, FAAN, APNP
Dean and Professor
University of Milwaukee
Milwaukee, Wisconsin

Holly Ma, MS, RN, BSN, CRN
Director of Nursing Professional
    Development and Education
Adult Academic Health Center at
    Indiana University Health
Indianapolis, Indiana

John McFadden, PhD, CRNA
Dean and Professor
College of Nursing & Health
    Sciences
Barry University
Miami Shores, Florida

Margaret Norton-Rosko, DNP, RN, NEA-BC
Regional Chief Nursing Officer
Loyola Medicine
Chicago, Illinois

Victor Ospina, DNP, APRN, ACNP-BC, CCRN
Corporate Director
Nursing and Health Sciences Research
Baptist Health South Florida
Miami, Florida

Barbara J. Patterson, PhD, ANEF, FAAN
Professor, Director PhD Program
Associate Dean for Scholarship & Inquiry
Widener University
Chester, Pennsylvania

Veronica Rankin, MSN, NP-C, CNL, RN-BC, CMSRN
Clinical Nurse Leader Program Coordinator
Carolinas Medical Center
Charlotte, North Carolina

Sean M. Reed, PhD, APN, ACNS-BC, ACHPN
President, National Association of Clinical Nurse Specialists
Assistant Professor
University of Colorado
Denver, Colorado

Sarah Rhoads, PhD, DNP, WHNP-BC, FAAN
Professor, The University of Tennessee Health Science Center
Memphis, Tennessee

Victoria L. Rich, PhD, RN, FAAN
Dean of Nursing, University of South Florida College of Nursing
Tampa, Florida
Retired Chief Nurse Executive for The University of Pennsylvania Healthcare System
Philadelphia, Pennsylvania

Jacqueline S. Rowles, DNP, MBA, MA, CRNA, ANP-BC, FNAP, DAIPM, FAAN
President, Meridian Adult Health, PC
President and Co-Founder, Our Hearts Your Hands
Associate Professor of Professional Practice
Director Advanced Pain Management Fellowship
Texas Christian University School of Nurse Anesthesia
Fort Worth, Texas

Marcella M. Rutherford, PhD, MBA, MSN
Dean, Ron and Kathy Assaf School of Nursing
Nova Southeastern University
Davie, Florida

Rose E. Sherman, EdD, RN, NEA-BC, CNL, FAAN
Professor Emeritus
Christine E Lynn College of Nursing
Florida Atlantic University
Boca Raton, Florida

Bobbi Shirley, MS, RN, CNL, OCN
Clinical Nurse Leader
Maine Medical Center
Portland, Maine

Mary Stachowiak, DNP, RN, CNL
Founding President of the Clinical
  Nurse Leader Association
Assistant Professor and Director of
  the MSN in Clinical Leadership
  Program
Rutgers School of Nursing
Newark, New Jersey

Katie Swafford, DNP, RN, CNS-BC,
CCRN
Director, Infection Prevention &
  Control
Eskenazi Health
Indianapolis, Indiana

Anne Thomas, PhD, RN, AGNP, FAANP
Former Associate Professor
Michigan State University
East Lansing, Michigan

Patricia E. Thompson, EdD, RN, FAAN
Former CEO Sigma Theta Tau
  International
Indianapolis, Indiana

Joan M. Vitello-Cicciu, PhD, RN,
NEA-BC, FAHA, FAAN
Dean of the Graduate School of
  Nursing
University of Massachusetts Medical
  School
Worcester, Massachusetts

Sharon M. Weinstein, MS, RN, CRNI-R,
FACW, FAAN, CSP
Chief Executive Officer of SMW
  Group and the Global Education
  Development Institute
Chicago, Illinois

Edward E. Yackel, DNP, FNP-C, FAANP
Deputy Executive Director
VHA National Center for Patient
  Safety and Healthcare Quality
Veterans Health Administrations
National Center for Patient Safety
Ann Arbor, Michigan

Reviewers

Cailen Baker, DNP, MSN, RN
Chief Nurse Administrator
University of the Cumberlands
Williamsburg, Kentucky

Kimberly Balko, PhD, MSN, RN
Associate Professor
Empire State College
Saratoga Springs, New York

Teri Berry, DNP, FNP-C
Graduate Nursing Professor
Herzing University
Carlyle, Illinois

Christine M. Berté, EdD, APRN, FNP-BC
Chairperson School of Nursing
Director of Graduate Programs
Mount Saint Mary College
Newburgh, New York

Anne Watson Bongiorno, PhD,
APHN-BC, CNE
Associate Professor of Nursing
SUNY Plattsburgh
Plattsburgh, New York

Kwaghdoo Atsor Bossuah, DNP, MSN,
MPA, FNP-C, RN
Associate Professor
Tennessee State University
Nashville, Tennessee

Holly Bradley, DNP, MS, ANP-BC, APRN
Clinical Assistant Professor
Sacred Heart University
Fairfield, Connecticut

Kathleen M. Burke, PhD, RN
Assistant Dean in Charge of Nursing
Professor of Nursing
Ramapo College of New Jersey
Mahwah, New Jersey

Deborah Busch, DNP, CRNP
Assistant Professor
Johns Hopkins School of Nursing
Baltimore, Maryland

Daniel Crawford, DNP, RN, CPNP-PC,
CNE
Director, Clinical Assistant Professor
Arizona State University Edson
    College of Nursing and Health
    Innovation
Phoenix, Arizona

Kristina Currier, DNP, FNP-C
Associate Professor
Indiana Wesleyan University
Marion, Indiana

Doris Davenport, DSN, RN, PNP
Professor
Austin Peay State University
Clarksville, Tennessee

Bridget Drafahl, PhD, CNL, RN-BC
Chair for DNP and Healthcare
  Programs
American Sentinel University
Aurora, Colorado

Dorothy J. Dunn, PhD, RNP, FNP-BC,
AHN-BC
Associate Professor
Northern Arizona University
Flagstaff, Arizona

Anne Marie Fink, PhD, RN, CNE
Assistant Dean for College and
  Student Services Director
Villanova University
Villanova, Pennsylvania

Julie S. Gayle, DNP, WHNP-BC
Associate Professor, Coordinator
  of Women's Health Nurse
  Practitioner Program
Northwestern State University
  College of Nursing
Shreveport, Louisiana

Mary E. Hancock, PhD, RNC-OB
Associate Professor of Nursing
Shepherd University
Sheperdstown, West Virginia

Annette Hines, PhD, RN, CNE
Associate Professor and Chair of
  Graduate Studies
Queens University of Charlotte
Charlotte, North Carolina

Catherine M. Hogan, PhD, MPH, RN
Assistant Professor
Maryville University
St. Louis, Missouri

Cheryl Jackson, DNP, FNP-C
Assistant Professor
Bloomsburg University
Bloomsburg, Pennsylvania

Cheryl Jusela, DNP, ANP-BC, NP-C
Assistant Professor
Oakland University
Rochester, Michigan

Carol Klamser, DNP, FNP-BC, AFN-BC,
SANE-A
Associate Professor, UAA
University of Alaska, Anchorage
Anchorage, Alaska

Angela Lukomski, DNP, RN, CPNP
Associate Professor
Eastern Michigan University
Ypsilanti, Michigan

Susan J. McFarlan, DNP, RN, NE-BC
Assistant Professor
Webster University
St. Louis, Missouri

Charman Miller, DNP, CNP, CNE
Associate Professor and Associate
    Director, Graduate Division
Ohio University
Athens, Ohio

Kimberlee Miller-Wenning, DNP, CNP,
ANP, FNP, PMHNP
Assistant Professor
Ohio University
Athens, Ohio

Abigail Mitchell, DHEd, MSN, RN, CNE,
FHERDSA
Professor & Director of Nursing
    Management
D'Youville College
Youngstown, New York

Bridget Moore, DNP, MBA, NEA-BC
Professor
University of South Alabama
Mobile, Alabama

Gloria Nwagwu, PhD, RN, FNP-BC
Director of RN-BSN Program
Mount St. Mary's University
Los Angeles, California

Kathleen T. Ogle, PhD, RN, FNP-BC,
CNE
Associate Professor
Towson University
Towson, Maryland

Theresa M. Parenteau, DNP, MSN,
RN-BC
Adjunct Professor
Nova Southeastern University
Fort Lauderdale, Florida

Valerie Pauli, EdD, MSN, RN, ACNS-BC,
CNE
Associate Professor
Mercy College of Ohio
Toledo, Ohio

Angela Phillips, DNP, APRN, FNP-BC
Associate Professor of Nursing
West Texas A&M University
Canyon, Texas

Marlena Seibert Primeau, DNP,
FNP-BC, NHDP-BC, BSHECS
Clinical Associate Professor
University of Alabama in Huntsville
    College of Nursing
Huntsville, Alabama

Rosalina Rivera-Rodríguez,
EdD, MSN, RN
Faculty
Pontifical Catholic University of
    Puerto Rico
Ponce, Puerto Rico

Marylou V. Robinson, PhD, FNP-C
Associate Professor
Pacific Lutheran University
Tacoma, Washington

Jennifer Savage, DNP, APN, FNP-BC
Assistant Professor of Nursing/
    Director of FNP Program
Lincoln Memorial University
Harrogate, Tennessee

G. Serdynski, FNP-BC
Adjunct Professor
Alverno College
Milwaukee, Wisconsin

Deborah Shirey, DNP, APRN, FNP-BC
Adjunct Professor
University of Arkansas
Fayetteville, Arkansas

Shelly Smith, DNP, ANP-BC
Clinical Assistant Professor
Virginia Commonwealth University
Richmond, Virginia

Heidi M. Smolka, DNP, FNP-BC
Graduate FNP Program Director
University of Saint Joseph
West Hartford, Connecticut

Beth R. Steinfeld, DNP, WHNP-BC,
FNYAM
Assistant Professor, WHNP Program
    Director
Chair Grad Programs, SUNY
    Downstate Medical Center
Brooklyn, New York

Ayman Tailakh, PhD, RN
Associate Professor of Nursing
California State University,
    Los Angeles
Los Angeles, California

Phyllis D. Thomson, PhD, RN, CNE
Assistant Professor
OSF Saint Anthony College of
    Nursing
Rockford, Illinois

Barbara Wilder, PhD, CRNP
Director of Graduate Programs
Auburn University
Auburn, Alabama

Patricia Wright, PhD, CRNP, ACNS-BC,
CHPN, CNE
Assistant Professor of Nursing
University of Scranton
Scranton, Pennsylvania

Theresa R. Wyatt, PhD, RN, CCM, CFN,
CCRE, FACFEI
Assistant Professor
University of Detroit Mercy
Detroit, Michigan

Aleksandra Zagorin, DNP, AGPCNP-
BC, RN
Assistant Professor/Clinical Advisor
    Hartford Institute for Geriatric
    Nursing
Wagner College Evelyn L. Spiro
    School of Nursing
Staten Island, New York

Preface

Nurses are increasingly drawn to roles beyond the baccalaureate degree and recognize that advanced education can provide new challenges and open doors to increased career opportunities. Career pathways include options in educational, administrative, and clinical roles. As technology continues to change the face of healthcare and nursing role opportunities multiply, it becomes increasingly important for nurses to understand the complexities of the differing advanced practice (APN) roles, including the advanced practice registered nurse (APRN) roles to make informed career choices. The recent pandemic is just one example of how APNs and APRNs are necessary in an ever-changing practice environment and why they must advance not only their clinical skills, but their leadership skills as well.

Career pathways are not finite—educational institutions have been attuned to the desires of nurses to have career mobility. While the BSN provides a generalist degree—nurses must know something about everything—graduate degrees provide nurses with focused educational programs that lead to advanced roles. Nurses also have options beyond their master's degree and can either seek a terminal degree or a second certification and advanced practice registered nurse licensure or a total switch from clinical to administrative or educational roles.

This textbook allows students to consider a longer career trajectory with immediate goals for the next 5 years as well as long-term goals that foster continued professional development opportunities. Providing an overview of educational, administration, and clinical roles offers students the ability to compare and contrast the essential competencies, challenges, and opportunities of these roles.

Understanding Advanced Practice Roles

Advancing Nursing Practice: Exploring Roles and Opportunities for Clinicians, Educators, and Leaders provides a framework for educating nursing students to the professional standards and expectations for roles as an educator, administrator, clinical nurse leader, or clinician. Frequently, advance practice nursing textbooks focus on the clinician role, including such options as a certified nurse anesthetist (CRNA), nurse practitioner (NP), certified nurse midwife (CNM), clinical nurse specialist (CNS), and clinical nurse leaders (CNL). The roles of nurse educators and administrators warrant special attention when discussing professional options requiring advanced education. *Advancing Nursing Practice* was created to address the absence of in-depth content recognizing nurse educator and administrator roles as advanced professional choices with certification and practice competencies from a professional organization. This is an especially valid argument as an increasing number of doctorate in nursing practice (DNP) programs offer education or leadership as specialization options.

Introduction to *Advancing Nursing Practice*

This text will serve as a significant resource for nurses seeking to advance their career or for faculty teaching undergraduate students or graduate nurses. *Advancing Nursing Practice* was created to provide nurses with an authoritative source for not only knowing what career choices are available but to gain insight into and appreciation for the realities of the role. As a role-driven text, *Advancing Nursing Practice* provides instructors with a valuable resource in teaching how competencies are applied and then individualized by incorporating professional standards.

This textbook was written with the understanding that most graduate nursing programs either are accredited by Commission on Collegiate Nursing Education (CCNE) or subscribe to the American Association of Colleges of Nursing's essential competencies, the building blocks for a program's curriculum. As such, content related to these essential competencies is provided in a succinct, introductory manner throughout the textbook, recognizing that stand-alone courses will be offered such as health policy, translational research, and technology and informatics. Not only does *Advancing Nursing Practice* address the essential competencies, but it also includes competencies of professional organizations as well as leadership skills that all APNs/APRNs have in common including leading change, achieving conflict resolution, building teams, developing as a scholar in their roles, allocating funds for their quality improvement projects, becoming an entrepreneur, and seeking and then serving as a mentor.

With its clear and concise writing style that fosters understanding of complex topics, this text is designed for any nurse who is involved in lifelong learning and is open to expanding their current practice or desiring to progress into a "newer" role. It is also appropriate for instructors who require an authoritative text to help present content related to advanced professional roles. The text can be used in a menu-driven fashion, exploring those chapters that are applicable to individual needs or course outcomes. Chapters related to specific roles include the historical background of the role, role competencies, certification and/or licensure requirements, and role challenges and opportunities.

Organization

Advancing Nursing Practice is organized across three major role categories, spanning five parts: educators, administrators, and clinicians, which covers roles that require advanced RN licensure (CRNA, CNM, NP, CNS), clinical roles that do not require licensure (CNL), and nonclinical roles that require advanced education (administrators and educators).

The Text

Part I presents an overview of advanced nursing roles. Chapters 1 to 3 provide an introduction to address the driving forces for advanced professional roles and challenges within the U.S. health system that increase the needs for nurses with advanced degrees. The intent of Part I provides background and context for understanding subsequent units. Content includes

- Differentiation of competencies that are required as the nurse moves from a generalist, undergraduate role to a specialized graduate-prepared role
- An introduction to clinical specialties, faculty, and leadership roles of administrator and clinical nurse leader
- Content from the American Association of Colleges of Nursing's (AACN) *Essentials of Master's Education for Advance Practice Nursing* (2011) and *Essentials of Doctoral Education for Advance Nursing Practice* (2006)
- Educational pathways, licensure and certification requirements for each advanced practice role

Parts II presents content related to the advanced practice roles of nurse educator and leadership roles of administrator and clinical nurse leader, providing the historical background for these roles, expected competencies, and challenges.

These advanced practice roles are in high demand across many sectors. Educators are needed in the classroom and in clinical education. Educators are also needed in other professional areas, such as practical nursing or certified nursing assistant programs. Opportunities exist outside of academe, with opportunities in the community as well as in staff or patient education. Advances in technology and the growth of online education add to the need for qualified educators.

Nurses are increasingly assuming administrative roles at the highest levels. Most healthcare institutions have a chief nursing executive (CNE) and these nurses are now assuming positions as the chief executive officer (CEO). At the unit level, nurse managers are responsible for multimillion-dollar budgets and must have expertise in business administration and management. Their administrative counterparts in education require much of these same skills in the oversight of academic units.

Clinical nurse leaders are a crucial response to improving patient outcomes. Their leadership skills affect direct care services, promote patient safety, and assure evidence-based practices are utilized by nursing staff. They are the newest of advanced practice roles and balance their role as director caregiver with the leadership demands of promoting best practices.

Part III explores the four APRN roles (NP, CNS, CRNA, and CNM). Within each of the role-specific chapters, the format is ordered around the content of role definition, history, role specifics, and professionalism. Also addressed are the specific competencies as a means of identifying scope and standards of practice.

Part IV introduces the leadership journey as an advanced practice nurse. This section of the text assists the reader in self-identifying strengths and understanding where they are in terms of engaging in new learning and using feedback to reach goals. The concept of finding and using a mentor is emphasized as is how to identify and use opportunities. Leading change is presented as a critical component of advanced professional practice. Included in this section is content on influencing and managing change.

Part V presents concepts of scholarship for the advanced practice nurse. Nurses are lifelong learners, and much of this content is a guidebook on how to grow into leaders who assume advanced professional roles. An important section not often covered in typical texts includes content related to becoming a scholar. In this chapter, students will explore the application of Boyer's Model of

Scholarship in their development within any of the three roles as well as practical information on dissemination of scholarly work. Related to change implementation is the challenge to find suitable funding for innovative solutions in education, administration, and clinical arenas. This is an often-overlooked competency that is increasingly needed by nurses with an advanced education.

Part VI presents the future expectations of the leadership journey. Readers will learn about entrepreneurial and alternative opportunities for advanced practice nurses in any of the three roles. Students reading this section will recognize that attaining advanced professional roles is an evolving process and not a destination. The final chapters introduce concepts that are germane to nurses as they move from novice to expert, including collaboration, reflective practice, preparing for an interview, and negotiating a contract.

Features

To provide the nurses and educators with an exciting and user-friendly text, a number of recurring features have been developed to facilitate student learning and support instructor learning strategies.

Key Terms

Each chapter contains a list of terms common to advanced practice nurses. Key terms appear with definitions at the beginning of each chapter to promote student understanding.

Learning Objectives

The provision of learning objectives for each chapter helps to guide advanced practice nurses toward prioritizing and evaluate their understanding of the presented materials.

In Their Own Words

Each chapter has "In Their Own Words" vignettes in which professionals share what inspires them, what challenges they face, and explain how expected competencies affect their daily practice. The personal accounts provide respective insight into advancing nursing practice roles.

Internet Resources

Within each chapter is a list of internet resources carefully selected to introduce students to authoritative sources for information that support and expand content. Many of these resources, including professional organizations, are intended to support lifelong learning and to be of value over the lifespan of a career.

Chapter Highlights

Chapter authors provided key points at the end of each chapter to emphasize important aspects of the chapter.

Tables, Boxes, and Figures

Each chapter includes tables, boxes, and figures to summarize key content areas throughout the book. The text's figures and charts help the student to visualize the content and gain quick accessibility to information.

Questions to Ask Yourself

Each chapter contains at least one list of questions students should ask themselves regarding the content presented. This builds a practice of reflection and self-guided learning.

References

A comprehensive list of references that were used in the development of the text are provided at the end of each chapter. The listings allow the students and nurses to further pursue topics of interest.

Teaching-Learning Package

Instructor's and Student Resources

Chapter-specific ancillary activities: Various active learning activities are included to support graduate-level education. Higher order thinking (application, analysis, synthesis) are emphasized. Instructor resources can also be used to support a rich and engaging remote learning experience for students. A variety of ancillaries are provided including:

- Chapter learning activities—An array of evaluation activities, short answer, and matching that encourage application of knowledge.
- Multiple-choice questions—A set of five in each chapter to foster knowledge retention.
- Student discussion boards—Opportunities of students to delve deeper into role aspects, opportunities, or challenges. Student discussion questions/activities are provided to encourage face-to-face and online students to engage with classmates. These questions can be used as active learning strategies to engage students with content and allow them to apply their learning to case studies or scenarios.
- Internet Resources are provided—Selected online sites are utilized to augment textbook materials. Students access short videos, articles, or professional websites to explore additional information related to individual chapters.
- PowerPoint presentations—Provided for each chapter to enhance chapter material and augment classroom discussion.
- Sample syllabi are also provided for 15- and 8-week courses. These syllabi, while designed for remote learning, are also appropriate for in-person courses.

Student Resources

An exciting set of free resources (when purchasing a new copy of the text) is available to assist students and nurses review the material and become more familiar advancing the practice of nursing.

Journal Articles, offer access to current research available in Wolters Kluwer journals.

Voice of the Expert videos: Provides insight and a deeper appreciation for the uniqueness of advanced practice nurses in various settings.

Acknowledgments

We are very grateful to our contributors. By sharing their expertise and experiences as reviewers and authors for chapters, In Their Own Words, and Voice of the Expert recordings, they have provided support and insight to nurses beginning a new stage of their career. We also wish to acknowledge the team at Wolters Kluwer, who believed in the need for a text that addressed all advanced practice roles and shepherded us through the publishing process.

We want to thank our husbands, Tim Hart and Tex Bell, for standing by us while we endlessly researched, wrote, edited, and labored over all details. They were supportive when we needed to spend evenings writing and patiently sat by over working lunches. Tim and Tex became dear friends along the way, bringing joy to our work. Without their support, we could not have completed this journey.

Contents

PART ONE

Role Preparation and Expectations

1

Introduction to Advanced Nursing Roles

Carolyn Hart · Pegge L. Bell

LEARNING OBJECTIVES

After completing this chapter, you will be able to:

1. Examine factors affecting advanced practice roles in nursing.

2. Identify the need for lifelong learning among nurses.

3. Compare three professional roles—educator, administrator, and clinician—requiring advanced education.

4. Analyze components of American Association of Colleges of Nursing (AACN) Essentials and contrast differences between BSN, MSN, and DNP competencies.

KEY TERMS

Affordable Care Act: The comprehensive healthcare reform laws enacted in 2010 designed to increase availability of healthcare insurance. Also called Obamacare or the Patient Protection and Affordable Care Act.

Advanced practice role: Collectively, nursing roles that require master's or doctoral education and have specific professional competencies.

Advanced practice registered nurse (APRN): Advanced practice nurse holding a separate RN license in an advanced clinical role.

Chief Nursing Officer (CNO): Functions at the executive level and is responsible for oversight of all nursing and patient-service activities within a healthcare organization.

Competencies: The measurable knowledge, skills, and attitudes that will broadly prepare graduates for successful transition into the workplace.

Certified registered nurse practitioner (CRNP): A registered nurse with advanced education and certification in providing healthcare to individuals. They are responsible for the evaluation, management, and treatment of patient and their practice includes prescriptive authority. Specialty areas exist such as family practice, acute care, and women's health.

Essentials: The American Association of Colleges of Nursing established the *Essentials* for each level of nursing education. These **Essentials** establish a framework for building nursing curricula by outlining the necessary curriculum content and expected competencies of graduates from baccalaureate, master's, and doctor of nursing practice programs.

Generalist role: At the undergraduate and graduate levels, refers to roles that are broad in skill set, populations served, or settings.

Primary care provider (PCP): Healthcare providers who manage and coordinate patients for wellness and maintenance of health as well as common medical problems. PCPs are involved in the total health of the patient and may work with specialists as needed.

Introduction

Healthcare reform and innovation in practice fueled by technology are changing the way in which we work and deliver care, which makes this a motivating time for nurses While these conditions create a wide array of opportunities, they also create the imperative for nurses to carefully consider the advanced educational pathway that will lead to their optimal career choice. Nurses who desire to advance their education are faced with a variety of choices regarding role (educator, administrator, and clinician), specialization, program environment (face-to-face, hybrid, online), full- or part-time status, and degree choice (master's vs. doctorate). The wealth of choices makes careful consideration all the more important. This chapter presents an overview of the healthcare system and the Affordable Care Act, the need for lifelong learning, and introduction to nursing roles for educators, leaders and administrators, and clinicians.

Questions to Ask Yourself

1. What is my overall professional goal?
2. Which degree will best help me achieve that goal?
3. What is the cost and how will I finance my studies?
4. Do I have the necessary social and professional support to complete my studies?
5. Am I willing to relocate if needed?
6. What is the reputation of the university or college? Is the program accredited?
7. How long until I complete my studies?
8. Am I suited to online learning, or do I need face-to-face classes?
9. Will a job be available in my locale after I graduate?
10. Is an accelerated program available and is that a realistic option for me?
11. Do I have the necessary time to complete any required practicum hours?

Understanding the Healthcare System

The American healthcare landscape is in a period of rapid transition and uncertainty. In 2010 during the Obama administration, the Affordable Care Act (ACA) was enacted to address many of the structural inequities present in the delivery of healthcare and within healthcare insurance, particularly that of access. The ACA was intended to serve three goals: (1) to make affordable health insurance readily available, (2) to expand the Medicaid program to cover low-income adults, and (3) to support creative medical care delivery models that would lower healthcare costs (Healthcare.gov, n.d.). Under this law, individuals were granted several rights, including coverage with no additional costs due to preexisting illnesses or conditions, free preventative care, increased coverage plans for young adults, and protection against insurance company cancellation of policies. Garrett and Gangopadhyaya (2016) report an additional 20 million Americans gained insurance coverage since enactment of the ACA. Box 1.1 presents a summary of the provisions of the original ACA. However, many concerns persist, and as regulations evolve, a deeper understanding is necessary for nurses to effectively function within the complex healthcare delivery system.

In 2017, major efforts were undertaken to repeal and replace ACA, but these initiatives were not able to pass through the U.S. Senate. In 2018, Congress passed a tax bill eliminating the tax penalty for those who do not maintain

BOX 1.1

▶ OVERVIEW OF KEY FEDERAL PROVISIONS

- Require employers to cover workers with exceptions for small employers
  - Provide tax credits to certain small businesses that cover specified costs of health insurance for their employees
  - Require individuals to have insurance
  - Require creation of state-based (or multistate) insurance exchanges to help individuals and small businesses purchase insurance
  - Expand Medicaid to cover people with incomes below 133% of federal poverty guidelines
  - Require insurance plans to cover young adults on parents' policies
  - Establish a national, voluntary long-term care insurance program for "community living assistance services and supports" (CLASS)

- Enact consumer protections to enable people to retain their insurance coverage
  - Increase consumer insurance protection
  - Prohibit lifetime monetary caps on insurance coverage and limit use of annual caps
  - Prohibit insurance plans from excluding coverage for children with preexisting conditions
  - Prohibit insurance plans from canceling coverage, except in cases of fraud
  - Establish state-based rate reviews for "unreasonable" insurance premium increases
  - Establish an office of health insurance consumer assistance

- Emphasize prevention and wellness
  - Establishes a Prevention and Public Health Fund to provide grants to states for prevention activities
  - Creates the National Prevention, Health Promotion and Public Health Council to coordinate federal prevention efforts
  - Requires insurance plans to cover certain preventive care without cost-sharing, such as immunizations; preventive care for children; and specified screening for certain adults for conditions such as high blood pressure, high cholesterol, diabetes, and cancer
  - Increases the federal share of Medicaid payments by 1% point for certain preventive services, for which states do not charge a copayment
  - Increases Medicare payments for certain preventive services
  - Establishes a federal home-visiting initiative to help states foster health and well-being for children and families who live in at-risk communities
  - Requires restaurant chains with 20 or more locations to label menus with calorie information and to provide other information, upon request, such as fat and sodium content

- Improve health quality and system performance
  - Comparative research to study the effectiveness of various medical treatments
  - Demonstration projects to develop medical malpractice alternatives and reduce medical errors
  - Demonstration projects to develop payment mechanisms to improve efficiency and results

- Investments in health information technology
  - Improvements in care coordination between Medicare and Medicaid for patients who qualify for both
  - Options for states to create "health homes" for those enrolled Medicaid with multiple chronic conditions to improve care
  - Data collection and reporting mechanisms to address health disparities among populations based on ethnicity, geographic location, gender, disability status, and language

- Promote health workforce development
  - Reforms in graduate medical education training
  - Increases in health profession scholarship and loan programs
  - Support for training programs for nurses

- Support for new primary care models, such as medical homes and team management of chronic diseases
  - Increased funding for community health centers and the National Health Service Corps
  - Support for school-based health centers and nurse-managed health clinics

- Curb rising health costs
  - Increased oversight of health insurance premiums and practices
  - Emphasize prevention, primary care, and effective treatments
  - Reduce healthcare fraud and abuse
  - Reduce uncompensated care to prevent a shift onto insurance premium costs
  - Foster comparison shopping in insurance exchanges to increase competition and price transparency

- Implement Medicare payment reforms

Courtesy of the National Conference of State Legislatures, 2020.

health insurance. Judge Reed O'Connor of the Federal District Court in Fort Worth, Texas, ruled that it is unconstitutional to require individuals to carry health insurance. He further determined that because this individual mandate could not be severed from the rest of the ACA, the entire law should be repealed. In December 2019, a federal appeals court ruled that while the requirement that individuals have health insurance is unconstitutional, the rest of the ACA must be reviewed to determine what parts can survive without the mandate.

Significant changes and political debate continue to bring into play questions about the future of the ACA and healthcare policy in the United States. Our nation faces the challenge of funding ACA-driven changes that were intended to provide insurance options for Americans who were underinsured or without insurance coverage (American Institute for Economic Research, 2014). Although evidence exists that the ACA was able to decrease the number of Americans without insurance and increase access to care (Glied et al., 2017), challenges remain with understanding how to finance, sustain, and close the gap between what is affordable to individuals and what can be publicly funded.

As debates continue for repeal or modification of the ACA, three points will be of paramount interest: (1) access to healthcare across the lifespan, (2) affordable healthcare insurance, and (3) control over rising healthcare costs while increasing quality (American Medical Association, 2017). As the solution to this quandary is not readily apparent, what is clear is that this is a pivotal time for nurses to make a difference in increasing the availability and accessibility of healthcare services offered, particularly to at-risk populations. Nurses have the opportunity to serve in advanced professional roles that provide direct healthcare services, educate those who provide services, or administer healthcare and educational entities.

While these conditions create a wide array of opportunities, they also create the imperative for nurses to carefully consider the advanced educational pathway that will lead to their optimal career choice. Nurses who desire to advance their education are faced with a variety of choices regarding role (i.e., clinician, educator, administrator), specialization, program environment (e.g., face-to-face, hybrid, online), full- or part-time status, and degree choice (master's versus doctorate) (Box 1.2). The wealth of choices makes careful consideration even more important.

BOX 1.2

▶ NURSING DEGREE OPTIONS

BSN	Considered a generalist degree; graduates are prepared to practice across the lifespan within a variety of settings.
MSN	Depending on program of study, graduates specialize in several areas including nurse practitioner specialties, clinical nurse leader, clinical nurse specialist, education, informatics, or administration. Some institutions also offer an MSN as entry to practice; although these graduates obtain a master's degree, because it is entry to practice, it is still considered a generalist degree.
DNP	The DNP is a terminal practice degree as well as the entry into practice for CRNAs. The focus of the scholarly or capstone project is typically on improving health systems or patient outcomes through the application of evidence-based practice.
PhD	The PhD is the terminal degree most widely recognized in research and education; the dissertation is focused on generation of new nursing knowledge.

Mandate for Lifelong Learning

Advances in technology and an increasing body of clinical research place new demands on practicing nurses. The Tri-Council of Nursing (2020) is an alliance of five autonomous nursing organizations, each focused on leadership for education, practice, and research—the American Association of Colleges of Nursing (AACN), the American Nurses Association (ANA), the American Organization for Nursing Leadership (AONL) (formerly American Organization of Nurse Executives [AONE]), the National Council of State Boards of Nursing (NCSBN), and the National League for Nursing (NLN). The Tri-Council released a consensus report indicating the imperative for nurses to continually add to their skills and education to build a stronger workforce. The Institute of Medicine (IOM) and the ANA (ANA, 2017) reinforced the need for RNs to engage in ongoing learning as a means of seeking knowledge and competence. Finkelman (2017) identifies three types of learning opportunities:

- Academic education: academic courses
- Staff development: in-service activities
- Continuing education: professional development events/courses

Lifelong learning, as a dynamic process, allows nurses to gain new ideas and appreciate different perspectives (Qalehsari et al., 2017). The recent coronavirus pandemic resulted in immediate changes for nursing education and nursing practice. The focus on social distancing and need for personal protection equipment to qualm the virus' spread reshaped nursing education and nursing practice. It also underscored the importance of knowing how to obtain reliable and up-to-date information from a variety of online sources. These evolving health threats along with advances in how we deliver patient care require a nursing workforce that engages in lifelong learning (Figure 1.1).

As nurses gain experiential knowledge and expertise, many seek formal education as a means of expanding scope of practice or opening new career pathways. The advanced roles beyond Bachelor of Science in Nursing (BSN) preparation presented in this text can be divided into three broad categories: clinician, educator, and administrator. Advanced practice clinical roles include the four advanced practice RN (APRN) roles of nurse practitioners, clinical nurse specialists (CNSs), nurse midwives, and nurse anesthetists; clinical nurse leaders (CNLs); educators including nursing faculty; and administrators in clinical and educational settings. These roles are briefly introduced in this chapter to provide

Lifelong Learning

- Professional expectation
- Must be consistent and self-motivated
- Improves patient care
- Increases competitiveness and employability
- Enhances personal and professional development
- All licenses require continuing education
- Can occur through reading, conference attendance, and formal course work

Figure 1.1. Lifelong learning.

context and background for the fuller discussion presented in the following units. While nurses can assume other roles (e.g., staff educator, sexual assault nurse examiner), this textbook focuses on the roles that require a graduate nursing degree. Flexibility in academic progression allows for individualization of the educational journey. This journey should be strategic and based upon long-term goals and personal circumstances. The nurse selecting an educational pathway (Boxes 1.3 and 1.4) should bear in mind that while a master's degree will

BOX 1.3

▶ EDUCATIONAL PATHWAYS TO ADVANCED PRACTICE DEGREES

RN-MSN	May or may not be awarded a BSN
RN-DNP	May or may not be awarded an MSN; less common pathway
BSN-MSN	Most common pathway
BSN-DNP	Would not typically earn an MSN
BSN-PhD	May or may not be awarded an MSN
Post-Masters Certificate	Prepares the MSN to obtain specialized certification or knowledge; no additional degree is awarded
MSN-DNP	Obtains terminal clinical degree
MSN-PhD	Obtains terminal academic degree

BOX 1.4

▶ ADVANCED ROLES FOR NURSES

	APRN	Requirement	Education	Setting
Administrator	No	Certification optional	MSN; Doctorate optional	Everywhere in healthcare
CNL	No	Certification	MSN; Doctorate optional	Acute care; community
CNM	Yes	Certification	MSN; DNP optional	Independent practice, community, birthing centers, acute care
CNS	Yes	Certification	MSN; DNP optional	Independent practice, community, acute care
CRNA	Yes	Certification	DNP	Independent practice, community, acute care
Educator	No	Certification optional	MSN; PhD preferred in Academe	All settings that provide health- and nurse-related educational services
NP	Yes	Certification	MSN; DNP preferred	Independent practice, community, acute care

CNL, clinical nurse leader; CNM, certified nurse midwife; CNS, clinical nurse specialist; CRNA, certified registered nurse anesthetist; NP, nurse practitioner.

allow them to teach in an academic setting, it will most likely be within licensed practical nurse (LPN), associate's degree in nursing (and), or BSN programs. Similarly, while the majority of advanced practice registered nurses (APRNs) have a master's degree, in 2010, AACN endorsed the Doctor of Nursing Practice (DNP) as the most fitting degree for APRNs and encouraged the transition of master programs to the doctoral level.

Faculty Shortages

The United States has a critical need for nurses who are educationally and experientially prepared to assume roles in clinical specialties, educational settings, and as leaders within organizations and in policy-creating arenas. The Institute of Medicine (IOM, 2010), in *The Future of Nursing: Leading Change, Advancing Health*, has stressed the importance of doubling the number of doctorally prepared nurses by 2020. IOM further suggests that one step in reaching this goal is approaching private and public funders to increase financial support for nursing programs offering accelerated graduate degrees. These initiatives are needed to ensure that educational pathways attract at least 10% of all baccalaureate-prepared nurses (BSN) into a graduate program (MSN, DNP, PhD) within 5 years of graduation.

Lippincott Solutions (2018a) reports an increase in the number of BSN-prepared nurses (49% in 2010 to 54% in 2016). Although this is a significant increase, it has not reached the goal of 80%. However, Lippincott further reports that the number of nurses with a doctoral degree more than doubled (8,267 in 2010 to 22,454 in 2016), meeting the targeted goal. Progress has also been seen in the number of states removing barriers to practice for nurse practitioners.

The reality of needing to increase the number of nurses enrolled in graduate programs is at odds with the significant shortage of master's and doctorally prepared faculty. AACN's (2019a) report "2018 to 2019 Enrollment and Graduations in Baccalaureate and Graduate Programs in Nursing" indicates that more than 75,000 qualified applicants were denied admission to nursing programs largely due to a faculty shortage. AACN (2019b) further reported more than 1,700 faculty vacancies in 2018 with a faculty vacancy rate of almost 8%. This same study identified the need to create an additional 138 doctorally prepared faculty positions to accommodate student demand.

The inability to attract nurses into graduate programs that prepare them for faculty roles placed more strain on graduating nurses in all areas of practice. Impending faculty retirements, faculty turnover, and noncompetitive salaries compared with their clinical counterparts add to the difficulties in attracting and retaining faculty and encouraging nurses to pursue education as a specialty (American Association of Colleges of Nursing, 2019b).

Nurse Administrator Shortages

Retirement, an aging workforce, and inadequate succession planning contribute to a lack of nurses who are educationally and experientially prepared to assume leadership roles. In a survey of almost 300 nurse managers, Warshawsky and Havens (2014) found that while almost 70% of managers were satisfied or very satisfied with their job and would recommend leadership as a career choice, 72% of these leaders were planning on leaving their positions within the next 5 years. Reasons for leaving included burnout, retirement, career change, and promotion.

As employment of registered nurses (RNs) grows and the proportion of healthcare administered by nurses increases, the need for highly educated nurse leaders rises. The nurse leader plays a large role in creating healthy work environments that contribute, in a very crucial way, to the satisfaction and retention of bedside nurses (Lippincott Solutions, 2018b). In addition, understanding of financial data and workforce needs leads to a well-staffed, well-functioning healthcare institution.

In Their Own Words

Joanne Cochran, PhD, CNS, RN , CEO and President, Keystone Health
"No one cares how much you know until they know how much you care."
—Unknown

The key points in understanding my role are… Major changes in the U.S. healthcare system and practice environment have required equally profound changes in my role as CEO of a healthcare organization and system.

(Continued)

My experience has led me to a better understanding of concepts such as care management, quality improvement methods, systems-level change management, and the reconceptualized role of nurses and CEOs in a reformed healthcare system. My nursing education has served as a platform for continued lifelong learning and has included opportunities for seamless transition to new roles and mastery of new skills and competencies. I have had to become much more diverse to respond to the inequality of the healthcare system.

What keeps me coming back every day is… I see such tremendous need all around me: medical needs, dental needs, and behavioral health needs. I see sick children, poor children, lonely children, and children being abused. I see elderly men and women sick and no one to take care of them. I see HIV/AIDS patients with nowhere to go but Keystone Health. I want to make things better for all these individuals.

It may sound surprising, but it takes courage to keep pushing oneself, and it also demands creativity. It means tapping into our creative intelligence in order to stay ahead of the crowd and to inspire those around you to push themselves too. It means rattling cages, starting with my own. Courage to not let circumstances dictate life for me and my neighbors.

There are things we know to be true but there are also things we feel to be true. Most of us have problems balancing logic with using one's intuition. But the truth is that those faculties are not opposed to one another. Intellect without intuition makes for a smart person without impact, and intuition without intellect makes for a spontaneous person without direction. Leaders need to figure out how to get these two faculties working together. Conviction is rare because our longing for stability and security is so strong. We make the mistake of looking outside ourselves for direction when we should be looking inside. There is something very compelling about a person with conviction. The secret is to find something you feel you are meant to do and give yourself to it totally. There is something out there that only we can do, and our job is to find it.

My greatest challenge is… Balancing the needs of the business—growth, cash flow, new opportunities—with the needs of employees is the biggest challenge I face and have faced for the last 15 years. Working with younger employees has presented a whole new set of challenges and opportunities that go back to having a culture of growth that everyone buys into. Keystone's culture

(Continued)

was formed early on by the founding members and key management staff and board. Those of us who worked very closely together made it relatively easy to maintain company culture. Keystone now has 500 employees. We have added not only new employees but many new locations, and it has become a real challenge to assimilate all of these individuals into one culture. This impacts capacity. We have increasingly been able to build our demand, but ensuring we have the right people to execute on this demand is difficult. There are brilliant potential employees, but truly understanding what kind of hires we need and how to get people up and running quickly, effectively, and productively, is our biggest challenge.

I wish someone had told me… Looking back over the years, I never would have predicted how hard it would be to manage growth and the inevitable culture changes that occur. It is so important to establish a culture that can evolve as you grow, but still maintain the core tenets (or soul) of the original founder's vision. Creating a great culture is all about setting clear company goals, clear individual goals, transparency as to how each employee is con-tributing, and then giving your employees the autonomy to do what they were hired to do.

I need to be a lifelong learner because… Keystone is only as strong as the people behind it. There is a direct correlation between individuals who strive for growth in their personal lives and those who strive in their professional lives. This can only be accomplished by committing to the concept of lifelong learning. In an ever-changing market and world, it is more important than ever to stay current, competitive, and up to date. Through lifelong learning, you stimulate a perpetual hunger that drives both your personal and profes-sional life.

Another point to understand is… Pay attention to what you are supposed to do and do what comes easily to you. This does not mean being lazy or refusing to work. What opportunities are finding you? Pay close attention to your emails, your friends, your conversations, your new acquaintances; pay attention to all those things that come to you that you did not solicit, these words and individuals inviting you to a chance meeting, a chance project. That is where you are supposed to operate. That is the sweet spot. When you acknowledge and take action on the bonuses that find you and you swell with the idea of all the potential loaded in those emails, in that phone call, in that meeting, answer the call. Embrace the gift of your purpose finding you.

> The more you do that, the more that you allow an open mind and heart to receive success and emotional and financial prosperity, the sharper your frequency becomes because you are finally in tune with identifying everything that is meant for you.

Clinical Provider Shortages

U.S. nurse practitioners, considered midlevel providers, number more than 290,000 (American Association of Nurse Practitioners, 2020). Of these, almost 90% are certified in an area of primary care as presented in Table 1.1.

Table 1.1. Fast Facts for NP Practice			
Certification[a]		**Percent of NPs**	
Family[b]	65.4	Adult-gerontology acute care	3.4
Adult[b]	12.6	Women's health	2.8
Adult-gerontology[b]	7.8	Psychiatric/mental health-family	1.8
Acute care	5.5	Gerontology[b]	1.7
Pediatrics-primary care[b]	3.7	Hospice and palliative care	1.5
Total % in primary care	89.7%	% NPs who accept Medicaid	80.2%
% NPs who accept Medicare	82.9%	% who prescribe medications	95.7%
% NPs who hold hospital privileges	41.7%	% NPs who hold long term care privileges	11.7%

[a]NPs may be certified in more than one area.
[b]Primary care focus.
Adapted from American Association of Nurse Practitioners®, 2020.

Despite strides in attracting nurses into primary care areas of practice, shortfalls in coverage continue to be a significant concern. The Association of American Medical Colleges (AAMC, 2004) cited a need for 25,000 primary care physicians in 2013 and predicted that number would grow to 45,000 by 2020. In 2019, AAMC confirmed this shortage, reiterating a need for up to 55,200 primary care physicians by 2032, largely due to a growing and aging population. Changes in health policies may also increase the need for primary care providers (PCPs). This leads to an increased demand for **PCPs**, and the question becomes, will nurse practitioners be able to fill this gap?

This shortage in primary care is mirrored in other clinical specialty areas of practice. In a 2019 Issue Brief, the National Rural Health Association (NRHA) reports less than half of all U.S. rural counties have obstetrical services and areas without this care experience a doubling of infant mortality rates (Anderson et al., 2019). Centers for Medicare & Medicaid Services (CMS) also identifies more than 10% of rural women drive 100 miles or more for obstetrical services. Furthermore, American College of Nurse-Midwives Board President Lisa Kane Low asserts that 40% of counties in the United States do not have access to either a certified nurse midwife (CNM) or obstetrician. The U.S. Bureau of Labor Statistics reports job growth for certified registered nurse anesthetists (CRNAs) is projected to be 26% between 2018 and 2028, well above the national average.

Differentiating Generalist and Advanced Professional Roles

Given the wealth of opportunities and the need for nurses with advanced educational preparation, it is important to review differences between practice expectations across roles. Baccalaureate-prepared nurses (BSNs) are considered **generalists**, as the BSN is a foundational degree that is conceptually broad. As such, BSN graduates are expected to competently provide professional nursing care across the lifespan and in a wide variety of settings (American Association of Colleges of Nursing, 2008). Graduates of AACN accredited programs must meet the standards outlined in AACN's Essentials (AACN, 2008). Postgraduation clinical experiences assist the BSN in moving from novice to an expert clinician, all within the scope of practice of an RN. To move beyond the standards of practice for an RN, many nurses will seek a graduate degree to increase career opportunities.

Practice-focused graduate degrees, such as the Master of Science (MSN) and clinical doctorate (DNP), offer the ability for nurses to gain new knowledge and skills or to specialize in a particular area or type of nursing. The PhD degree focuses on development of research-based skills. Graduate degrees expand the scope of practice for nurses by adding a complexity to expected practice. Educationally, AACN articulates this progression of expected practice within the Essentials (see Chapter 3).

As one progresses educationally, while the Essentials are similar, the expectation of practice increases. AACN delineates the expected outcomes for these different levels of nursing education in their *Essentials* as identified in Table 1.2.

Overview of Roles

Having an overview of each of the three main advanced practice roles—educator, administrator, and clinician—increases an understanding of what is to come in the next chapters of this text. It will also increase your understanding of how the various roles complement each other. Although the setting and scope of practice vary widely, these advance roles do share commonalities. One such commonality is leadership, as leadership expectations are present among the three main advanced practice role competencies. Nurses with advanced education are prepared to lead effective teams, resolve conflict, influence change, possess an entrepreneurial spirit, develop and disseminate scholarship, successfully seek funding for their projects, and bring value to their professional practice. Thus, chapters for each of these leadership skills are included in the text.

Table 1.2. AACN Essentials With Competency Examples

Content Area	BSN Essentials (AACN, 2008)	MSN Essentials (AACN, 2011)	DNP Essentials (AACN, 2006)
Educational Foundation	Liberal Education for Baccalaureate Generalist Nursing Practice • Use humanities, ways of knowing, and ethics in care of patients	Background for Practice From Science and Humanities • Integrate nursing and related sciences into the delivery of advanced nursing care	Scientific Underpinnings for Practice • Integrate nursing science with knowledge from ethics, sciences, and humanities
Leadership	Basic Organizational and Systems Leadership for Quality Care and Patient Safety • Apply leadership skills • Participate in safety initiative • Apply principles of quality improvement	Organizational and Systems Leadership; Quality Improvement and Safety • Assume a leadership role in implementing patient safety and quality improvement initiatives • Participate in the design of new models of care delivery	Organizational and Systems Leadership for Quality Improvement and Systems Thinking • Ensure accountability for quality of healthcare and patient safety • Develop and evaluate care delivery approaches
Scholarship and EBP	Scholarship for Evidence-Based Practice • Participate in the process of retrieval, appraisal, and synthesis of evidence • Collaborate in the collection, documentation, and dissemination of evidence	Translating and Integrating Scholarship Into Practice • Analyze information and design systems to sustain improvements • Lead quality improvement initiatives that integrate sociocultural factors • Conduct root cause analysis of errors	Clinical Scholarship and Analytical Methods • Design and implement processes to evaluate outcomes • Analyze data from practice • Predict and analyze outcomes • Identify gaps in evidence for practice

Informatics	Information Management and Application of Patient Care Technology • Demonstrate skill in patient technologies • Use technology to document patient care	Informatics and Healthcare Technologies • Analyze technologies to support safe practice environments • Provide oversight in the integration of documentation technologies • Promote policies that incorporate ethical principles and standards	Information Systems Technology and Patient Care Technology for the Improvement and Transformation of Healthcare • Design, select, use, and evaluate programs to evaluate and monitor outcomes including use of consumer information systems
Policy and Advocacy	Healthcare Policy, Finance, and Regulatory Environments • Describe state and national rules and regulations • Explore impact of factors influencing healthcare delivery • Advocate for consumers and nursing profession	Health Policy and Advocacy • Participate in development of institutional, local, and state and federal policy • Interpret research for policy-makers and stakeholders • Advocate for policies that improve the health of the public and nursing profession	Healthcare Policy for Advocacy in Healthcare • Analyze health policy proposal, health policies, and related issues from the perspective of consumers, nursing, and others • Advocate for social justice

(Continued)

Table 1.2.   AACN Essentials With Competency Examples   (continued)

Content Area	BSN Essentials (2008)	MSN Essentials (2011)	DNP Essentials (2006)
Interprofessional Education	Interprofessional Communication and Collaboration for Improving Patient Health Outcomes • Build relationships with team members • Use interprofessional communication • Participate in decision-making	Interprofessional Collaboration for Improving Patient and Population Health Outcomes • Advocate for the value of the professional nurse as a member of interprofessional teams • Use effective communication to develop and lead interprofessional teams	Interprofessional Collaboration for Improving Patient and Population Health Outcomes • Employ leadership skills with intra-/interprofessional teams • Lead interprofessional teams in the analysis of complex practice and organizational issues
Clinical Prevention and Population Health	Clinical Prevention and Population Health • Conduct a health history • Assess health and illness beliefs • Use clinical judgment • Employ evidence-based prevention strategies	Clinical Prevention and Population Health for Improving Health • Use social determinants of health to deliver evidence-based, culturally relevant prevention interventions • Develop culturally relevant and linguistically appropriate health education, communication, and interventions	Clinical Prevention and Population Health for Improving the Nation's Health • Analyze scientific data related to individual and population health • Develop, evaluate, and implement interventions that address health promotion and disease prevention efforts

	Professionalism and Professional Values (across all levels of education)		
Professional Values	• Demonstrate professional values and standards of conduct • Protect patient privacy and confidentiality		
Nursing Practice	Baccalaureate Generalist Nursing Practice	Master's Level Nursing Practice	Advanced Nursing Practice
	• Implement holistic, patient-centered care • Provide appropriate patient-teaching • Implement evidence-based nursing interventions	• Conduct a comprehensive and systematic assessment as a foundation for decision-making • Advance patient education through information technologies • Use leadership skills to teach, coach, and mentor	• Design, implement, and evaluate therapeutic interventions • Educate and guide individuals and groups through complex health situations • Guide, mentor, and support other nurses to achieve excellence

AACN, American Association of Colleges of Nursing; EBP, evidence-based practice.
Modified from American Association of Colleges of Nursing.

In Their Own Words

Cathy Catrambone, PhD, RN, FAAN
Associate Professor, Adult Health and Gerontological Nursing
Rush University College of Nursing
Past President, Sigma Theta Tau International

The role of a leader… The role of nurse leaders is essential in addressing the rapidly unfolding health challenges across the globe. The power of the 19.4 million nurses and midwives worldwide to influence and shape healthcare is profound and unprecedented. The message of the global Nursing Now Campaign (2018–2020), a collaborative effort between the World Health Organization and the International Council of Nurses, addresses the importance of nurses' voices being heard as well as to the importance of nurses being recruited into key leadership positions. Early in my professional career, I realized that I had a deep commitment to serving in a leadership role and advocating for both quality healthcare systems and the advancement of the nursing profession. My vision was to take a path where I would serve an organization with a local health mission and to work as a leader in a national or international organization with a health mission and commitment to developing next generation nurse leaders. As I reflect on my path I realized how three guiding principles have shaped my journey and I offer these for others to consider:
1.

- **first**, discover your passion;
- **second**, be intentional about your journey; and
- **third**, do not wait to be asked, put yourself at the table.

Discovering passion: The principle of discovering one's passion requires conscious work. Commit defined time to reflect on where you get great joy and what generates a deep sense of fulfillment in your work and life. What is it that motivates you? Let your passion fuel your commitment and expand your ability to influence. When you connect to your passion, it provides energy and strengthens your ability to persist in making a difference and to address the many challenges encountered along the way.

(Continued)

As a pulmonary critical care nurse, the American Lung Association's "tag line" which speaks as deeply to me today as it did upon entering the profession is "when you can't breathe, nothing else matters." I realized this vision for respiratory health was my passion, and I took on serving as an advocate for lung health and promoting the well-being of vulnerable populations. I continue to serve as a Board and Executive Committee member for the Respiratory Health Association. The organization's mission focuses on prevention of lung disease and clean air with an emphasis on education, research, and policy change. I continue to be actively engaged in advocacy and policy work related to lung health, clean air, tobacco control, and asthma management in the school setting.

Intentional journey: The second principle is to **be intentional about your journey.** As with pursuing any goal, it takes planning and intent to achieve what we want. Consider mapping out your goals—both personal and professional. Commit to creating a timeline that helps you visualize and prioritize the steps to take. Use this timeline as your map to help you define areas where you will increase your skills and capacity so that you are prepared to achieve your goals. Throughout my journey, I have greatly benefitted from the mentor relationships I have developed. I strongly suggest that you seek mentors throughout your career—mentors that will be able to provide guidance in a variety of areas.

The Honor Society of Nursing, Sigma Theta Tau International, or Sigma's mission is advancing world health and celebrating nursing excellence in scholarship, leadership, and service. Currently there are over 135,000 members in more than 90 countries worldwide. Given the scope and complexity of the organization, my journey during the past decade was intentional both in preparing to seek certain elected positions and in organizing my personal and professional life to achieve my most deeply held goals. The journey included creating a path that would provide me with the opportunities to develop the depth of insight into the organization locally, regionally, and internationally, and prepare me well to serve as President and to lead the international organization.

Putting yourself at the table: Finally, and equally important is the principle of **do not wait to be asked, put yourself at the table.** Today healthcare desperately needs innovation, compassion, and transformational leadership.

(Continued)

We have the opportunity and responsibility to create systems that promote the safety of our patients and significantly advance positive health outcomes. You do not have to wait for someone to invite you to the table. Be comfortable with being out of your comfort zone. We each have valuable knowledge of current science and possess the skills and ability to influence others and to advocate for and contribute to better health for those entrusted to your care.

Funded by the Illinois Department of Public Health (IDPH), my research focused on the burden of asthma in Illinois and asthma management consistent with national guideline recommendations. Given my commitment to improving asthma care, I was intentional about pursuing a position at the table to influence asthma care in Illinois. As a volunteer and pulmonary nurse leader and scientist, I continue to serve as cochair of the Illinois Asthma Partnership (IAP) Executive Committee. The IAP provides oversight for implementation of Illinois state asthma plan and advising the organization on asthma-related issues in Illinois.

Another point to understand is… As you aspire to develop your influence as a leader, it is essential to be aware of your brand. Your brand defines you as a leader both personally and professionally. Your brand is a reflection on your leadership style and core values. Brand projects an image of what is important to you as a leader, your ability to drive results, and to successfully and strategically manage change. It is essentially to reflect thoughtfully on your brand and to be intentional about living daily.

Educators

While generalist nurses at the baccalaureate level are expected to teach individuals, families, and communities, education as a scholarly endeavor requires graduate-level preparation with a focus in education. Billings and Halstead (2019) argue that specific academic preparation in the educator role is necessary to adequately prepare nurses to teach. The need for nurses with advanced knowledge and skills related to education makes this an advanced practice role recognized by the NLN (2020). The NLN has developed competencies for the academic nurse educator which establish nursing education as a specialty area of practice.

Nurses who precept other staff nurses or students may determine that teaching would be a rewarding role and can choose from opportunities in community, clinical, or academic settings. In addition to these different settings, academic teaching roles encompass various levels and types of students. Undergraduate, graduate, and doctoral programs all present possibilities, as do opportunities within LPN and certified nurse assistant (CNA) programs. Clinical instructors who specialize in teaching practicum experiences at the undergraduate level may teach with an MSN, preferably with content specific to education; within graduate and doctoral programs, the expected preparation is a doctorate. While the settings and educational levels of audiences may change, role preparation and responsibilities of the educator are similar. Educational preparation typically includes content in curriculum development, teaching and learning practices, assessment, and outcome evaluation. While novice instructors tend to start at the undergraduate level, opportunities also exist at the graduate master's and doctoral programs in both face-to-face and online modalities. Educators for staff development may be responsible for dissemination of information about changing policies, new technologies, and compliance issues. Regionally, qualifications for educators in staff development and community education vary, with some institutions requiring an MSN and others accepting a BSN. Educators may also obtain certification as a nurse educator through NLN. Additional information about the educator role is presented in Chapter 4.

Administrators

Leadership and administrative roles abound in healthcare and academic settings. Although differences exist in job descriptions, salaries, and details of role responsibilities, many competency domains are shared. Administrators are responsible for safe, timely, and efficient work practices that promote best practices. In clinical settings, this may mean establishing a multidisciplinary approach to patient safety (AONL, 2019). In the academic setting, the focus is on student and faculty practices.

The American Organization for Nursing Leadership (AONL, formerly AONE) promotes the knowledge and abilities that are needed to guide leaders in healthcare settings. This model, as presented in Figure 1.2, identifies the leadership competencies under five major concepts that capture the practice of nurse executives. These concepts include leadership, communication and relationship

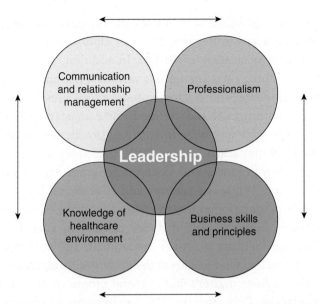

Figure 1.2. American Organization for Nursing Leadership (AONL) competencies. (Reprinted with permission from American Organization for Nursing Leadership [AONL], 2019. All Rights Reserved.)

management, professionalism, business skills and principles, and knowledge of healthcare environments (AONL [AONE], 2007). Within this text, these competencies are adapted to reflect the role of the academic nurse administrator, as no universal model exists.

In clinical settings, leaders exist at the unit, department, and executive levels. **Chief Nursing Officers (CNOs)** are typically responsible for supervising nurse managers and influencing the design and implementation of patient care. They are very involved in meeting the complex challenges of patient safety, quality of patient care, patient and family experiences, nurse employee satisfaction, and fiscal responsibility (Ingwell-Spolan, 2018). In the academic settings, educational administrators must also possess the competencies that are required of nurse executives. These leaders will oversee educational units and require business skills, knowledge of healthcare environments, communication and relationship management, and professionalism. These roles can include program coordinators, department chairs, assistant/associate deans, and deans.

Clinicians

Improvements in decreasing practice barriers make the role of an advanced practice nurse increasingly attractive. IOM's 2010 report released key messages regarding nursing practice, including

- Practice to the full extent of their education and training
- Achieve higher levels of education and training through seamless academic progression

The recommendation related to scope of practice has been strongly supported by the Robert Wood Johnson Foundation (RWJF). RWJF (2017) argued that regulations established by states' practice acts or federal statutes calling for physician oversight of APRNs limit public access to quality healthcare and undermine efforts to improve the state of healthcare in the United States. In the 6 years following IOM's 2010 report, 21 states have enacted regulations which grant full practice rights to APRNs (Figure 1.3). An additional 16 states have increased practice rights for APRNs, but they continue to have one or more elements restricted. Only 13 states require supervision by another health profession, resulting in restricted practice.

The family nurse practitioner (FNP) is the generalist among nurse practitioner roles. The FNP helps to manage acute and chronic illnesses across the lifespan. Population-based specialist roles among nurse practitioners include women's health, geropsychiatry, neonatal/pediatrics, and adult/acute care. These practitioners also manage acute and chronic illnesses but within the context of their specific population. Practice settings for these roles may also vary and can include primary and ambulatory care, community settings, schools, and acute care. Collectively, these roles are referred to as APRNs or a **certified registered nurse practitioner (CRNP)**.

Specialty clinical roles also exist, including CNS. The CNS provides care to patients in a range of specialties that may include pediatrics, geriatrics, emergency care, oncology, and neurology. CNSs may serve as consultants to bedside nurses or work with patients and families to manage health, illness, and disease states. Primarily, CNSs work in acute care. Because the CNS is subject to state boards' regulations for APRNs, they too can prescribe independently or with physician collaboration. Though the typical CNS may not prescribe medications, prescriptive authority for CNSs allows them to write orders for laboratory and diagnostic tests, durable medical equipment, and discharge instructions. Only nine states do not allow prescriptive authority for CNSs (NACNS, 2020).

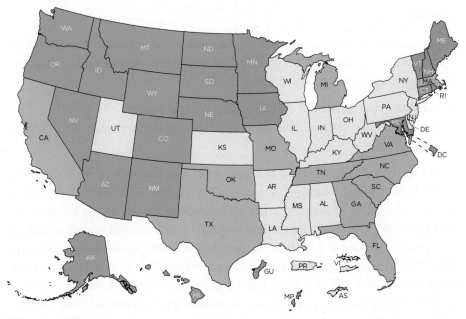

Full Practice
State practice and licensure laws provide for nurse practitioners to evaluate patients, diagnose, order and interpret diagnostic tests, initiate and manage treatments – including prescribe medications and controlled substances – under the exclusive licensure authority of the of the state board of nursing. This is the model recommended by the National Academy of Medicine, formerly called the Institute of Medicine and National Council of State Boards of Nursing.

Reduced Practice
State practice and licensure law reduces the ability of nurse practitioners to engage in at least one element of NP practice. State requires a career-long regulated collaborative agreement with another health provider in order for the NP to provide patient care or limits the setting of one or more elements of NP practice.

Restricted Practice
State practice and licensure law restricts the ability of a nurse practitioner to engage in at least one element of NP practice. State law requires career-long supervision, delegation or team-management by another health provider in order for the NP to provide patient care.

Figure 1.3. State practice environment. (Reprinted with permission from American Association of Nurse Practitioners®, 2020.)

The CNLs' role was developed by AACN to be a generalist role that would oversee the care coordination of a group of patients. The CNL functions as part of an interdisciplinary team to communicate, plan, and implement care while assessing risk. While many similarities exist between the CNS and CNL, the main difference is that the CNS functions as an expert clinician in a specialty or subspecialty, while the CNL functions as a generalist (Spross, 2004).

The scope of practice for a certified nurse midwife (CNM) includes primary care for women across the lifespan as well as for newborns. While many may think of the CNM role in terms of monitoring mother and baby during the labor and delivery process and ensuring healthy outcomes for both, their role can encompass so much more. CNMs are involved with health promotion and disease prevention for women in addition to primary, preconception, gynecologic, antepartum, intrapartum, and postpregnancy care.

CRNAs provide anesthesia and related care before and after surgical, therapeutic, diagnostic, and obstetrical procedures. In some cases, they may also provide services in pain management. CRNAs have specific skills in airway management including intubation. CRNAs function with a high degree of autonomy; they are often the main provider of anesthesia services rurally as well as for the armed services.

Summary

This chapter provided an introduction to advanced practice roles. There is a need in the United States for advanced practice nurses who are educators, administrators, and clinicians. Shortages in all these areas have been documented and are projected to become more acute. Nurses who desire to grow into an advanced practice role have an opportunity to explore the expectations of these roles and consider if they are prepared for the increased responsibility and autonomy of these positions.

The mandate for lifelong learning is especially important in the healthcare field. New discoveries in every aspect of healthcare challenge all healthcare providers to stay up-to-date with the latest findings. Advanced practice nurses are in a key position to identify areas that need further investigation and to apply new strategies to address existing problems.

Encouragement to seek advanced practice degrees abound for nurses. Not only are professional nursing organizations supportive of continued education, but the Institute of Medicine (IOM) also encourages nurses to practice to the fullest scope of their educational preparation. While barriers still exist for some advanced practice nurses, effectiveness and support for these roles become increasingly clear as research findings evolve.

Chapter Highlights

- Advanced practice roles require a higher level of education and include educators, administrators, and clinicians.
- Nurse educators, nurse administrators, and clinical nurse leaders are APNs who do not need a license to practice.
- Advanced practice registered nurses (APRNs) are licensed to practice within a scope of practice that includes prescriptive authority.
- APRNs include nurse practitioners, nurse anesthetists, nurse midwives, and clinical nurse specialists.
- Shortages in all areas of advance practice have been documented and are projected to become more acute.
- Advanced practice nurses are in a key position to identify areas that need further investigation and to apply new strategies to address existing problems.
- While barriers still exist for some advanced practice nurses, effectiveness and support for these roles become increasingly clear as research findings evolve.

Web Resources

- American Association of Nurse Practitioners: https://www.aanp.org/
- American Association of Nurse Practitioners State Practice Environment: https://www.aanp.org/advocacy/state/state-practice-environment
- Affordable Care Act Summary: https://www.kff.org/health-reform/fact-sheet/summary-of-the-affordable-care-act/
- American Association of Colleges of Nursing: http://www.aacnnursing.org/
- American Organization for Nursing Leadership (AONL): https://www.aonl.org/
- Institute of Medicine *Future of Nursing: Leading Change, Advancing Health*: http://nationalacademies.org/hmd/reports/2010/the-future-of-nursing-leading-change-advancing-health.aspx
- Understanding the Affordable Care Act: https://www.aier.org/research/understanding-affordable-care-act

References

American Association of Colleges of Nursing (AACN). (2006). *The essentials of doctoral education for advanced nursing practice.* https://www.aacnnursing.org/Portals/42/Publications/DNPEssentials.pdf

American Association of Colleges of Nursing (AACN). (2008). *The essentials of baccalaureate education for professional nursing practice.* https://www.aacnnursing.org/Portals/42/Publications/BaccEssentials08.pdf

American Association of Colleges of Nursing (AACN). (2011). *The essentials of master's education in nursing.* https://www.aacnnursing.org/Portals/42/Publications/MastersEssentials11.pdf

American Association of Colleges of Nursing. (2019a). *2018–2019 Enrollment and graduations in baccalaureate and graduate programs in nursing.* https://www.aacnnursing.org/Portals/42/News/Factsheets/Faculty-Shortage-Factsheet.pdf

American Association of Colleges of Nursing. (2019b). *Fact sheet: Nursing faculty shortage.* https://www.aacnnursing.org/Portals/42/News/Factsheets/Faculty-Shortage-Factsheet.pdf

American Association of Nurse Practitioners. (2020). *NP fact sheet.* https://www.aanp.org/about/all-about-nps/np-fact-sheet

American Institute for Economic Research. (2014). *Executive Brief: Understanding the affordable care act.* https://www.aier.org/research/understanding-affordable-care-act

American Medical Association. (2017). *AMA vision on health reform.* https://www.ama-assn.org/delivering-care/patient-support-advocacy/ama-vision-health-care-reform?ad_seg=Influencers

American Nurses Association (ANA). (2017). *Recognition of a nursing specialty, approval of a specialty nursing scope nursing scope of practice statement, acknowledgment of specialty nursing standards of practice, and affirmation of focused practice competencies.* https://www.nursingworld.org/~4989de/globalassets/practiceandpolicy/scope-of-practice/3sc-booklet-final-2017-08-17.pdf

American Organization for Nursing Leadership. (2020, AONE, 2007). *Guiding principles for the role of the nurse executive in patient safety.* https://www.aonl.org/guiding-principles-role-nurse-executive-patient-safety

Anderson, B., Gingery, A., McClellan, M., Rose, R., Schmitz, D., & Schou, P. (2019). *NRHA policy paper: Access to rural maternity care.* https://www.ruralhealthweb.org/NRHA/media/Emerge_NRHA/Advocacy/Policy%20documents/01-16-19-NRHA-Policy-Access-to-Rural-Maternity-Care.pdf

Association of American Medical Colleges. (2004). *COGME report predicts physician shortage.* http://www.aamc.org/newsroom/reporter/nov04/cogme.htm

Billings, D. M., & Halstead, J. A. (2019). *Teaching in nursing: A guide for faculty* (6th ed.). Elsevier.

Conover, C. (2015). *A faster, better, cheaper path to filling the doctor shortage.* https://www.forbes.com/sites/theapothecary/2015/03/16/a-faster-better-cheaper-path-to-filling-the-doctor-shortage/#3eab4c3e5996

Finkelman, A. (2017). *Professional nursing concepts: Competencies for quality leadership* (4th ed.). Jones & Bartlett Learning.

Garrett, B., & Gangopadhyaya, A. (2016). *Who gained health insurance coverage under the ACA, and where do they live? (Robert Wood Johnson Foundation report).* http://www.urban.org/sites/default/files/publication/86761/2001041-who-gained-health-insurance-coverage-under-the-aca-and-where-do-they-live.pdf

Glied, S. H., Ma, S., & Borja, A. A. (2017). Effect of the affordable care act on health care access. *Commonwealth Fund, 13,* 1–11.

Healthcare.gov. (n.d.). *Affordable care act (ACA).* https://www.healthcare.gov/glossary/affordable-care-act/

Ingwell-Spolan, C. (2018). Chief nursing officers' views on meeting the needs of the professional nurse: How this can affect patient outcomes. *Healthcare, 6*(2), 56. https://www.ncbi.nlm.nih.gov/pmc/articles/PMC6023280/

Institute of Medicine (US); Committee on the Robert Wood Johnson Foundation Initiative on the Future of Nursing, at the Institute of Medicine. (2010). *The future of nursing: Leading change, advancing health.* National Academies Press.

Lippincott Solutions. (2018a). *Update on future of nursing report: Are we there yet?* http://lippincottsolutions.lww.com/blog.entry.html/2018/02/13/update_on_futureof-q5jh.html

Lippincott Solutions. (2018b). *For better or worse, nurse managers influence outcomes.* http://lippincottsolutions.lww.com/blog.entry.html/2018/03/20/for_better_or_worse-yALW.html

National Association of Clinical Nurse Specialists (NACNS). (2020). *Scope of practice.* https://nacns.org/advocacy-policy/policies-affecting-cnss/scope-of-practice/

National League for Nursing (NLN). (2020). *Certified nurse educator 2020 candidate handbook.* http://www.nln.org/docs/default-source/default-document-library/cne-handbook-sept-2020.pdf?sfvrsn=2

Qalehsari, M. Q., Khaghanizadeh, M., & Ebadi, A. (2017). Lifelong learning strategies in nursing: A systematic review. *Electronic Physician, 9*(10), 5541–5550. https://www.ncbi.nlm.nih.gov/pmc/articles/PMC5718860/

Robert Wood Johnson Foundation. (2017). The case for removing barriers to APRN practice. *Charting Nursing's Future, 30,* 1–3. http://www.rwjf.org/content/dam/farm/reports/issue_briefs/2017/rwjf435543

Spross, J. A. (2004). *Working statement comparing the CNL and CNS roles.* http://www.aacn.nche.edu/cnl/CNLCNSComparisonTable.pdf

The Tri-Council for Nursing. (2020). *Welcome.* https://tricouncilfornursing.org/

Warshawsky, N. E., & Havens, D. S. (2014). Nurse manager job satisfaction and intent to leave. *Nurse Economics, 32*(1), 32–39.

2

Education and Licensure Considerations

Carolyn Hart · Pegge L. Bell

LEARNING OBJECTIVES

After completing this chapter, you will be able to:

1. Explain the purpose of nursing accreditation.

2. Review degree and postgraduate certificate options in advanced nursing education.

3. Compare PhD and DNP options in doctoral education.

4. Discuss licensure and certification requirements.

5. Recognize standard APRN terminology as presented in the Consensus Model.

KEY TERMS

Accreditation: Certification that an educational institution or program of study has met standards set by an external evaluator.

Advanced practice nurse (APN): Nurse holding a graduate degree who may work within the broad roles of educator, administrator, or clinician (including APRN roles).

Advanced practice registered nurse (APRN): Advanced practice nurse holding a separate RN license in an advanced clinical role, including certified nurse midwives (CNMs), clinical nurse specialists (CNSs), certified registered nurse anesthetists (CRNAs), and nurse practitioners (NPs).

Bridge programs: Academic programs designed to allow nurses to obtain a higher level of education in a more streamlined fashion.

Certification: Credentials earned after passing a psychometrically evaluated examination offered by a professional nursing organization.

Certificate: Issued after completing a course, series of courses, or continuing education event.

Consensus Model: A document that defines APRN practice, describes the APRN regulatory model, and defines specialties and titles.

Doctor of nursing practice (DNP): The advanced terminal nursing degree with a practice focus.

Doctor of philosophy (PhD): The advanced terminal nursing degree with a research focus.

Master of Science in Nursing (MSN): The advanced nursing degree that follows the bachelor's degree in nursing.

Specialization: A focus area or track in an advanced nursing practice program of study.

Terminal degree: The highest level of education awarded in a particular field. In nursing, this is a doctoral degree.

Introduction

The decision to pursue graduate nursing education requires appropriate consideration, as formal education is both expensive and time consuming. Nurses must be very careful to select an institution that will provide the appropriate advanced degree (master's, DNP, or PhD) relevant to their goals. They also must consider the advanced practice nurse (APN) role so that the program of study matches the certification and licensure requirements of the role. Lastly, they must consider if the educational program has national accreditation by a nursing organization. If not, they may not have further educational mobility, as most Doctor of Nursing practice (DNP) and Doctor of Philosophy (PhD) programs require their master's-prepared applicants to graduate from an accredited program. The information below will aid in decisions regarding educational and career choices.

Accreditation

Accreditation is the process of evaluating educational institutions and programs of study to ensure that they meet standards and quality indicators as determined by an authorized external evaluator. Accreditors are authorized by the U.S. Department of Education (2020) and serve the public by assuring that programs adhere to published standards.

In advanced practice, accreditation is layered. As with undergraduate education, the institution must first be accredited; this is typically done through regional accreditation as presented in Figure 2.1. In some instances, universities

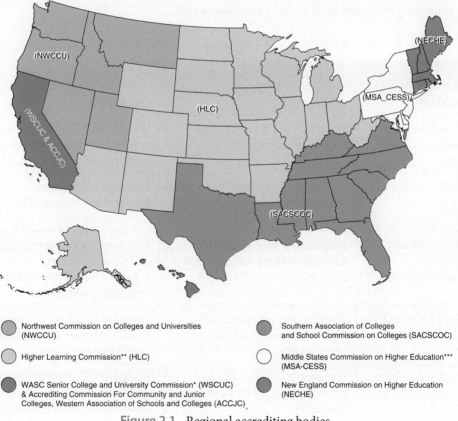

Northwest Commission on Colleges and Universities (NWCCU)

Higher Learning Commission** (HLC)

WASC Senior College and University Commission* (WSCUC) & Accrediting Commission For Community and Junior Colleges, Western Association of Schools and Colleges (ACCJC)

Southern Association of Colleges and School Commission on Colleges (SACSCOC)

Middle States Commission on Higher Education*** (MSA-CESS)

New England Commission on Higher Education (NECHE)

Figure 2.1. Regional accrediting bodies.

may seek to obtain national rather than regional accreditation. Although regional accreditation is widely recognized and credits are easily transferred to other institutions, credits can be more expensive compared with those obtained at an institution with national accreditation. The U.S. Department of Education reports approximately 85% of colleges and universities maintain regional accreditation. This process accredits the institution and not individual programs.

Nursing programs must also be accredited. Undergraduate and graduate programs must be accredited by one of the three agencies: the National League for Nursing's Commission for Nursing Education Accreditation (CNEA), the American Association of Colleges of Nursing's Commission on Collegiate Nursing Education (CCNE), or the Accreditation Commission for Education in Nursing (ACEN). Although the requirements for meeting standards of accreditation vary by agency, they generally focus on mission and governance, curriculum, faculty standards, evaluation, and the student experience. Table 2.1 presents a comparison of accreditation standards.

Table 2.1. Comparison of Accreditation Standards

ACEN (2017)	CCNE (2013)	CNEA (2016)
Standard 1: Mission and Administrative Capacity	Standard I: Program Quality: Mission and Governance	Standard II: Culture of Integrity and Accountability—Mission, Governance, and Resources
Standard 6: Outcomes	Standard IV: Program Effectiveness: Assessment and Achievement of Program Outcomes	Standard I: Culture of Excellence—Program Outcomes
Standard 2: Faculty and Staff Standard 3: Students	Standard II: Program Quality: Institutional Commitment and Resources	Standard III: Culture of Excellence and Caring—Faculty Standard IV: Culture of Excellence and Caring—Students
Standard 4: Curriculum	Standard III: Program Quality: Curriculum and Teaching-Learning Practices	Standard V: Culture of Learning and Diversity—Curriculum and Evaluation Processes
Standard 5: Resources	Standard II: Program Quality: Institutional Commitment and Resources	Standard II: Culture of Integrity and Accountability—Mission, Governance, and Resources

The final layer to accreditation is for specific advanced practice specialties, which may use other accreditation standards. While some certified nurse anesthetist (CRNA) programs also carry nursing accreditation, they are required to maintain accreditation by the Council on Accreditation (COA). Certified nurse midwife (CNM) programs are accredited by the Accreditation Commission for Midwifery Education (ACME). The CNM and CRNA programs that do not use CCNE, CNEA, or ACEN for accreditation still provide a curriculum that is a good match with the essential competencies of American Association of Colleges of Nursing's (AACN's) "*Essentials for Nursing Education*." Nurse practitioner programs also comply with the standards set by the National Organization of Nursing Practitioner Faculty (NONPF).

 In Their Own Words

Judith Halstead, PhD, RN, FAAN, ANEF
Executive Director, National League for Nursing (NLN) Commission for Nursing Education Accreditation (CNEA)

What Is the Purpose of Accreditation?
The primary purpose of program accreditation is to protect the interests of the public and demonstrate the program's accountability to the public. Nursing programs are accountable to students, employers, funders, the profession, and ultimately the patients who are recipients of nursing care. Achieving accreditation demonstrates this accountability and provides the program with a public mark of quality.

How Does Accreditation Relate to Quality?
Quality improvement is the core concept underpinning the accreditation process. Engaging in continuous quality improvement can help bring a faculty together to collectively address its program's outcomes, strengths, and areas for improvement.

How Are Faculty Involved in Accreditation?
The faculty role in accreditation is one of shared responsibility with program administrators, built upon a spirit of collaboration and mutual decision-making, in partnership with the program's stakeholders. When thinking about

(Continued)

accreditation, I wish faculty would consider it to be an opportunity to reach out and build relationships with these stakeholders. It is an opportunity to share the program's success stories and efforts at improvement with others and to invite others to share their unique perspective about the program's accomplishments and areas to grow.

I wish someone had told me ... Early in my nursing education career, I wish someone had told me that participating in the accreditation process is not something to fear. Instead, it is a means by which nurse educators can increase their knowledge about the educational process and develop their leadership skills, thus positively impacting not only the students in their program but also their own career development.

Degree Options

Multiple degree pathways are available to nurses seeking an advanced education. Although navigating the options can seem difficult, understanding the purpose of the degrees and trends in nursing education can help simplify the choice. Just as various entry points are available for licensure as a registered nurse (i.e., diploma, associate, or baccalaureate), different academic pathways exist for nurses wishing to advance their education. However, in contrast to undergraduate education where all pathways lead to licensure as a registered nurse, at the advanced practice level different pathways lead to different roles.

Graduate-level degrees generally include all degrees above the baccalaureate level, including master's and doctoral options. Graduate degrees usually are obtained to further a career or create new job opportunities. Requirements for entry into a graduate program vary based upon the program but generally include a minimum grade point average (GPA) for admission. Some institutions also may request references, a resume, or results from the Graduate Record Examination (GRE). The GRE is a test that, much like the SAT and ACT, is a broad measure of ability in critical thinking, analytical writing, verbal reasoning, and quantitative skills.

Master of Science in Nursing

The **Master of Science in Nursing (MSN or MS)** is a graduate degree consisting of a variable number of credits and taking 2 to 3 years to complete. The length of time needed to complete an MSN depends on the student's ability to attend on a full- or part-time basis. Full-time graduate work is typically a credit load of 9 semester hours including summers, while part-time students will carry about 6 semester hours. MSN programs are offered in a variety of settings including online, hybrid, or face-to-face. Accredited MSN programs will adhere to the competencies required by their accrediting body. The AACN's *Essentials for Master's Education in Nursing* (2011) is used by accredited nursing programs to guide the course content of individual programs. In some cases, such as the CRNA or CNM, an alternate professional accrediting body is used. The curriculum of CRNA and CNM programs addresses the professional organization's competencies and also can include the AACN's *Essentials for Master's Education in Nursing*.

While the BSN is considered a generalist degree, MSN programs typically have **specializations**. These areas may be broad, including nursing education, administration, and leadership, or specifically focused on a population or setting. **APRN** educational preparation categories include nurse anesthetists, CNSs, nurse practitioners, and nurse midwives. Further specialization for nurse practitioners may address primary or acute care settings or population foci (see Chapter 1, Table 1.1). CNS tracks also include a specialty area either by clinical focus (e.g., medical-surgical, perinatal, critical care, pediatric) or by diagnosis (e.g., wound care, ostomy care, diabetes).

Universities or colleges may offer **bridge programs** that do not require a BSN for admission to the graduate program. The purpose of a bridge program is to allow nurses to earn a higher degree without having to pursue a BSN. The term *bridge* refers to those courses that may substitute for bachelor-level courses or courses that prepare students for graduate-level study. These accelerated programs may or may not grant a BSN at some point in the curriculum. Additionally, some programs have a clear distinction between courses that are considered part of a bridge and those that are part of graduate coursework. Common bridge programs include RN-MSN, RN-DNP, or BSN-Doctorate (PhD or DNP).

Doctoral Education

Doctoral degrees are either research-focused or practice-focused. The research-focused doctoral degree is the PhD, while the practice-focused degree is the DNP. The PhD and DNP are each considered a **terminal degree** for nurses. While both types of programs emphasize a scholarly approach to professional practice as nurses, differences do exist between their educational preparation and practice, as identified in Table 2.2. Nurses may opt to complete both the PhD and the DNP degree programs to better match their career goals.

The research-focused PhD degree prepares nurses with the skills needed to design, conduct, and lead independent research studies. The Doctor of Philosophy title refers to the Greek derivation of the term *philosophy*—meaning love of wisdom—and implies expertise in one's field of study (Waddle, 2015). Many PhD-prepared nurses will assume faculty roles; however, clinical entities that value their contribution to clinical research—from large healthcare corporations to the Veterans Administration—will also employ PhD-prepared nurses. The PhD curriculum largely focuses on philosophy, theory, research methods, as well as quantitative and qualitative data collection methods. Most PhD programs require completion of coursework in a defined area of study that supports research or career interests through the completion of electives.

Practice-focused DNP programs can lead to **certification** and thus have specific course requirements. In their seminal publication, *Crossing the Quality Chasm: A New Health System for the 21st Century*, the Institute of Medicine (IOM, 2001) advocated for an increased emphasis in nursing education to (1) translate evidence into practice, (2) apply technology to safety, and (3) work

Table 2.2. Comparison of PhD and DNP Degrees		
	PhD	**DNP**
Program type	Research focus	Practice focus
Emphasis	Theory and research methodology	Clinical practice
Program outcome	Dissertation: Original research that adds to nursing knowledge	Clinical project: Validates impact or significance of research on practice

DNP, Doctor of Nursing Practice.

within interdisciplinary teams. The AACN (2004) developed criteria for the DNP to align with these recommendations and to further improve patient outcomes. Careers supported by this terminal degree include nurses with a clinical practice focus such as nurse practitioners, nurse anesthetists, and nurse midwives. Some programs also have a leadership track that is appropriate for nurse administrators, nurse educators, and other specialty areas such as informaticists.

Not all nursing faculty are PhD prepared; many faculty have completed the DNP degree or other terminal degrees related to education. DNP preparation is likely for faculty members who hold certification as an APN and have an active practice. They can combine their interest in practice with their role as educator, administrator, or clinician. Although credentialed degrees such as doctor of nursing science (DNSc, DNS) exist, this text is consistent with AACN's recommendation that the DNP be the practice-focused doctoral credential.

Questions to Ask Yourself

1. Is my career goal to be research-focused or practice-focused?
2. How much time am I able to devote to my studies?
3. Do I meet the clinical requirement of practice hours before admission?
4. Do I need help in scholarly writing?
5. What graduate education options are available in my area?
6. Is an online program a realistic option for me?
7. Does my employer offer educational benefits?
8. What scholarships or fellowships might help finance my education?
9. Is the GRE required, and what preparation do I need?

DNP Program Outcomes and Expectations

DNP programs are the result of the AACN expressing a need for a terminal clinical degree and the National Organization of Nurse Practitioner Faculty (NONPF) recommending that the DNP be the entry level to practice for nurse practitioners. The AACN reports significant growth in the number of DNP programs over the past decade, outpacing the growth of PhD programs in that same period. DNP programs meet the standards prescribed by the AACN's "*Essentials of Doctoral Education for Advanced Nursing Practice*" (2006; see Chapter 3). Figure 2.2, prepared by the AACN task force (2017), visually demonstrates the growth pattern of these two programs.

Growth in doctoral nursing programs: 2006-2018

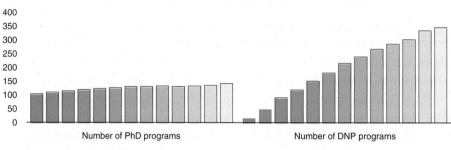

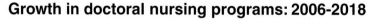

Figure 2.2. Growth of DNP (doctor of nursing practice) and PhD (doctor of philosophy) nursing programs. DNP Fact Sheet (2019), American Association of Colleges for Nursing (AACN). https://www.aacnnursing.org/News-Information/Fact-Sheets/DNP-Fact-Sheet.

In 2004, the AACN recommended that all nurse practitioner programs transition to the DNP and that this become the entry level into advanced practice roles. Several reasons exist for this emphasis on doctoral education. Education at the doctoral level would be more in line with the degree requirements in other fields such as medicine, pharmacy, physical therapy, and audiology. The number of hours required for a practice specialty in nursing at the master's level is higher than that of other fields. Research indicates that higher nurse education is linked to better care and improved outcomes. While nurses may still become certified as practitioners at the master's level, this will likely change in the future.

In June 2007, the American Association of Nurse Anesthetists' (AANA) board adopted a position statement to support doctoral education for entry into nurse anesthesia practice by 2025. The Council on Accreditation of Nurse Anesthesia Educational Programs (COA) voted in 2009 to require nurse anesthesia educational programs to transition to a doctoral degree no later than 2022. All entry into practice graduates from CRNA programs will be required to possess a doctoral degree as of January 1, 2025, and most programs have already begun the transition from master's to doctoral degrees for educational preparation into the role. As of November 2017, 67 nurse anesthesia programs were approved to offer entry-level doctoral degrees and 23 programs offered post-master's doctoral degree completion programs. Fifty-three programs remain to be approved at the doctoral level by the deadline of January 1, 2022.

In Their Own Words

Sarah Rhoads, PhD, DNP, WHNP-BC, FAAN
Professor, The University of Tennessee Health Science Center

How Do You Relate Your Educational Journey Since Receiving Your BSN? (Degrees/Specializations and Dates or Number of Years Later?)

As a nurse, I have always been driven to be the best provider I could be for my patients. The drive to provide excellent care, fueled my passion to further pursue my education. When I was a nurse on labor and delivery, I cared for so many women with high-risk pregnancies. Although I enjoyed my experiences as a labor and delivery nurse, I felt the need to care for women earlier in their pregnancy ideally preventing severe complications. During graduate school, I was able to broaden my career options, upon graduation with my Master's of Science in Nursing (WHNP).

What Were Your Professional Goals and/or Impetus for Completing Each of These Degrees?

In 2000 with my MSN with a specialization as a women's health NP, I became an undergraduate faculty member in the College of Nursing. I was very fortunate to have wonderful mentors as a new faculty member. They guided me to further pursue my education. I applied for the Doctorate of Nursing Science (DNSc) program at the University of Tennessee Health Science Center for several reasons. I had thought a practice focus doctorate was more in line with my career goals and UTHSC was a different university than my other two degrees. I felt the need to broaden my perspective with a new university setting and faculty members. Just as I was starting the DNSc program, the Doctorate of Nursing Practice program was approved by AACN, so current DNSc students had the option of completing a DNSc or a DNP. I chose to graduate with a DNP in 2006. I did not delay in pursuing a PhD and applied and was accepted for the part-time PhD program in 2007 and graduated 2013. For me, the dual doctoral degree has allowed me to see the importance of both degrees and the specific role each has in improving healthcare.

How Do You Think Your Current Faculty Role Has Been Enhanced With the Completion of the DNP?

Many people ask me what I use more, my PhD or my DNP. I always say that I use both! My experiences and educational background have allowed me to look at clinical issues and see the research opportunities. When I am planning a

(Continued)

research study, I am able to see the clinical issues related to feasibility. Many of my research studies examine the usability and feasibility of technology in the healthcare setting.

What Steps Do You Take to Maintain Certification and Licensure for Your APRN Role?
As a women's health nurse practitioner, I am able to maintain my certification through testing and continuing education. When I transitioned to less of a clinical role into an administrative role, I gave up my clinical practice as a WHNP. I do miss working with individual patients, but I feel in my current role that I am able to impact healthcare on a systems and public health level.

What Advice Do You Have for Other Nurses Who Want to Advance Their Nursing Education?
The best thing you can do is continue to work on your degrees. Do what fits into your personal and professional life. Whether that be taking one course a semester or going to school full time. Make sure you have a support network of peers, mentors, and people who care for you.

Clinical Hours

Clinical requirements vary across the advanced practice programs (MSN and DNP) for admission to the program and during the program. Students in a BSN-DNP program may complete at least 1,000 clinical hours during their program of study (AACN, 2015). BSN-prepared RNs who enter a graduate program may be required to complete a minimum of 500 practice hours before admission to the program. BSN students who graduate from their program and successfully pass the NCLEX-RN examination may be required to work full time (40 hours per week for almost 13 weeks) to be eligible for admission to a clinical graduate program.

DNP Project

The AACN (2015) uses the term "DNP project" to distinguish this requirement from other programs that require a final project before graduation. This project reflects the translation of evidence into practice and should follow AACN's DNP *Essentials*. These *Essentials* clarify that the DNP project should successfully integrate key components identified in Box 2.1.

BOX 2.1

▶ DNP PROJECT REQUIREMENTS

Focus on a change that impacts healthcare outcomes through either direct or indirect care
Have a system's (micro-, meso-, or macrolevel) or population/aggregate focus
Demonstrate implementation in the appropriate area of practice
Include a plan for sustainability (financial, systems, or political realities)
Include an evaluation of processes and/or outcomes (formative or summative)
Provide a foundation for future practice scholarship

American Association of Colleges of Nursing. (2015). *The doctor of nursing practice: Current issues and clarifying recommendations.* http://www.aacnnursing.org/Portals/42/News/White-Papers/DNP-Implementation-TF-Report-8-15.pdf?ver=2017-10-18-151758-700

PhD Program Outcomes and Expectations

The PhD is a globally recognized degree offered in a wide variety of disciplines and, on average, takes more than 3 years to complete. Because those with this level of education are expected to be experts in their field, the PhD is traditionally considered the required degree to teach nursing students at all levels. A PhD program requires completion of a dissertation or doctoral thesis. PhD students complete courses in theory, research, statistics, and philosophy to prepare for their dissertation and role of researcher upon graduation. Graduates of these programs primarily assume nursing faculty or research positions. PhD-prepared faculty may engage in writing grant proposals, securing funding to support their research projects, conducting research that has been approved by an Internal Review Board (IRB), and disseminating findings in publications and by presentations, which leads to the development of their scholarship in an identifiable area of research.

PhD nursing programs currently are not required to seek nursing accreditation. Prospective PhD students should be diligent in selecting a program that has resources in place to support research endeavors. Prospective students should also inquire about the availability of educational courses that support the development as a faculty member if a faculty role is the goal upon graduation.

PhD Dissertation

The dissertation is the final step of doctoral education and consists of a new and valuable contribution to the field of study, typically in the form of research. The steps leading to the dissertation include development of a sound methodology that is appropriate to the proposed study, collection of data, and analysis and reporting of results. Although no one clear definition of original research exists (Edwards, 2014), Phillips and Pugh (2010) developed a framework for understanding originality (Box 2.2).

The dissertation is the process of defending one's research, results, and conclusions before a board of faculty. During the defense, the doctoral student is expected to present a clear rationale for choices and decisions made during the research process. Although some variation may exist, the dissertation typically includes the following chapters: introduction, literature review, methods, results, discussion, and references (Box 2.3).

Postgraduate Certificates

At the completion of the master's degree, graduates can gain additional expertise or second advanced practice specializations through a postgraduate certificate. Postgraduate certificates build on the knowledge and clinical experiences

---

BOX 2.2

▶ RESEARCH ORIGINALITY

- New empirical research
- Original synthesis of information or data
- New interpretation of an existing material
- Application of a previous study to a different population
- New application of an existing technique
- New evidence for an existing issue
- Research into unexplored topics
- Adding to knowledge in a new way

Adapted from Phillips, E. M. & Pugh, D. S. (2010) *How to get a PhD: A handbook for students and their supervisors* (5th ed.). Open University Press.

BOX 2.3

▶ ORGANIZATION OF A TYPICAL DOCTORAL DISSERTATION

1. Introduction
   a. Significance
   b. Problem statement
   c. Research questions and hypothesis

2. Literature review
   a. Historical background and current relevant information
   b. Theoretical framework

3. Method
   a. IRB approval
   b. Sample
   c. Research design
   d. Data analysis

4. Results
   a. Statistical analysis to answer research questions
   b. Presentation of data

5. Discussion
   a. Summary
   b. Conclusions
   c. Limitations
   d. Recommendations for future research

6. References

provided in the original master's degree program of study. This helps reduce the number of required credit hours for the certificate as nonclinical courses are similar across the master's programs. What varies are the actual advanced nursing theory and clinical courses to support the role or specialization. These courses and clinical experiences are required for certification in a specific role or specialization. However, APNs seeking a postgraduate certificate should be aware that clinical hours completed during the master's program will not apply to clinical hours required for the additional role or specialization.

For example, an APRN in clinical practice may obtain a postgraduate certificate in administration to support a transition to a leadership role. Similarly, a nurse with an MSN in education may opt to complete a postgraduate certificate as a nurse practitioner. APRNs also may add an additional area of specialization. For example, a master's-prepared family nurse practitioner can obtain a postgraduate certificate as a psychiatric mental health nurse practitioner. CRNAs may complete the Advanced Pain Management Certificate Program, accredited by the COA, and take a certification examination on Nonsurgical Pain Management offered by the National Board of Certification and Recertification for Nurse Anesthetists.

Certification

Nurses who graduate from an APRN educational program in one of the four clinical categories (CRNA, CNM, CNS, and certified nurse practitioner [NP]) are eligible to sit for the appropriate certification examination. Nurses seeking initial certification must pass the certification to apply for APRN licensure in their respective state. Additional information on APRN certification is provided in Part III of this book. Graduates of other advanced nursing programs (educator, administrator, and clinical nurse leader [CNL]) do not require licensure but may obtain certification as part of career growth (Chapters 4, 5, and 10).

Each APRN professional organization has specific requirements for initial certification and for maintenance of that certification with numerous professional organizations offering APRN certification. The American Nurses Credentialing Center (ANCC) allows APRN candidates to test before graduation and conferral of their degree, provided they have completed all coursework and faculty-supervised clinical practice hours for the degree (ANCC Newsletter, 2018). Candidates for certification must match the appropriate certifying body with their educational preparation, as provided in Table 2.3.

Licensure

When certification in one of the four APRN roles is achieved, the CRNA, CNM, CNS, or certified NP can apply to their state for licensure as an APRN.

Table 2.3. Certification and Certifying Bodies

Certifying Body	Role
American Midwifery Certification Board (AMCB)	CNM
American Nurses Credentialing Center (ANCC)	CNS
The National Board of Certification and Recertification for Nurse Anesthetists (NBCRNA)	CRNA
American Academy of Nurse Practitioners National Certification Board (AANP)	NP

CNM, certified nurse midwife; CNS, clinical nurse specialist; CRNA, certified registered nurse anesthetists; NP, nurse practitioner.

Nurses must be certified by a national organization to apply for a state APRN license. As the RN license is renewable, so is the APRN license. These are separate licenses; both will need to be renewed for continued practice. For renewal of the APRN license, ARPNs must demonstrate continued education and clinical practice as defined by their certifying professional nursing organization.

Nurses who have completed graduate programs (MSN or DNP) with a focus on education, administration, and clinical leadership can assume advanced nursing roles as educators, nurse administrators, or clinical nurse leaders upon graduation. They may also sit for a certification examination in these advanced nursing roles, but certification in these advanced practice roles is not required for practice. There is no licensure requirement above the RN licensure for these advanced nursing roles. Therefore, these roles are not given the designation of APRN.

Consensus Model

Each state has laws regarding the title and scope of practice for APNs, which can cause barriers for APRNs who wish to relocate to other states. Unfortunately, there were inconsistent standards across states regarding

APRN education, practice, and licensure. In 2008, the National Council of State Boards of Nursing (NCSBN) proposed a Consensus Model for APRN regulation with the goal of having consensus across all states with respect to APRN title, roles and recognition of APRNs, licensure and titles, education at the graduate level, advanced certification, independent practice, and full prescriptive authority.

At the time of the original Consensus Model, four categories of APRNs were identified: CRNA, CNM, CNS, and NP (NCSBN, 2008). The clinical nurse leader role had not yet been envisioned nor were existing roles, such as nurse educator and nurse administrator, considered advanced nursing practice (AACN, 2008). In assessing compliance of state boards of nursing in meeting Consensus Model goals, language issues were identified. For example, *licensure* was not uniformly applied to APRNs, with some states instead referring to certification, approval to practice, authorization, and APN registry.

In 2014, a review of states' compliance with the Consensus Model found the APRN title was adopted by 60% of the states (Cahill et al., 2014). Fifty-two percent of states issued an APRN license, and three states (South Dakota, Minnesota, and Indiana) did not require graduate education for one or more of the APRN roles (p. 8). Certification was required by all states except four in one or more of the APRN roles (California, Kansas, Indiana, and New York). Fourteen states granted independent practice to all four APRN roles, with 21 states that required collaboration or direct supervision of all roles (p. 9). Fourteen states granted independent prescriptive authority to all four APRN roles, but 33 jurisdictions did not grant independent prescribing privileges to any of the roles (Cahill et al., 2014, p. 9).

In 2018, the NCSBN provided an update on how states have moved legislation to be more uniform as outlined in the Consensus Model. Only two states (South Dakota and Indiana) do not require a graduate degree or postgraduate certificate to practice as an APRN. Twelve states and one territory do not include all four APRN groups (CNP, CRNA, CNS, and CNM) under the APRN title. Nineteen states and one territory do not use the term "license" in authoring APRN practice. National certification was not a requirement to practice as an APRN in California, Kansas, Indiana, and New York.

Tracking the success of the Consensus Model is important for APRNs who want to practice at their full capacity. With healthcare becoming more specialized, it is important to remember that APRNs may need to add a specialization or even a post-master's certification in another APN role to legally practice with their population of interest. This additional education will enhance marketability, but also requires additional certification and licensure. An algorithm can be helpful in making decisions about the patient population(s) of interest, practice focus (e.g., provide anesthesia, educate, focus on a specialty area or acute illness), and primary care vs. acute care considerations (Doherty et al., 2018). More information about the Consensus Model is presented in Chapter 7.

Figures 2.3 and 2.4 present the Consensus Model for nurse practitioners and CNSs, respectively. In addition to role regulation, the Consensus Model aligns educational programs and areas of study by providing standard terminology for population foci and specialization (Thomas et al., 2017).

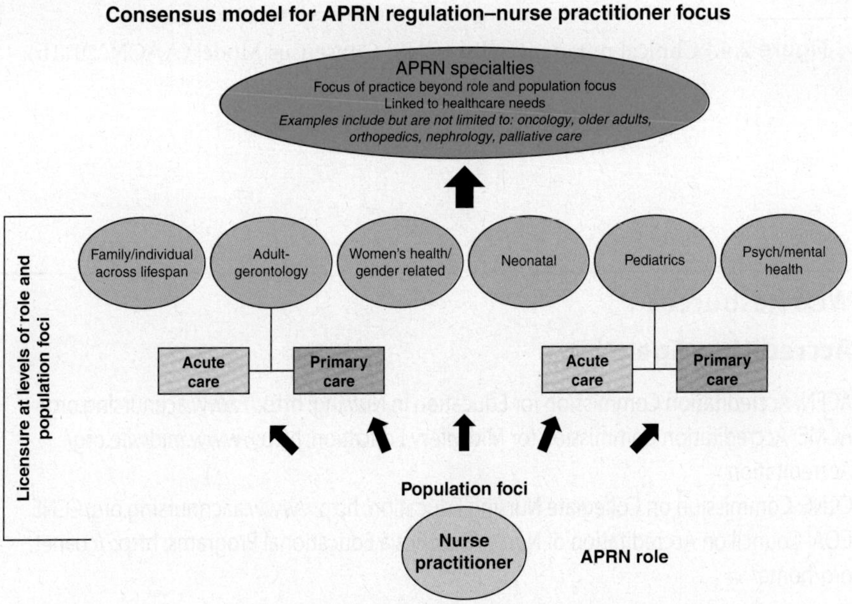

Consensus model for APRN regulation–nurse practitioner focus

Figure 2.3. Nurse practitioner Consensus Model (AACN, 2011a).

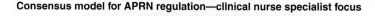

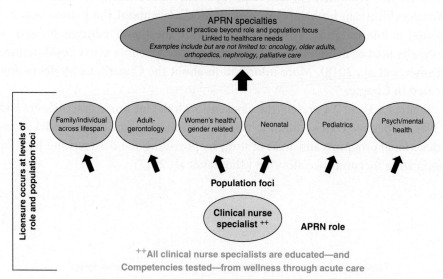

Figure 2.4. Clinical nurse specialist (CNS) Consensus Model (AACN, 2011b).

Web Resources

Accrediting Agencies

ACEN: Accreditation Commission for Education in Nursing: http://www.acenursing.org/
ACME: Accreditation Commission for Midwifery Education: http://www.midwife.org/
Accreditation
CCNE: Commission on Collegiate Nursing Education: http://www.aacnnursing.org/CCNE
COA: Council on Accreditation of Nurse Anesthesia Educational Programs: http://coanet.
org/home/

> **Professional Organizations**
>
> - AACN: American Association of Colleges of Nursing (oversees CCNE): http://www.aacnnursing.org/
> - AANA: American Association of Nurse Anesthetists: https://www.aana.com/
> - AANP: American Association of Nurse Practitioners: https://www.aanp.org/
> - AONL: American Organization for Nursing Leadership (formerly AONE): https://www.aonl.org/
> - NLN: National League for Nursing (Oversees ACEN): http://www.nln.org/
> - ANA: American Nurses Association: https://www.nursingworld.org/
> - NLN: National League for Nursing: http://www.nln.org/
> - Sigma: Sigma Theta Tau International: https://www.sigmanursing.org/

Summary

This chapter provides an overview of the educational and licensure aspects related to APN. Future APNs should carefully select an educational program that is the best match for their career goals, is accredited by a nursing organization, and meets their needs for work-school balance. Choosing an accredited educational program—particularly at the master's level—will provide educational mobility for doctoral degrees. Additionally, accreditation also provides graduates with the assurance their program provided the necessary curriculum to be successful in their career choice. Certification is available for all advanced practice roles but are required for the four APRN roles (CNM, CNS, CNP, and CRNA) to seek APRN licensure. Recertification demonstrates a commitment to lifelong learning, as most certifying bodies require recertification every 5 years. The Consensus Model provides APRNs with important information regarding individual states' compliance with title, licensure, and scope of practice. The ability to practice to one's full scope lies at the state level.

Chapter Highlights

- Certification by a professional organization and licensure by one's individual state are necessary steps in achieving the APRN role.

- Certification for nonclinician APNs can validate their competencies of educator and administrator roles.
- Future APNs should carefully select an educational program that is the best match for their career goals and is accredited by a nursing organization.
- Recertification demonstrates a commitment to lifelong learning, as most certifying bodies require recertification every 5 years.
- The Consensus Model provides APRNs with important information regarding individual states' compliance with title, licensure, and scope of practice.

References

American Association of Colleges of Nursing (AACN). (2004). *AACN position statement on the practice doctorate in nursing.* https://www.aacnnursing.org/Portals/42/News/Position-Statements/DNP.pdf

American Association of Colleges of Nursing (AACN). (2008). *Consensus model for APRN regulation: Licensure, accreditation, certification & education.* https://www.aacnnursing.org/Portals/42/AcademicNursing/pdf/APRNReport.pdf

American Association of Colleges of Nursing (AACN). (2011a). *Consensus model for APRN regulation – nurse practitioner focus.* https://www.aacn.org/~/media/aacn-website/nursing-excellence/standards/aprnconsensusmodelnpoverlay.pdf?la=en

American Association of Colleges of Nursing (AACN). (2011b). *Consensus model for APRN regulation – clinical nurse specialist focus.* https://www.aacn.org/~/media/aacn-website/nursing-excellence/standards/aprnconsensusmodelcnsoverlay.pdf?la=en

American Association of Colleges of Nursing. (2015). *The doctor of nursing practice: Current issues and clarifying recommendations.* http://www.aacnnursing.org/Portals/42/News/White-Papers/DNP-Implementation-TF-Report-8-15.pdf?ver=2017-10-18-151758-700

American Nurses Credentialing Center. (2018). Yes, that's correct! APRN candidates may test before graduation with ANCC. *APRN Faculty Newsletter.* https://contentsharing.net/actions/email_web_version.cfm?ep=0P6KaqAM6P1D2n6WLoXUNjXae6JmOE2lrUG3dSLrki-YWpO6wkK6WSLk4WVtO9Z1Ha9wevVRz4imqNdJHqeIgWvBSUHtOwtkblQQgjtgKUB4C4lsm-P5-EPYrRLjB-ZN

Cahill, M., Alexander, M., & Gross, L. (2014). The 2014 NCSBN consensus report on APRN regulation. *Journal of Nursing Regulation, 4*(4), 5–12. http://www.journalofnursingregulation.com/article/S2155-8256(15)30111-3/pdf

Doherty, C. L., Pawlow, P., & Becker, D. (2018). The consensus model: What current and future NPs need to know. *American Nurse Today, 13*(1), 65–67. https://npwomenshealthcare.com/wp-content/uploads/2018/01/ant1-Consensus-1222.pdf

Edwards, M. (2014). What does originality in research mean? A student's perspective. *Nurse Researcher, 21*(6), 8–11.

Institute of Medicine. (2001). *Crossing the quality chasm: A new health system for the 21st Century.* National Academies Press. http://www.ihi.org/resources/Pages/Publications/CrossingtheQualityChasmANewHealthSystemforthe21stCentury.aspx

National Council of State Boards of Nursing (NCSBN). (2008). *Consensus model for APRN regulation: Licensure, accreditation, certification & education.* https://www.ncsbn.org/Consensus_Model_for_APRN_Regulation_July_2008.pdf

NCSBN. (2018). *Consensus model implementation status.* https://www.ncsbn.org/5397.htm

Phillips, E. M. & Pugh, D. S. (2010) *How to get a PhD: A handbook for students and their supervisors* (5th ed.). Open University Press.

Thomas, A., Crabtree, M. K., Delaney, K., Dumas, M. A., Kleinpell, R., Marfell, J., Nativio, D., Udlis, K., & Wolf, A. (2017). *Nurse practitioner core competencies content.* https://cdn.ymaws.com/www.nonpf.org/resource/resmgr/competencies/20170516_NPCoreCompsContentF.pdf

U.S. Department of Education. (2020). *Accreditation in the United States.* https://www2.ed.gov/admins/finaid/accred/index.html

Waddle, W. (2015). *Overqualified/underqualified: What will your education (and life experience) be worth to you?* Wheatmark.

3

Educating Nurses: Standards and Competencies

Pegge L. Bell · Carolyn Hart

LEARNING OBJECTIVES

After completing this chapter, you will be able to:

1. Examine the history and purpose of the Essentials developed by the American Association of Colleges of Nursing (AACN).

2. Explore the underpinning of ethics throughout the Essentials.

3. Differentiate MSN- and DNP-prepared advanced practice nurse roles.

4. Evaluate the need for a common classification of competencies of practice for health professionals.

5. Discuss future entry-into-practice educational requirements for nursing.

6. Evaluate the impact of Essentials and competencies on the advanced practice role (educator, administrator, and clinician).

KEY TERMS

AACN Essentials: Elements defined by AACN that provide a framework for nursing education by outlining expected professional behaviors and skills specific to a generalist or advance practice role.

Clinical prevention: Health-promotion and disease-prevention activities.

Competency-based education: To progress, students must meet objectively defined performance-based standards; because the focus in on demonstration of content and skill mastery, competency-based education may be independent of time-centered traditional teaching methods as students progress when they are able to demonstrate content mastery.

Educational competencies: Observable indicators of knowledge, skills, and attitudes that can be measured.

Health determinants: Personal, social, economic, and environmental factors that determine the health status of individuals or populations.

Healthy People 2030: A national initiative that targets clinical prevention and health activities to improve the health status of U.S. citizens.

Leading health indicators: Targets for the Healthy People 2030 designed to help achieve goals.

Population-based health: An approach that treats the population as a whole as the patient with care and services that are responsive to unique cultural, ethnic, socioeconomic, emotional, and spiritual needs and values.

Risk management: Activities, processes, or policies used to reduce liability exposure and improve the quality of patient care within a healthcare institution.

Introduction

Educational competencies set expectations for baccalaureate, master's, and doctorally prepared nurses and are typically based upon the American Association of Colleges of Nursing's (AACN) Essentials of Nursing Education. However, as the science of learning evolves, so must the approach for educating nurses to excel in today's complex healthcare system and to adapt to changing technology (Fawaz et al., 2018). Similarly, we must find new ways to help professionals maintain necessary competencies and acquire new competencies throughout their career. Thus, AACN is involved in moving toward identifying the standards needed to support competency-based education for nursing. This chapter presents information related to role competencies, AACN's *Essentials* as standards of nursing education, and insight into competency-based education. Because the *Essentials* speak to expectations of practice, this foundational knowledge is important for educators, administrators and leaders, and clinicians.

Role Competencies and the Essentials

Role competencies are defined by an ethical code of conduct, professional organizations, and accrediting bodies. This chapter provides an overview of common themes and expected outcomes of educational programs. Within parts II and III of this text, specific role competencies are further delineated. Because the AACN (AACN, 2006, 2011, 2013) provides more detail in the progression of outcomes across levels of education, the *Essentials* are used to highlight differences between levels of education and advanced nursing practice roles.

History

AACN developed a series of *Essentials* documents that establish expectations and competencies for nursing education within baccalaureate, master's, and Doctor of Nursing Practice (DNP) programs. Colleges and universities use the *Essentials* to demonstrate how they meet these standards and accreditation guidelines. The organization was established in 1969 to be the national voice for baccalaureate and graduate degree nursing education programs. This is accomplished through the creation of essential competencies that are expected outcomes for graduates of the three program levels.

The *Essentials* were created in a broad manner, to facilitate evolving expectations of advanced practice roles. The *Essentials* themselves may remain the same across time, but the expected competencies for each can be adapted with advanced practice nurses' (APNs') expanded scope of practice, new treatment modalities, or advances in technology. The *Essentials* provide consumers and stakeholders with knowledge of the nurse's expected practice and skills. Nurses can use the *Essentials* to negotiate specific aspects of their job description upon graduation, while employers can use the *Essentials* to create the job description that matches the desired educational preparation.

The *Essentials* were introduced in Chapter 1 as a beginning understanding of the educational differences for Bachelor of Science in Nursing (BSN), Master of Science in Nursing (MSN), and DNP graduates. Expectations within each Essential increase as nurses move from a generalist to an advanced practice role. As nurses gain knowledge with academic progression, higher levels of performance are possible within each competency. While the *Essentials* are the same for all advanced practice roles, definite differences exist in how the competencies are applied to practice.

Although all advanced practice roles share a common educational framework as outlined in AACN's **Essentials**, each specialty role has specific competencies as defined by their certifying body or professional organization. These differences and similarities are captured in discussions of each essential. The inclusive tables of all essentials by degree and professional organization are found in Appendix A and B (pp. 611-614) where the four broad categories of advanced practice registered nurse (APRN) roles (certified registered nurse anesthetist [CRNA], clinical nurse specialist [CNS], certified nurse midwife [CNM], and nurse practitioner [NP]) as well as the advanced practice roles of administrator, clinical nurse leader (CNL), and educator will be depicted. This chapter addresses each competency, providing further definition and explanation.

Clinical Prevention and Population Health for Improving Health

MSN- and DNP-prepared APNs have an educational foundation in clinical prevention and population health. As leaders in their respective roles, APNs contribute to the nation's health. This is particularly important in addressing the health disparities that exist among various populations. Population health is defined for each advanced practice role, as their practice focuses on the gender, diagnosis, setting, or age of the populations they serve.

Healthy People

For more than 30 years, Healthy People, an entity in the Office of Disease Prevention and Health Promotion housed in the U.S. Department of Health and Human Services, maintains a focus to improve the health status of U.S. citizens in the form of Healthy People goals. The initiative began in 1979 following the release of "Healthy People: The Surgeon General's Report on Health Promotion and Disease Prevention." Part of this report included national health promotion and disease prevention goals for the United States within a 10-year period (by 1990) that would reduce preventable death and injury. Since that initial report, 10-year Healthy People goals and objectives—Health People 2000, 2010, 2020, and 2030—have identified national health objectives that target actions and efforts to improve health across the country. Each decade, these national health goals are updated to reflect specific objectives, including individual and population health. These focused efforts have allowed the United States to make significant progress in improving health outcomes such as reducing major causes of death such as heart disease and cancer and reducing infant and maternal mortality (HealthyPeople.gov, 2020). Healthy lifestyle efforts have successfully improved outcomes for people with hypertension and elevated cholesterol as well as increasing compliance with childhood vaccinations and smoking cessation (ODPHP, 2020). During these decades, the importance of collaborating across agencies at the national, state, local, and tribal levels, and with the private and public health sectors has been demonstrated.

Healthy People 2030 is the fifth edition of Healthy People and builds on lessons learned in the first 4 decades to address new challenges. The goals of Healthy People 2030 (ODPHP, 2020) are presented in Figure 3.1.

Health Promotion

The World Health Organization (WHO, 2016) describes health promotion as a process that allows people to increase control over their own health. Rather than concentrating on treatment and cure, the focus is on preventing the cause of illness through social and environmental interventions that will benefit and protect people. The WHO (2018) defines health as "a state of complete physical, mental, social well-being and not merely the absence of disease or infirmity." These definitions have implications for all healthcare providers, particularly nurses.

Attain healthy, thriving lives and well-being, free of preventable disease, disability, injury, and premature death.	Eliminate health disparities, achieve health equity, and attain health literacy to improve the health and well-being of all.	Create social, physical, and economic environments that promote attaining full potential for health and well-being for all.

Engage leadership, key constituents, and the public across multiple sectors to take action and design policies that improve the health and well-being of all.	Promote healthy development, healthy behaviors, and well-being across all life stages.

Figure 3.1. Healthy People 2030 goals.

Nurses are integral to the success of health promotion efforts through their focus on creating healthy environments and optimizing health outcomes in cases of chronic disease or disability (Pender et al., 2015). Just as Healthy People targets leading health indicators for the national population, APNs have the skills and knowledge to use similar methods of identifying and tracking health determinants for their unique population foci.

Health disparities among populations can occur at the national, state, city, and community or neighborhood level. Disparities result when a segment of the population has more risk for disease or less resources for health promotion initiatives compared to others. Factors that contribute to health disparities are referred to as health determinants and include age, gender, occupation, income, health insurance, ethnicity or culture, primary language spoken, educational and literacy level, and sexual orientation (Huff et al., 2015).

The growing diversity within the United States challenges APNs to provide culturally responsive care in the delivery of health promotion interventions and disease prevention services. The U.S. Census Bureau projects that by 2030, one in five Americans will be 65 years of age and older and by 2044, more than half of all Americans will belong to a minority group or self-identify as being multi-racial (Colby & Ortman, 2015). Colby and Ortman (2015) assert that the United States will be defined as a plurality of racial and ethnic groups by the end of 2060, with no ethnic group having a majority share of the total U.S. population.

The following sections will describe educational and role differentiation regarding the essential of health promotion and disease prevention. Consider your educational aspirations and career goal when reviewing these sections.

Questions to Ask Yourself

1. What is my comfort level with promoting health among my patient clientele, their families, and their community?
2. Will my degree give me the skills necessary to make an impact among the population I wish to serve?
3. Are the professional competencies noted by my future professional organization applicable to my career goals?
4. What personal and professional challenges will I face in addressing this essential at the MSN or DNP level in my chosen role?

Educational Differentiation

In the competencies related to population-based health promotion and disease prevention, APNs build upon previous learning and expand their scope of practice. Table 3.1 includes AACN's MSN (2011) and DNP (2006) competencies related to population-based health promotion and disease prevention to highlight the progression between levels of education. Regardless of educational level, all nurses have the responsibility to view patients in terms of their family and community and move beyond an individualistic focus of care (Kent, 2018). Preparation for all nursing roles includes population concepts and is specifically addressed within AACN's *Essentials*. Furthermore, many practice competencies also target population health as defined in role differentiation. For example, nurse leaders are expected to advocate for improvements in the health of their communities through a focus on positive health outcomes and a culture of continuous improvement. Nurse midwives are expected to be able to promote public health and provide care to vulnerable populations.

Role Differentiation

The comparison of MSN and DNP competencies related to population-based health promotion and disease prevention in Table 3.2 provides the expected competencies for MSN-prepared APNs but also demonstrates where the DNP-prepared APN has competencies that extend their practice. The MSN competencies reflect more involvement with synthesizing data on health determinants, designing interventions that are culturally responsive and population-based, and evaluating the effectiveness and equity of interventions. The inclusion of patient education considers culture, literacy, and communication strategies. The

Table 3.1. MSN and DNP Population-Based Health Promotion Disease Prevention Essentials

MSN Essential: Clinical Prevention and Population Health for Improving Health Competencies	DNP Essential: Clinical Prevention and Population Health for Improving the Nation's Health Competencies
Synthesize broad determinants of health, principles of genetics, and epidemiologic data to design and deliver evidence-based, culturally relevant clinical prevention interventions and strategies.	Synthesize concepts related to clinical prevention and population health (psychosocial dimensions and cultural diversity) in developing, implementing, and evaluating interventions to address health promotion/disease prevention efforts, improve health status/access patterns, and/or address gaps in case of individuals, aggregates, and populations.
	Analyze scientific data (epidemiological, biostatistical, environmental, and other appropriate scientific data) related to individual, aggregate, and population health.
Evaluate the effectiveness of clinical prevention interventions that affect individual and population-based health outcomes, using health information technology and data sources.	Evaluate care delivery models and/or strategies using concepts related to community, environmental and occupational health, and cultural socioeconomic dimensions of health.
Design patient-centered and culturally responsive strategies in the delivery of clinical prevention and health promotion interventions and/or services to individuals, families, communities, and aggregates/clinical populations.	
Advance equitable and efficient prevention services; and promote effective population-based health policy through the application of nursing science and other scientific concepts.	
Integrate clinical prevention and population health concepts in the development of culturally relevant and linguistically appropriate health education, communication strategies, and interventions.	

Table 3.2. Population-Based Health Promotion Disease Prevention by Professional Organization

Professional Organization	Competency/Practice Standard	Examples
Nurse Practitioner (NONPF, 2017)	Provides the full spectrum of healthcare services to include health promotion, disease prevention, health protection, anticipatory guidance, counseling, disease management, palliative, and end-of-life care. Provides patient-centered care recognizing cultural diversity and the patient or designee as a full partner in decision-making.	Educate patients and families to increase their participation in their health decisions.
Certified Nurse Midwife (ACNM, 2014)	Applies knowledge, skills, and abilities to manage (1) primary health screening, health promotion, and care of women preconception, gynecologic, antepartum, intrapartum, and postpregnancy care; perimenopausal and postmenopausal and (2) the care of newborns immediately after birth and up to 28 days for well newborns.	Develops best practice models by using relevant data and analyzing health outcomes.
Clinical Nurse Specialist (NACNS, 2017)	Use relationship-centered communication to promote health, healing, self-care, comfort, and peaceful end of life. Conducts an evidence-based comprehensive health and psychosocial, functional history, and physical assessment considering issues that may well affect wellness, health promotion, and illness in the patient/population in diverse care settings.	Collaborate with health team members to meet caregiving needs of clients.
Clinical Nurse Leader (AACN 2007)	Design and provision of health promotion and risk reduction services for diverse populations.	Facilitate a culture of safety and enhance safety of care.
Certified Nurse Anesthetist	Perform a comprehensive history and physical; conduct a preanesthesia evaluation.	Prepare patients for anesthesia process.
Nurse Administrator	Establishes an environment that values diversity and promotes cultural competency.	Ensure patients' welfare with policies that are evidence-based.
Nurse Educator	Participates in curriculum design.	Participates in design of curriculum to reflect community and societal needs.

DNP-prepared APN has gained more experience with synthesizing and analyzing epidemiological, biostatistical, occupational, and environmental data sets. They use these data sets to plan, develop, implement, and evaluate interventions while addressing gaps in the care of individuals, aggregates, or populations (AACN, 2006). They evaluate care delivery models and strategies using concepts related to health.

Health Policy and Advocacy

APNs may not choose their role based on the responsibility and opportunity to shape policies that affect the nation's health. Nevertheless, they are key to promoting health, providing patients with safe and quality care, and serving as advocates for the profession, patient populations, and themselves. As APNs, they can influence health policy as an individual or as a member of professional organizations. In other words, policy and politics are an aspect of the APN role that cannot be ignored (Goudreau & Smolenski, 2018).

Policy Process

Because nurses represent the largest segment of healthcare providers, they can improve patient care services and outcomes through application of their knowledge to healthcare policy. Goudreau and Smolenski (2018) present Anderson's (2011) five stages of policy making to guide this process as depicted in Figure 3.2. While nurses may not be involved in every stage, contributions can be made at any phase of this process.

Policy Advocacy

Williams and associates (2018) argue that "Advocating for evidence-based, effective policies can ensure healthier communities and address the lack of access to social and material resources that form the root of health inequities. Nurses can advocate for the right social policies to promote justice, fairness, and health equity and adequately address [the social determinants of health]." Essential competencies related to health policy and advocacy demonstrate the educational foundation for APNs to advocate for their patients in the creation of health policy or in the revision of existing health policy. Examples of APN effort in influencing policy changes include efforts for independent practice and prescriptive authority, continuation of the Nurse Faculty Loan Program, and increased penalties for violence against nurses. As a profession and individually, nurses

Stage 1: Agenda setting

The policy and the problem being addressed are placed on the public agenda. The problem must be clearly defined so that the policy is successful in gaining the attention of individuals, organizations, and legislators. Nurses can play a role in this stage by helping to explain the issues involved and the impact on individuals or society. Nurses can also drive agenda setting by raising public awareness related to healthcare needs or problems.

Stage 2: Policy formulation

Various policy options are weighed and debated to solidify the problem and the solution. Nurses may be called upon to provide a compelling story that humanizes the issues involved, the impact of legislation, or to advocate for the rights and needs of patients.

Stage 3: Adoption or decision-making

Decisions are made about the approaches to be taken to solve the problem. Nurses can help inform those decisions by giving voice to the impact of legislation on individuals, families, and communities.

Stage 4: Implementation

The parameters of policy implementation are resolved, as policy makers have considered the actual effects of the policy on its ability to achieve the overall objective, the complexity of the problem, magnitude of expected change, human and financial resources, and administrative structures and regulations. Nurses can help ensure that policies are carried out in an appropriate manner that meets intended outcomes.

Stage 5: Policy evaluation

The evaluation stage is necessary to make sure the effects of the policy are aligned with the initial objectives for creating the policy. Nurses can be involved in creating and monitoring the internal mechanisms to measure the policy's outcomes.

Figure 3.2. Five stages of policy making.

have and should continue to have an impact on improving health conditions for underserved populations and advancing the profession.

APNs can remain aware of policy challenges, changing regulations, and advocacy efforts by remaining involved in professional organizations. For example, Sigma and the American Nurses Association (ANA) are two professional nursing organizations that have advocacy as an integral part of their mission. Nurses should also consider information from their state boards of nursing as they often release information about pending proposals of interest to nurses. Finally, do not forget the impact made by professional organizations that represent individual groups of APNs. Nurse practitioners, nurse leaders, nurse anesthetists, and all other APN groups have a professional organization specifically dedicated to advancing the interests of that particular group. Active involvement in these orga-nizations is one way of remaining in touch with policy challenges and ongoing efforts and can assist individual APNs in knowing how to have an active voice.

Examples of Policy Challenges

All APNs—educators, clinicians, and leaders—face some type of policy challenge with which individuals and professional organizations are actively engaged. APRNs lack full autonomous practice in most of the 50 states, as only 20 states and the District of Columbia provide full scope of practice in licensure regulations as presented in Chapter 1, Figure 1.3. The other 30 states require some degree of physician oversight or collaboration. Despite the National Academies of Science, Engineering, and Medicine (NASEM; formerly the Institute of Medicine [IOM]) recommendations that APRNs should be allowed to practice at the full extent of their education and training, APRNs continue to face barriers to full-practice authority. Some states require a collaborative practice agreement or supervision arrangement with a physician (Goudreau & Smolenski, 2018). We have yet to see the full impact of COVID-19 on independent practice as during the pandemic, some states waived the required practice agreements (see Figure 3.3).

Another barrier to APRN practice is reimbursement for services. For exam-ple, reimbursement rates vary between physicians and NPs who provide care to residents in long-term care facilities. NPs are reimbursed at 85% of the Medicare physician rate for the same services when billed under the APRNs National Provider Identifier (NPI) number; however, when billed under the supervis-ing physician's NPI as an "incident to" charge, reimbursement is at 100% of the Medicare physician rate (MedPac, 2019). Under the "incident to" model, Medicare is unable to determine who actually provided care to the patient.

APRN prescriptive authority continues to evolve. Many states are in the process of reviewing legislation to expand prescriptive authority. Historically, physicians have been opposed to expanding prescriptive authority for APRNs (Brown, 2012). However, support has been increasing with the publication of the American College of Physicians position paper recognizing the value of APRNs in meeting the demand for healthcare services (Azar et al., 2018).

The following sections will describe educational and role differentiation regarding the essential of health policy. Consider your educational aspirations and career goal when reviewing these sections.

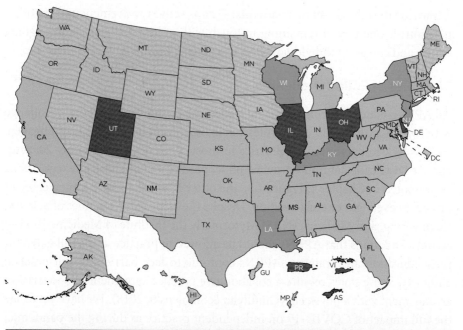

Temporary suspension of all practice agreement requirements

Temporary waiver of select practice agreement requirements

Currently no action on this issue

Full Practice Authority states

Figure 3.3. State licensure regulations.

Questions to Ask Yourself

1. What is my comfort level with advocating for my patient clientele, their families, and their community?
2. Will my degree give me the skills necessary to make an impact with health policy among the population I wish to serve?
3. Are the professional competencies for health policy noted by my future professional organization applicable to my career goals?
4. What personal and professional challenges will I face in addressing this essential at the MSN or DNP level in my chosen role?

Educational Differentiation

While both MSN and DNP graduates are expected to assume leadership roles with health policy and advocacy, there are some educational differences in how these APNs are prepared to engage in this competency. Table 3.3 provides a comparison of MSN and DNP competencies with the essential of health policy. Table 3.4 compares those competencies between MSN and DNP graduates of APN programs. Although all APNs have a component of health policy within

Table 3.3. MSN and DNP Health Policy and Advocacy Essentials	
MSN Essential (AACN, 2011)	**DNP Essential (AACN, 2006)**
Analyze how policies influence the structure and financing of healthcare, practice, and health outcomes.	Critically analyze health policy proposals, health policies, and related issues from the perspective of consumers, nursing, other health professions, and other stakeholders in policy and public forums.
Participate in the development and implementation of institutional, local, and state, and federal policy.	Demonstrate leadership in the development and implementation of institutional, local, state, federal, and/or international health policy.
Examine the effect of legal and regulatory processes on nursing practice, healthcare delivery, and outcomes.	Develop, evaluate, and provide leadership for healthcare policy that shapes healthcare financing, regulation, and delivery.
Interpret research, bringing the nursing perspective, for policy makers and stakeholders.	Influence policy makers through active participation on committees, boards, or task forces at the institutional, local, state, regional, national, and/or international level to improve healthcare delivery and outcomes. Educate others, include policy makers at all levels, regarding nursing, health policy, and patient care outcomes.
Advocate for policies that improve the health of the public and the profession of nursing.	Advocate for the nursing profession within the policy and healthcare communities. Advocate for social justice, equity, and ethical policies within all healthcare arenas.

their educational preparation, the focus and exact nature of this education varies by role. For example, nurse educator content may include details regarding the Federal Educational Rights and Protection Act and other regulatory responsibilities. APRN content will most likely include information regarding prescriptive authority and collaborative practice.

Table 3.4. APN/APRN Roles With Health Policy Competencies

Professional Organization	Competency/ Practice Standard	Examples
Nurse Practitioner (NONPF, 2017)	Policy Competencies	Contribute in the development of health policy; evaluate the impact of globalization on healthcare policy development; advocate for policies for safe and healthy practice environments.
Certified Nurse Midwife (ACNM, 2014)	Professional Responsibilities	Analyze the process for health policy development, influential factors, and the impact of policy on clinical practice; support of legislation and policy initiatives that promote quality healthcare; knowledge of issues and trends in healthcare policy and systems.
Clinical Nurse Specialist (NACNS, 2017)	Nurses/Nursing Sphere Organization/ System Sphere	Analyze legislative, regulatory, and fiscal policies as they impact nursing practice and patient/population outcomes. Advocate for equitable healthcare by participating in professional organizations or public policy activities
Clinical Nurse Leader (AACN 2013)	AACN Essential 6: Health Policy and Advocacy	Advocate for policies that leverage social change, promote wellness, improve care outcomes, and reduce costs. Advocate for the integration of the CNL within care delivery systems.

(Continued)

Table 3.4. APN/APRN Roles With Health Policy Competencies   (continued)

Professional Organization	Competency/ Practice Standard	Examples
Certified Nurse Anesthetist (COA, 2018)	Professional Responsibility	Function within appropriate legal requirements as a registered professional nurse, accepting responsibility and accountability for own practice.
Nurse Educator (NLN, 2020)	Engage in Scholarship	Advocate for nursing, nursing education, and higher education in the political arena.
Nurse Administrator (AONE, 2015)	Knowledge of the Healthcare Environment: Healthcare Economics and Policy	Use knowledge of federal and state laws and regulations that affect the provision of patient care; interpret impact of legislation at the state and federal level on nursing and healthcare organizations.

AACN, American Association of Colleges of Nursing; APN, advanced practice nurse; APRNs, advanced practice registered nurses; CNL, clinical nurse leader.

Role Differentiation

Professional organizations, as well as accreditation standards of practice, provide information on how various APN/APRN roles demonstrate competency in health policy and advocacy. Table 3.4 depicts the professional organization and/or practice standard for health policy and advocacy, along with examples of how APNs engage in this competency. Nurse administrators including chief nursing officers (CNOs) and nurse managers along with CNLs play a particularly important role in shaping policies that are intended to safeguard patients and promote positive outcomes (Steusse, 2014). CNOs must ensure patient safety and access to appropriate services by collaborating with hospital management and stakeholders to acquire the right infrastructure and resources. CNOs are also responsible for formulating and implementing new nursing strategies. CNLs are involved in delivery of healthcare across all settings, evaluating outcomes, and assessing cohort risk.

Quality Improvement and Safety

The Joint Commission defined quality and safety as, "the degree to which care, treatment, or services for individuals and populations increases the likelihood of desired health or behavioral health outcomes; considerations include the appropriateness, efficacy, efficiency, timeliness, accessibility and continuity of care, the safety of the care environment and the individual's personal values, practices and beliefs" (AHRQ, 2018). Quality and safety measures are the means of improving patient outcomes by decreasing errors and ensuring that appropriate services and actions are provided at the correct time (Pestotnik & Lemon, 2019). Within the U.S. healthcare system, changes have been adopted to create a culture of safety in which providers are supported in disclosing errors and maintaining professional accountability while seeking systems solutions for decreasing errors (Haviley et al., 2014).

The Quality and Safety Education for Nurses (QSEN) initiative was developed to assist in preparing nurses with the knowledge needed to continuously improve healthcare delivery (QSEN, 2020). Quality improvement (QI) is the process of using data to improve healthcare outcomes and the practice of healthcare delivery. Data are used to measure the success or failure of an intervention or to determine intervention steps in a process (D'Eramo & Puckett, 2018). In a QI environment, all staff are involved in continuous improvement (CQI) to understand and improve patient outcomes (Finkelman, 2019). The Institute for Healthcare Improvement (IHI) notes that "While all changes do not lead to improvement, all improvement requires change" (2018). Thus, nurses involved in application of quality care will continue to evolve their practice based on new findings and information. Chapter 13 provides further detail about change and change theory.

Healthcare outcome measures are a key component of quality improvement—the ability to measure patient responses to interventions is necessary to demonstrate success or failure of quality improvement interventions. Outcome measures are defined and prioritized by major health organizations such as CMS (Centers for Medicare and Medicaid Services), The Joint Commission, and the National Association for Healthcare Quality (Tinker & Falk, 2016). Among the most commonly measured patient outcomes are mortality, safety of care, readmissions, patient experiences, effectiveness of care, timeliness of care, and efficient use of medical imaging. Set by the IHI, the Quadruple Aim of healthcare as presented in Figure 3.4 is designed to optimize health system performance.

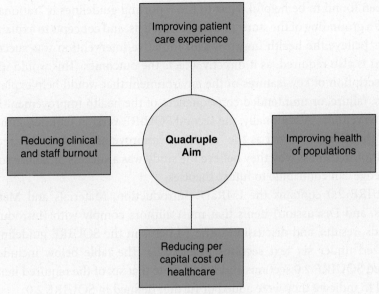

Figure 3.4. Quadruple Aim.

Quality Improvement Reporting

Guidelines were introduced in 2005 to assist in the reporting of health-care improvement projects. These guidelines became known as SQUIRE 1.0 (Standards for Quality Improvement Reporting Excellence). Later, the guidelines were updated for a second version as educational programs began to focus on healthcare improvement, considering it a standard competency. The SQUIRE 2.0 version was released in 2016 based on feedback from focus groups and resulted in the compilation of 18 items that should be addressed when healthcare providers disseminate their findings of quality improvement endeavors (Ogrinc et al., 2016). The SQUIRE guidelines provide a framework for preparing publications that allows author to provide relevant content.

While the first SQUIRE version contained specific subitems, the second version accepts that there are multiple ways of approaching health improvement (Ogrinc et al., 2016). Thus, the 18 items are included, but authors are encouraged to address only those that apply to their studies. A glossary of terms is provided to assure that terms and their definitions are useful to the broadest audience. It is important to note that "improvement" is no longer used as a term, but remains in the SQUIRE title, because well-conducted studies with negative results have also been found to be helpful. New to the reporting guidelines is "rationale" to require a grounding of the study to theories, models, and concepts to explain why authors believe the health improvement initiative/intervention was successful. Context is also required, as it directly affects the outcomes. This would include the description of key features of the environment that would help explain the success, failure, or unintended consequences of the health improvement initiative/intervention. Additionally, the second SQUIRE version requires authors to report the "doing" as well as the "studying" improvement work. This requires the author to discuss why they believe the study was a success or failure so their knowledge can contribute to future theories.

SQUIRE 2.0 contains the IMRaD (Introduction, Materials and Methods, Results, and Discussion) items that most authors comply with (introduction, methods, results, and discussion). The 18 items in the SQUIRE guidelines are organized under six text sections (Table 3.5). The table below includes the required SQUIRE 2.0 sections and items. Note that six of the required items are bolded to indicate they were added or further defined in SQUIRE 2.0.

The following sections will describe educational and role differentiation regarding the essential of patient safety and quality of care. Consider your educational aspirations and career goal when reviewing these sections.

Questions to Ask Yourself

1. What is my comfort level with promoting safety and quality of care with my patient clientele, their families, and their community?
2. Will my degree give me the skills necessary to make an impact with assuring patient safety and quality of care among the population I wish to serve?
3. Are the professional competencies for quality and safety noted by my future professional organization applicable to my career goals?
4. What personal and professional challenges will I face in addressing this essential at the MSN or DNP level in my chosen role?

Educational Differentiation

Because quality and safety are high priorities for all levels of nursing education, many outcomes are shared between the MSN and doctoral level. These expectations are presented in Table 3.6. Education regarding quality and safety again

Table 3.5. SQUIRE Version 2.0: Required Items

Text Section	Required Items
Title and Abstract	Title and Abstract
Introduction	Problem description Available Knowledge **Rationale** Specific Aims
Methods	**Context** **Intervention(s)** **Study of the Intervention(s)** Measures Analysis Ethical Considerations
Results	Results/Findings
Discussion	**Summary** **Interpretation** Limitations Conclusions
Other Information	Funding Source(s)

SQUIRE, Standards for Quality Improvement Reporting Excellence.
Adapted from Ogrinc, G., Davies, L., Goodman, D., Batalden, P., Davidoff, F., Stevens, D. (2016). Squire 2.0 (Standards for Quality Improvement Reporting Excellence): revised publication guidelines froma detailed consensus process. *BMJ Quality & Safety, 25*, 986–992. https://qualitysafety.bmj.com/content/qhc/25/12/986.full.pdf

varies for each of the advanced roles. Nurse educators will learn techniques to instill values of quality and safety within students. Nurse leaders including CNOs and CNLs will learn their role in using big data to monitor, evaluate, and promote positive patient outcomes. In all APRN specializations, quality and safety content are integral parts of all education.

Role Differentiation

All nurses are responsible for the quality and safety of patients and the care that they deliver. Clinicians are direct caregivers who must deliver care in a safe, competent manner that promotes positive patient outcomes and quality

Table 3.6. Health Policy and Advocacy by Professional Organization

Professional Organization	Competency/ Practice Standard	Examples
Nurse Practitioner (NONPF, 2017)	Policy Competencies	Contribute in the development of health policy; evaluate the impact of globalization on healthcare policy development; advocate for policies for safe and healthy practice environments.
Certified Nurse Midwife (ACNM, 2014)	Professional Responsibilities	Analyze the process for health policy development, influential factors, and the impact of policy on clinical practice; support of legislation and policy initiatives that promote quality healthcare; knowledge of issues and trends in healthcare policy and systems.
Clinical Nurse Specialist (NACNS, 2017)	Nurses/Nursing Sphere Organization/ System Sphere	Analyze legislative, regulatory, and fiscal policies as they impact nursing practice and patient/population outcomes. Advocate for equitable healthcare by participating in professional organizations or public policy activities.
Clinical Nurse Leader (AACN, 2013)	AACN Essential 6: Health Policy and Advocacy	Advocates for policies that leverage social change, promote wellness, improve care outcomes, and reduce costs. Advocate for the integration of the CNL within care delivery systems.
Certified Nurse Anesthetist (COA, 2018)	Professional Responsibility	Function within appropriate legal requirements as a registered professional nurse, accepting responsibility and accountability for own practice.

Table 3.6.	Health Policy and Advocacy by Professional Organization (continued)	
Professional Organization	**Competency/ Practice Standard**	**Examples**
Nurse Educator (NLN, 2020)	Engage in Scholarship	Advocate for nursing, nursing education, and higher education in the political arena.
Nurse Administrator (AONE, 2015)	Knowledge of the Healthcare Environment: Healthcare Economics and Policy	Use knowledge of federal and state laws and regulations that affect the provision of patient care; interpret impact of legislation at the state and federal level on nursing and healthcare organizations.

AACN, American Association of Colleges of Nursing; CNL, clinical nurse leader.

experience for patients. Administrators must oversee the institutional policies, procedures, and resources that yield positive patient outcomes. Nurse educators must prepare the future nursing workforce with the necessary competencies to keep patients safe, while assuring there is minimal risk to patients. Each practitioner has a duty and responsibility to promote quality and safety among their colleagues and staff. While specific examples of how each advanced practice role might engage in quality and safety vary greatly, they are reflective of their differences in scope of practice. Table 3.7 presents specific advanced practice role expectations related to patient safety.

Informatics and Healthcare Technologies

Clinical informatics is the general term used to address the ways in which information systems enhance or impact the day-to-day care of patients and communities. These systems include electronic health records (EHRs), barcoding systems, digital imaging services, and many patient care devices (Alexander et al., 2019). While these tools can add to the quality of patient care and provide powerful clinical decision-making support, proper use is needed to improve patient outcomes (McGonigle & Mastrian, 2018). The need to communicate patient information electronically to members of the healthcare team is complicated

Table 3.7. MSN and DNP Informatics and Healthcare Technologies Essentials

MSN Essential (2011)	DNP Essential (2006)
Analyze current and emerging technologies to support safe practice environments and to optimize patient safety, cost-effectiveness, and health outcomes.	Design, select, use, and evaluate programs that evaluate and monitor outcomes of care, care systems, and quality improvement including consumer use of healthcare information systems.
Provide oversight and guidance in the integration of technologies to document patient care and improve patient outcomes.	Analyze and communicate critical elements necessary to the selection, use, and evaluation of healthcare information systems and patient care technology.
Evaluate outcome data using current communication technologies, information systems, and statistical principles to develop strategies to reduce risks and improve health outcomes.	Demonstrate the conceptual ability and technical skills to develop, execute, and evaluate an evaluation plan involving data extraction from practice information systems and databases.
Promote policies that incorporate ethical principles and standards for the use of health and information technologies.	Provide leadership in the evaluation and resolution of ethical and legal issues within healthcare systems relating to the use of information, information technology, communication networks, and patient care technology.
Use information and communication technologies, resources, and principles of learning to teach patients and others.	Evaluate consumer health information sources for accuracy, timeliness, and appropriateness.
Use information and communication technologies, resources, and principles of learning to teach patients and others.	

by patient privacy rights as information contained in the EHR is increasingly shared. Examples of data sharing include patient portals with access shared between family members, information released to schools, or patient information shared between providers. Solutions that allow a provider to "block" sensitive data from being shared have been proposed but also come with drawbacks that must be carefully evaluated (Galvin, 2019).

Health Literacy

The Centers for Disease Control and Prevention (CDC, 2019) agrees with the 2010 Patient Protection and Affordable Care Act of 2010, Title V, definition of health literacy as "the degree to which an individual has the capacity to obtain, communicate, process, and understand basic health information and services to make appropriate health decisions". Health literacy skills allow patients and their families to be more informed healthcare consumers, increasing treatment compliance and improving outcomes (Chilton, 2015). Because nurses are considered frontline providers in healthcare settings, they can play a critical role in increasing health literacy through the education of those within their care (Alexander et al., 2019).

Nursing Informatics

Nursing informatics, defined as the combination of computer science, information science, and nursing science, supports nursing practice through the management and processing of health data (Vasuki, 2016). Thus, nursing informatics is vital to nursing education, administration, and clinical practice. Educators need to ensure that all levels of nursing students understand how to use technology to communicate patient information, monitor and track patient outcomes, and help patients cope with disease and treatment plans; administrators can use nursing informatics to improve workflow and enhance and support budgetary decisions; clinicians find nursing informatics tools useful in evidence-based practices, decisional support, and identifying data trends (McGonigle et al., 2014).

General Data Protection Regulation

The European Union (EU) instituted regulations to ensure individual rights to data portability, called the General Data Protection Regulation (GDPR). GDPR requires that those entities that collect individual data, referred to as data controllers, be accountable to providing access and control of this information to the individual (Vanberg, 2018). These reforms are intended to address the realities of living in a technology-enhanced world, creating obligations surrounding how personal information, including names, credit card and social security numbers, date of birth, and addresses are collected and stored (Palmer, 2018).

Goddard (2017) identifies six general concepts addressed within the GDPR: fairness and lawfulness, purpose limitations, data minimization, accuracy, storage limitations, and integrity and confidentiality (p. 703). These principles are intended to provide the individual with the right to access personal information from data controllers as well as the right to transfer data from one controller to another (Vanberg, 2018). GDPR regulations also provide expectations for reporting and handling of data breaches.

Although the GDPR is an EU initiative, important implications exist for the United States where data portability varies by state. For the most part, these are guidelines rather than legally binding regulations. Vanberg (2018) reports that surveys from the Office of Science and Technology Policy (OSTP) indicate that increased data portability could heighten financial awareness and consumer confidence in technology-enhanced services. U.S. firms conducting business in the EU must also be GDPR compliant, increasing the need to address data portability policies and global data protection.

The following sections will describe educational and role differentiation regarding the essential of information technology. Consider your educational aspirations and career goal when reviewing these sections.

Questions to Ask Yourself

1. What is my comfort level with utilizing information technology with my patient clientele, their families, and their community?
2. Will my degree give me the skills necessary to make an impact with the application of information technology among the population I wish to serve?
3. Are the professional competencies for information technology noted by my future professional organization applicable to my career goals?
4. What personal and professional challenges will I face in addressing this essential at the MSN or DNP level in my chosen role?

Educational Differentiation

All APNs will receive information technology content as it relates to their specialty. Nurse practitioners, nurse midwives, nurse anesthetists, and CNSs may focus on patient privacy rights and use of technology in patient education or communication among healthcare team members. Nurse educators may focus on remote and virtual simulation learning opportunities. CNLs and nurse administrators may focus on the use of big data enabled by technology in decision-making. Table 3.8 illustrates the different expectations in information technology competencies for MSN and DNP nursing roles.

Table 3.8. Informatics and Healthcare Technologies by Professional Organization

Professional Organization	Competency/ Practice Standard	Examples
Nurse Practitioner (NONPF, 2017)	Technology and Information Literacy Competencies	Integrate appropriate technologies for knowledge management to improve healthcare; demonstrate information literacy skills in complex decision-making.
Certified Nurse Midwife (ACNM, 2014)	Professional Responsibilities	Utilize information systems and other technologies to improve the quality and safety of healthcare for women and newborns; knowledge of information systems and other technologies to improve the quality and safety of healthcare.
Clinical Nurse Specialist (NACNS, 2017)	Organization/ Systems Sphere	Lead the integration, management, and evaluation of technology to promote safety, quality, efficiency, and optimal health outcomes.
Clinical Nurse Leader (AACN, 2013)	AACN Essential 5: Informatics and Healthcare Technologies	Implement use of technologies to coordinate and laterally integrate patient care across settings and among providers; analyze current and proposed use of patient care technologies in the design and delivery of care in diverse settings.

Table 3.8. Informatics and Healthcare Technologies by Professional Organization (continued)

Professional Organization	Competency/ Practice Standard	Examples
Certified Nurse Anesthetist (COA, 2018)	Critical Thinking	Interpret and utilize data obtained from noninvasive and invasive monitoring modalities.
Nurse Educator (NLN, 2013)	Facilitate Learner Development and Socialization	Provide resources for diverse learners to meet their learning needs.
Nurse Administrator (AONE, 2015)	Business Skills: Information Management and Technology	Use technology to support improvement of clinical and financial performance; use data management systems for decision-making.

AACN, American Association of Colleges of Nursing.

Role Differentiation

Just as educational content related to informatics varies by specialization, so too does the way in which APNs use and interact with technology. Table 3.9 presents examples of competency standards across the various disciplines within advanced practices nursing. One can note the linkages between differing practices and the importance of nursing informatics and health literacy.

Interprofessional Collaboration for Improving Patient and Population Health Outcomes

The importance of interprofessional collaboration was included in the Institute of Medicine's report (2010) as an essential method of addressing accessibility, quality, and value of healthcare in the United States. Interprofessional collaboration occurs when all members of the healthcare team, including the patient, communicate and consider each other's unique perspectives that influence the health of the patient, whether that is an individual, family, or community (Sullivan et al., 2015). When interprofessional collaboration occurs, comprehensive services are provided to patients and patient care outcomes can be improved (Homeyer et al., 2018). Interprofessional care fosters the sharing of information and knowledge

Table 3.9. MSN and DNP Interprofessional Collaboration Essentials

MSN Essential (2011)	DNP Essential (2006)
Advocate for the value and role of the professional nurse as a member and leader of interprofessional healthcare teams.	
Understand other health professions' scopes of practice to maximize contributions within the healthcare team.	
Employ collaborative strategies in the design, coordination, and evaluation of patient-centered care.	Lead interprofessional teams in the analysis of complex practice and organizational issues.
Use effective communication strategies to develop, participate, and lead interprofessional teams and partnerships.	Employ effective communication and collaborative skills in the development and implementation of practice models, peer review, practice guidelines, health policy, standards of care, and/or other scholarly products.
Mentor and coach new and experienced nurses and other members of the healthcare team.	
Functions as an effective group leader or member based on an in-depth understanding of team dynamics and group processes.	Employ consultative and leadership skills with intraprofessional and interprofessional teams to create change in healthcare and complex healthcare delivery systems.

toward a common goal—improving patient outcomes (Hospitals, 2018). When the healthcare team works together, patient experiences are enhanced; they are satisfied with their treatment plan, their ability to access healthcare providers and information, and appreciate communication they have with healthcare providers.

Currently, medical errors are said to be the "third most common cause of death in the United States," and teamwork failures account for up to 70% to 80% of serious medical errors (Makary & Daniel, 2016). When healthcare team members do not collaborate, the patient's quality of care is diminished and their risk for errors is heightened. Failure to convey key information jeopardizes patient safety, contributing to gaps in the patient's treatment plan, loss of crucial information, or missed interventions. Poor team interactions contribute to medical errors, some very costly to patients (Rosen et al., 2018).

Interprofessional collaboration is a competency that requires development by all team members. The WHO released a blueprint in 2010 for implementing interprofessional education and collaborative practice (IPECP), giving healthcare students the opportunity to engage with students from other disciplines. The Interprofessional Education Collaborative Expert Panel (2016) published four competencies for interprofessional education and collaborative practice. Within the model, emphasis is placed on shared values and ethics by team members, role delineation for each team member, use of effective communication skills, and the promotion of teamwork (Figure 3.5).

Challenges continue to affect the full implementation of interprofessional education and collaborative practice. Many clinicians and educators were not educated or socialized to work in interprofessional teams that require collaboration. Therefore, they may not be prepared to create these educational and clinical opportunities for students. Scheduling logistics of the need to match curricular plans can also present barrier to interprofessional education. These barriers may prevent educational programs from fully

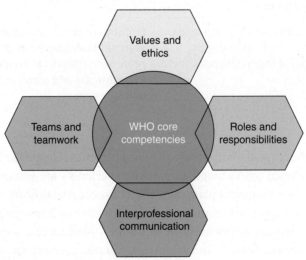

Figure 3.5. World Health Organization (WHO) competencies.

embracing interprofessional collaboration, creating a gap between student learning and the realities of practice requiring teamwork skills (Speakman & Arenson, 2015).

New models of care need to be created or implemented so that educational programs can help promote collaboration within health systems. Clinical environments in healthcare benefit greatly when teams have open communication and inclusive collaboration (Mayo & Wooley, 2016). The group's ability to work well with each other and see issues from the perspective of other team members can result in collective intelligence—a team's general ability to perform on a wide variety of tasks. Team members must share information by speaking up, especially if they have relevant information. Groups norms are established as team members become more comfortable speaking to the team, even when there are diverse professions represented. This enables the group to share information for critical thinking rather than consensus building. It encourages the team to include every member in the discussion, leading to better processing and integration of information.

The following sections will describe educational and role differentiation regarding the essential of interprofessional collaboration. Consider your educational aspirations and career goal when reviewing these sections.

Questions to Ask Yourself

1. What is my comfort level with incorporating interprofessional collaborative practice techniques to improve my advanced practice?
2. Will my degree give me the skills necessary to strategically collaborate with other professionals to improve the services I provide my target population?
3. Are the professional competencies for interprofessional collaboration noted by my future professional organization applicable to my career goals?
4. What personal and professional challenges will I face in addressing this essential at the MSN or DNP level in my chosen role?

Educational Differentiation

Education regarding collaboration takes many different forms depending on one's specialization. CRNAs will focus on the collaboration between surgeons, operating room nurses, postanesthesia recovery unit nurses, perfusionists, and other operating room personnel to ensure optimal care. Midwives may learn the collaborative skills needed to work with other healthcare providers, and social workers along with family and support system members. Differences between student learning outcomes for the MSN- and DNP-prepared APN as related to interprofessional collaboration are presented in Table 3.10.

Table 3.10. Interprofessional Collaboration by Professional Organization

Professional Organization	Competency/Practice Standard	Examples
Nurse Practitioner (NONPF, 2017)	Leadership competencies	Collaborates with multiple stakeholders (patients, community, healthcare team, policy makers).
Certified Nurse Midwife	Collaboration with other members of the interprofessional healthcare team	Collaborates with physician during obstetrical emergencies.
Clinical Nurse Specialist (AACN, 2013)	Interprofessional collaboration for improving patient and population health outcomes	Collaborates with other team members to facilitate transitions of care settings.
Clinical Nurse Leader (AACN, 2013)	CNL competencies	Collaborates with healthcare professionals to plan, implement, and evaluate an improvement opportunity.
Certified Nurse Anesthetist (COA, 2019	Communication	Uses interpersonal and communication skills to exchange information and collaborate with patients and their families and other healthcare professionals.
Nurse Educator (NLN, 2018)	Function effectively within the organizational environment and academic community	Integrates the values of respect, collegiality, professionalism, and caring to build an organizational climate that fosters the development of learners and colleagues.
Nurse Administrator (AONE, 2015)	Communication and relationship building	Collaborates with medical staff leaders, physicians, and other disciplines.

CNL, clinical nurse leader.

Role Differentiation

Collaboration between members of the healthcare team is an integral part of patient safety and promotion of positive outcomes. As with learning outcomes, differences exist across the APN professions in how collaboration influences population health. These differences are presented in Table 3.11 and provide insight into expectations of practice for each APN specialization.

Table 3.11. MSN and DNP Organizational and Systems Leadership Essentials

MSN Essential (2011)	DNP Essential (2006)
Apply leadership skills and decision-making in the provision of culturally responsive, high-quality nursing care, healthcare team coordination, and oversight/accountability for care delivery and outcomes.	Ensure accountability for quality of healthcare and patient safety populations with whom they work.
Assume a leadership role in effectively implementing patient safety and quality improvement initiatives within the context of the interprofessional team using communication skills.	Use advanced communication skills/processes to lead quality improvement and patient safety initiatives in healthcare systems.
Develop an understanding of how healthcare delivery systems are organized and financed and identify the economic, legal, and political factors that influence healthcare.	Employ principles of business, finance, economics, and health policy to develop and implement effective plans for practice initiatives in healthcare systems.
Demonstrate the ability to use complexity science and systems theory in the design, delivery, and evaluation of healthcare.	Develop and/or evaluate effective strategies for managing the ethical dilemmas inherent in patient care, the healthcare organization, and research.
Apply business and economic principles and practices to develop a business plan.	Develop and/or monitor budgets for practice initiatives.
Design and implement systems change strategies that improve the care environment.	Analyze the cost-effectiveness of practice initiatives accounting for risk and improvement of healthcare outcomes.
Participate in the design and implementation of new models of care delivery and coordination.	Develop and evaluate care delivery approaches that meet current and future needs of patient populations.

Organizational and Systems Leadership

APNs work and lead within micro- and macrosystems of care to meet the needs of patients (Metzger & Rivers, 2014) and therefore should play a critical role in leading changes in healthcare delivery and reform (Elliott, 2016). Development of leadership competencies ensures an active voice for the nursing profession in the healthcare delivery system (Finkelman, 2019). Nurses for a Healthier Tomorrow, a coalition of 45 nursing and healthcare organizations, views the role of nurse executives as a dynamic one, shifting from a single focus on nursing services to a broader concern and accountability for patient care services. Clinicians must also adopt a leadership mindset, as this provides increased skills in leading effective healthcare teams that improve patient outcomes (Rosen et al., 2018; Institute of Medicine [IOM], 2011). Healthcare leadership includes four key behaviors, as defined by Cosgrove (2016) for the Cleveland Clinic in Figure 3.6.

Risk Management

The Health and Human Resources and Services Administration (HRSA) views risk management policies as a key to the success of a quality improvement program.

Lead through change
- Communicate strategies
- Achieve consensus
- Move quickly to implement change
- Demonstrate character and integrity

Foster teamwork
- Inspire your team
- Work together toward a common vision

Demonstrate character and integrity
- Be compassionate and actively listen
- Communicate from the heart
- Show mutual respect at every interaction

Develop ourselves and others
- Create a learning environment that opens all caregivers to new skills and capabilities
- Inspire and uplift our teams
- Commit to professional growth and development of ourselves and others

Figure 3.6. Key leadership behaviors.

Quality of care has been loosely defined as "doing the right thing at the right time to achieve the best positive results" (Campbell et al., 2000) but may more specifically include the six concepts of effectiveness, safety, patient-centeredness, accessibility, equality, and knowledge-based care (Jangland et al., 2017).

- Effectiveness: providing the processes necessary in achieving outcomes supported by scientific evidence
- Safety: Avoiding harm to patients
- Patient-Centeredness: Respectful and responsive care that meets individual patient preferences, needs, and values
- Accessibility: Ensuring access to correct care, reducing waits and sometimes harmful delays for both those who receive and those who give care
- Equality: Providing care that does not vary by the social determinants of health
- Knowledge-Based Care: Evidence-based care that is appropriate to meet individual needs, to all who could benefit and refraining from providing services to those not likely to benefit

In the nursing role, risk managers have advanced knowledge of medical practices, treatments, and complications. They may proactively work to ensure that protocols are correctly implemented but also intervene to limit adverse patient outcomes and financial repercussions when situations do not progress as expected. As patient advocates, all nurses provide value in their daily operations as they identify inefficient or potentially hazardous aspects of healthcare treatment and procedures; within the acute care setting, risk management nurses work to understand the steps leading to an error and reduce the risk of recurrence (Decker, 2018).

Financing Care or Fiscal Resources

The United States spends more per capita per person on healthcare than any other country in the world. Yet, many U.S. citizens are without health insurance and we experience lower life expectancy and survival rates compared to other high-income countries (Petersen, 2015). The Patient Protection and Affordable Care Act, conceived during the Obama administration, was intended to provide coverage to more than 94% of Americans while staying under the $900 billion limit that President Obama established, bending the healthcare cost curve and reducing the deficit over the next 10 years and beyond (Rosenbaum, 2011). With pending changes in the Patient Protection and Affordable Care Act (PPACA), many citizens who initially enrolled in a national policy provided through the Affordable Care Act (ACA) were already dropping out (Trivedi, 2016). APRNs who can bill for their healthcare services are paid by private insurance, government insurance programs, or individual out-of-pocket funds. Government programs include Medicare, Medicaid, Tricare, Veterans Health Administration, Indian Health Service, and State Children's Health Insurance Program. Overall, about 30% of the population is covered by government insurance.

Three parties are involved in healthcare costs when the patient has insurance—the patient who receives the care, the clinician who delivers the care, and the insurance company that negotiates prices and pays all or some part of the medical bill (Bartol, 2018). The patient assumes that all the costs related to their care will be necessary, while the clinician chooses the tests and laboratory work with no knowledge of their actual costs. Insurance companies use language that is not understandable by patients and sometimes clinicians. The actual cost of care is revealed only after charges are filed. APRNs should be considerate of healthcare costs and choose only those measures that are necessary to the patient's care.

Systems Thinking

Systems thinkers are important in complex healthcare organizations, as systems are growing in number and complexity. The literal definition of systems thinking is a system of thinking about systems (Arnold & Wade, 2015). Systems theory is an approach to looking at the whole of the system as well as the parts of the system to solve problems (Cordon, 2013). Definitions of systems thinking have developed over the years. Squires and associates (2011) added defined systems thinking as "the ability to think abstractly to envision multiple perspectives, understand diverse operations and contexts of the systems, identify the inter and intra-relationships and dependencies, understand complex system behavior, and reliably predict the impact of change to the system" (p. 3).

The organization as a whole system needs to be considered; viewing only the parts of the organization (people, processes, and structures) in isolation will omit an important action of viewing the interrelationship among the parts (Cordon, 2013). Making organizational changes to one part of the system can affect other parts of the system and eventually the whole system. Rather than improving the overall system, this focus on the parts without considering the overall effect to the organization could result in more chaos.

Systems theories can provide frameworks for seeing the overall organization, as well as the smaller components of the organization. General systems theory was developed by Beralanffy (1968) for universal application to systems, regardless of their properties or elements (Cordon, 2013). This theory considers that systems are open or closed systems. Open systems interact with their environment, while closed systems do not. Equilibrium is a principle of this theory, as a system will make necessary adaptive changes to maintain equilibrium. Adjustments are made in the human body when sodium levels are low, just as a healthcare system makes adjustments when there are deficits in one of the patient support systems. Chaos theory developed by Wheatley (2006) describes how organic systems respond to change in a chaotic manner, as all parts are interrelated. When change begins, the organization looks chaotic and unpredictable, but the order and predictability to its boundaries maintain the system. These two forces are required for change to occur. A healthcare facility will continue to function despite the implementation of the electronic medical record (EMR). There may be chaos for a few weeks, but ultimately it will become the norm in the system.

Theories and models used to guide systems thinking help leaders explain how things work within the organization (Peters, 2014). Systems theories and models can also identify areas where more data should be collected or where more questions need to be asked. Additionally, using these theories and models can become a mindset for understanding organizational behavior. Systems thinking should become a habit—something the leader does to improve their understanding of how things work in the system and how theories and models can be applied to improve patient care outcomes.

The following sections will describe educational and role differentiation regarding the essential of organizational and systems leadership. Consider your educational aspirations and career goal when reviewing these sections.

Questions to Ask Yourself

1. What is my comfort level with applying systems thinking as I develop as healthcare leader?
2. Will my degree give me the skills necessary to make an impact on my ability to influence the necessary change to improve the services provided to the population I wish to serve?
3. Are the professional competencies for organizational and systems leadership noted by my future professional organization applicable to my career goals?
4. What personal and professional challenges will I face in addressing this essential at the MSN or DNP level in my chosen role?

Educational Differentiation

By virtue of a graduate degree, there will be leadership expectations of both MSN and DNP graduates. The ability to consider the effect of organizational or system changes on each entity in the system will facilitate the success of the proposed change. Effective leaders utilize systems theory to reduce resistance to change and facilitate the adoption and sustainment of change across all departments. Level of education influences the expectations of MSN and DNP graduates. These outcomes are presented in Table 3.12.

Table 3.12. Organizational and Systems Leadership by Professional Organization

Professional Organization	Competency/ Practice Standard	Examples
Nurse Practitioner (NONPF, 2017)	Leadership Competencies	Assumes complex and advanced leadership roles to initiate and guide change; applies knowledge of organizational practices and complex systems to improve healthcare delivery.
Certified Nurse Midwife (ACNM, 2014)	Hallmarks of Midwifery Professional Responsibilities	Advocates for informed choice; shared decision-making, and the right to self-determination. Evaluates healthcare finance and identifies appropriate use of resources for management of a healthcare practice.
Clinical Nurse Specialist (NACNS, 2017)	Organization/ System Sphere	Uses leadership, team building, negotiation, and conflict resolution skills to build partnerships within and across systems, including communities; evaluates system-level programs and outcomes based on the analysis of information from relevant sources.
Clinical Nurse Leader (AACN, 2013)	AACN Essentials 2: Organizational and Systems Leadership	Demonstrates working knowledge of the healthcare system and its component parts; uses systems theory in the assessment, design, delivery, and evaluation of healthcare within complex organizations.

Table 3.12. Organizational and Systems Leadership by Professional Organization   (continued)

Professional Organization	Competency/ Practice Standard	Examples
Certified Nurse Anesthetist (COA, 2018)	Communication Skills	Effectively communicates with individuals influencing patient care.
Nurse Educator (NLN, 2013)		Adapts to change in systems; implements strategies for change.
Nurse Administrator (AONE, 2015, 2016)	Leadership: Systems Thinking	Provides visionary thinking on issues that impact the healthcare organization; promotes systems thinking as an expectation of leaders and staff; adjusts to new models of care; shares leadership to improve interdisciplinary teams.

AACN, American Association of Colleges of Nursing.

Role Differentiation

Across the APN professions, examples of role differentiation related to systems thinking and leadership are presented in Table 3.13.

Translating and Integrating Scholarship Into Practice

The Institute of Medicine's Roundtable on Evidence-Based Medicine was convened in 2009 to aid in the transformation of how evidence on clinical effectiveness should be generated and used to improve health and healthcare (IOM, 2011). Participants set a goal that 90% of clinical decisions would reflect evidence-based practices (EBPs) by 2020. They estimated that in 2009 about 15% of clinical decisions were guided by evidence.

Translational Science

Evidence-based practice in nursing is desired for its ability to standardize healthcare practices with the latest, best scientifically available findings (Stevens, 2013). This application of evidence-based practice is intended to minimize variations

Table 3.13. MSN and DNP Quality and Safety Essentials

MSN Essential (AACN, 2011)	DNP Essentials (AACN, 2006)
Analyze information about quality initiatives recognizing the contributions of individuals and interprofessional healthcare teams to improve health outcomes across the continuum of care.	
Implement evidence-based plans based on trend analysis and quantify the impact on quality and safety.	
Analyze information and design systems to sustain improvements and promote transparency using high reliability and just culture principles.	
Compare and contrast several appropriate quality improvement models.	
Promote a professional environment that includes accountability and high-level communication skills when involved in peer review, advocacy for patients and families, reporting of errors, and professional writing.	Use advanced communication skills/processes to lead quality improvement and patient safety initiatives in healthcare systems.
Contribute to the integration of healthcare services within systems to affect safety and quality of care to improve patient outcomes and reduce fragmentation of care.	
Direct quality improvement methods to promote culturally responsive, safe, timely, effective, efficient, equitable, and patient-centered care.	Demonstrate sensitivity to diverse organizational cultures and populations, including patients and providers.
Lead quality improvement initiatives that integrate sociocultural factors affecting the delivery of nursing and healthcare services.	

in care while avoiding unintentional harm to patients. Evidence-based practice in nursing got its boost when the IOM in 2001 recommended that training and curriculum development of evidence-based practice be added to the core curriculum of healthcare professionals' educational programs (Correa-de-Araujo, 2016). As a result, the AACN added the following five competencies to nursing educational programs: patient-centered care, interdisciplinary teams, evidence-based practice, quality improvement, and information technology.

It is not enough for APNs to provide patient-centered care in a compassionate way; they must also have the skills to translate science into evidence-based practice. Evidence-based practice is not about conducting research; evidence-based practice is about applying the research findings to clinical situations in order to make evidence-based clinical decisions (Williamson, 2016). APNs must go beyond monitoring their patients for the presence of positive patient care outcomes; they should link the patient care outcomes to nursing interventions that have been found to be beneficial. This information leads to APNs ordering/administering effective treatments, patients expressing satisfaction with treatments, and payers providing coverage for effective treatments (White et al., 2016). APNs can adjust their care to "benchmark" their practice, thus improving the care they provide patients.

Numerous models can be used to guide the APN's quest to find not only evidence-based practices but to implement the best evidence-based practices in their own practice (White et al., 2016). Common to all these models are these six steps: (1) identify a clinical problem or question of practice, (2) search for the best evidence, (3) critically appraise the strength, quality, quantity, and consistency of the evidence, (4) recommend action based on appraisal findings: no change, change, further study, (5) implement the recommendation, and (6) evaluate the recommendation (p. 7). The following figure depicts the role these steps have in transforming knowledge to practice (Figure 3.7).

The identification of a clinical problem is the first step in developing a doctoral project. Nurses should continually monitor their practice environment for indications that there are lapses in patient or student outcomes. An inquisitive nature of nurses who continually survey these outcomes will lead to more substantial questions regarding how the clinical problem was created, why it is persisting, and what can be done to ameliorate its impact on outcomes.

Discussions with nurse leaders at a specific facility can easily lead to the identification of diagnostic groups that cause the most challenges with getting patients discharged in a timely manner. Nursing administrators are interested in studies

Pose questions to discover answers

- Identify clinical problem or issue in practice

Review existing evidence

- Conduct systematic reviews

Translate findings into action

- Critically appraise the findings of numerous studies

Integrate into practice

- Adopt findings that best match targeted population/diagnosis/condition

Evaluate impact on patients

- Measure impact on patient care outcomes, satisfaction with care, efficacy and efficiency of care, and changes in policy

Figure 3.7. Transforming knowledge to practice. Adapted from Stevens, K. R. (2013). The impact of evidence-based practice in nursing and the next big ideas. *Online Journal of Issues in Nursing, 18*(2), 4.

that focus on improving access to care, minimizing risks to patient safety, reducing barriers to improving patient care outcomes, and finding opportunities to reduce costs (Schub & Strayer, 2016). This is a good time to consider the demographics and characteristics of the patients most affected by this diagnostic group or clinical situation. Inquire about the situational factors that could be impeding positive outcomes—Are novice staff being assigned these patients? Are there patients who have communication challenges that make it difficult for them to comply with treatment protocols? Interview staff members to determine their challenges with caring for these patients to determine what aspect of their care causes the most challenges. Conversations with the quality assurance team can also reveal safety challenges for patients—Is there an increase in medication errors on a given unit, escalating falls in a segment of the population, or documentation errors that need attention? Inquire about the recent statistics related to incident reports as this department typically monitors infection rates, falls, extended length of stay, readmission rates, complications, mortality, and patient satisfaction surveys.

The next step is to find the most current research findings that relate to your clinical problem or question and appraise the studies for their strength, quality, number of participants, and consistency of evidence. Consider evidence-based practice as a means by which clinical decision-making can occur based on the best available evidence (Correa-de-Araujo, 2016). Look for studies where researcher(s) are testing an instrument or an innovation that you could replicate with your own population of interest. Is there a phone app that could promote communication between patient and caregiver that has been found to be effective in keeping patients from returning to the emergency room after discharge? Could that also be adapted to improve communication between nurses and physicians who are monitoring patients on telemetry? Identify interventions that have been effective with your population of interest. This review will provide insight into interventions that have been successful in improving outcomes and are evidence-based. Many studies provide a model or framework to assure important concepts are measured, contributing to the rigor of the study and allowing the results to be disseminated. Based on these findings, you can develop a project that will address a critical need in your institution and assure that your approach is evidence based.

Translate the findings of your literature review into action by developing an evidence-based practice guideline. This document incorporates the best practices and assures that nurses will provide this care to all patients who have this diagnosis/condition. As the new policy is developed, note the researcher(s) who have provided the findings to support your policy guidelines. This will allow others on the health-care team to review the research study should they have additional questions.

The next step is to integrate the new/revised policy into practice. The team is instrumental to the implementation of this phase. Consider all healthcare team members and other stakeholders who will be affected by this policy. For example, your findings suggest a computerized learning module can assist diabetic patients with dietary choices. Patients can provide valuable information during a test pilot to assure that the information is presented in an easily understood manner, that it applies to the age/ethnic/geographic target population, and that it is easily accessible. Otherwise, the intended population will have little interest or become frustrated and confused by verbiage they do not understand. Patients can benefit greatly from computerized educational resources, but if there is no technical support, they may have problems accessing or completing the modules. Consider the technical support that would be required for patients to complete these modules at home and include it in the plan prior to implementation or policy adoption.

Lastly, the outcomes of the evidence-based practice should be evaluated which means they are a key component to the application of evidence-based practices. One must know what will be measured before the research is utilized. Otherwise, it will be impossible to evaluate its ability to inform clinical decision-making. In this phase, the researcher should evaluate whether the evidence-based findings have the same results in the target population and meet quality indicators. The point of evidence-based practice is to inform quality improvement when providing care. The impact of evidence-based practice can be obtained by measuring the impact on health outcomes, patients' satisfaction with care, efficacy and efficiency of care, and changes in health policy (Williamson, 2016).

The following sections will describe educational and role differentiation regarding the essential of translational science. Consider your educational aspirations and career goal when reviewing these sections.

Questions to Ask Yourself

1. What is my comfort level with translating research findings to improve the care of my patient clientele, their families, and their community?
2. Will my degree give me the skills necessary to make an impact with the application of evidence-based practices among the population I wish to serve?
3. Are the professional competencies for translational science noted by my future professional organization applicable to my career goals?
4. What personal and professional challenges will I face in addressing this essential at the MSN or DNP level in my chosen role?

Educational Differentiation

Evidence-based practice is inherent in each of the APN essential competencies, as implementing best practices in each of these competencies relies heavily on the translation of research into practice. Table 3.14 matches the translation of research with APN essential competencies.

Role Differentiation

While nursing care is a key aspect of all advanced practice roles, what varies among advanced practice roles is whether the evidence-based care rendered to patients is direct or indirect. These differences are presented in Table 3.15.

Nursing Practice

The Gallup, 2017 Poll found, for the 16th consecutive year, Americans rated nurses the highest profession over 21 other occupations for honesty and ethical standards. All nurses, regardless of educational preparation, are socialized during their academic studies to practice according to the Code of Ethics developed

Table 3.14. Quality and Safety by Professional Organization

Professional Organization	Competency/Practice Standard	Examples
Nurse Practitioner (NONPF, 2017)	Quality Competencies	Uses best available evidence to continuously improve quality of clinical practice; evaluates the relationships among access, cost, quality, and safety and their influence on healthcare.
Certified Nurse Midwife (ACNM, 2014)	Professional Responsibilities Midwifery Management Process	Participates in self-evaluation, peer review, life-long learning, and other activities that ensure and validate quality practice; assumes responsibility for the safe and efficient implementation of a plan of care.
Clinical Nurse Specialist (NACNS, 2017)	Organization/Systems Sphere	Leads systematic quality and safety initiatives based on precise problem/etiology identification, gap analysis, and process evaluation.
Clinical Nurse Leader (AACN, 2013)	AACN Essential 3: Quality Improvement and Safety	Promotes a culture of continuous quality improvement strategies based on current evidence, analytics, and risk anticipation; performs a comprehensive microsystem assessment to provide the context for problem identification and action.
Certified Nurse Anesthetist (COA, 2018)	Patient Safety Professional Responsibility	Remains vigilant in the delivery of patient care. Refrains from engaging in extraneous activities that abandon or minimize vigilance while providing patient care. Participates in activities that improve anesthesia care.
Nurse Educator (NLN, 2013)	Pursue Continuous Quality Improvements in the Nurse Educator Role	Commits to maintaining competence in the role.
Nurse Administrator (AONE, 2015)	Knowledge of the Healthcare Environment: Patient Safety and Risk Management	Supports the development of an organization-wide patient safety program; leads/facilitates performance improvement teams to improve systems/processes that enhance patient safety/identifies early warning predictability indications for errors.

AACN, American Association of Colleges of Nursing.

Table 3.15. MSN and DNP Translating and Integrating Scholarship Into Practice Essentials

MSN Essential (AACN, 2011): Translating and Integrating Scholarship Into Practice	DNP Essential (AACN, 2006): Clinical Scholarship and Analytical Methods
Integrate theory, evidence, clinical judgment, research, and interprofessional perspectives using translational processes to improve practice and associated health outcomes for patient aggregates.	Design and implement processes to evaluate outcomes of practice, practice patterns, and systems of care within settings, organizations, or communities against national benchmarks to determine variances in practice outcomes and population needs.
Advocate for ethical conduct of research and translational scholarship—protect patients.	Use information technology and research methods appropriately in data collection, database design, data analysis, evidence-based practice design, outcomes analysis, examination of outcomes patterns, and identification of gaps in evidence.
Articulate to a variety of audiences the evidence base for practice decisions, including the credibility of sources of information and the relevance to the practice problem confronted.	Disseminate findings from evidence-based practice and research to improve health outcomes.
Participate, leading when appropriate, in collaborative teams to improve care outcomes and support policy changes through knowledge generations, knowledge dissemination, and planning and evaluating knowledge implementation.	Design, direct, and evaluate quality improvement methodologies to promote safe, timely, effective, efficient, equitable, and patient-centered care. Function as a practice specialist/consultant in collaborative knowledge-generating research.
Apply practice guidelines to improve practice and the care environment.	Apply relevant findings to develop practice guidelines and improve practice and the practice environment.
Perform rigorous critique of evidence derived from databases to generate meaningful evidence for nursing practice.	Use analytic methods to critically appraise existing literature and other evidence to determine and implement the best evidence for practice.

by the American Nurses Association (ANA, 2015). This code is foundational to the nursing profession as it influences nursing practice, nursing theory, and the application of knowledge and skills. Ethics is the underpinning for each of the essential competencies as presented in this chapter.

Ethical Principles

The ANA defines the fundamental principles for ethical nursing practice as including " …respect for the inherent dignity, worth, unique attributes, and human rights of all individuals" (ANA, 2015, p. 1). The ANA further stipulates that nurses must develop trust with their patients regardless of any personal biases they might have toward the patient. Patients have autonomy in their treatment; they have the right to make their own decisions. Nurses should understand that patients have the right to self-determination; patients can determine with informed consent their options to accept, refuse, or terminate any, and all treatment options (ANA, 2015).

Nurses are primarily responsible to patients in their care; this commitment can be to the individual, a family, group, community, or population (ANA, 2015). Nurses promote and advocate for the patient's health by protecting their rights, health, and safety. Nurses should report any healthcare provider—even if it is another nurse, who provides incompetent, unethical, illegal practices that could cause harm to patients.

APNs are challenged by patient autonomy, as in many cases, patients do not understand the implications or consequences of their actions (Grace, 2018). APNs must respect the patient's right to shared decision-making, as patients have legal rights to informed consent prior to invasive procedures therapeutic interventions (Farmer & Lundy, 2017). While APNs should respect a patient's right to make decisions concerning their care, there are patients who lack the cognitive or developmental skills necessary to make informed decisions. In this case, the APN can be unclear about how to proceed with a treatment plan. APNs must determine what a "reasonable person" would do in this situation. APNs must also consider the decision-making capacity of their patients, as patients should be competent enough to make difficult decisions.

The principles of nonmaleficence (do no harm) and beneficence (do good) also pose concerns for APNs. Nonmaleficence may come into question, as some treatments performed by APNs can be painful and expensive or cause distress for their patients (Grace, 2018). APNs may inadvertently harm their patients, particularly if they make a referral to a professional who causes harm to the patient, leaving them without the optimal care they need to improve their health. There is also the possibility of causing harm to a patient because the APN does not know the appropriate course of action, makes an error, or fails to understand the patient's unique needs and wishes. Beneficence in healthcare settings is the duty to maximize benefits and minimize harm to patients. APNs may need to provide services and care to patients who cannot make decisions for themselves. These services are performed for the good of the patient and are what "any reasonable" person would do in a similar situation.

Patient advocacy is a key principle of the APN's provision of ethical care. Advocacy is a core principle in the Nurses Code of Ethics (ANA, 2015), as it requires nurses to "promote, advocate for, and protect the rights, health, and safety of the patient" (p. 9). The APRN educational competencies, as well as professional core competencies, include patient advocacy in many of the essential competencies. However, how advocacy is used in practice across the APRN roles has not been fully examined (Hanks et al., 2018). A fuller understanding is needed of the APRN level of advocacy to improve educational preparation for more effective patient advocacy in clinical situations.

Ethical Research and Human Subject Protection

Nurses must assure that patients are protected when they participate in research. This includes providing patients with an informed consent document that explains the rationale for the study; provides the potential risks and benefits of the study; lists alternatives to participating in the study; provides an explanation of how the data will be used, managed, and protected; and discloses how the results will be reported (ANA, 2015). Nurses should always consider that vulnerable populations such as children, patients with cognitive impairments, disadvantaged or underserved individuals, fetuses, older adults, pregnant women, and prisoners require heightened vigilance. In these situations, the nurse must advocate for the patient to prevent harm during the research process.

APNs may encounter conflict with protecting patients when the APN is the one conducting research (Grace, 2018). Participants may not be aware that the APN not only provides health services but is also integral to the research for which they are being recruited as a human subject. APNs must be clear that the goal of the research project is to improve patient care not to promote the APN's personal or professional career goals.

Nurses who conduct or participate in research may be required to complete formalized training in ethical practice for the protection of human subjects.

These programs provide foundational training in research that involves human subjects. The training addresses how human subjects should be protected throughout the research process, ethical issues that can arise when using human subjects, and current regulating policies related to conducting research with human subjects (CITI Program, n.d.). These courses are for anyone involved in research studies with human subjects or who have responsibilities setting policies regarding research using human subjects. Examples of these types of courses include the Collaborative Institutional Training Initiative (CITI) or the National Institutes of Health (NIH) training modules.

The following sections will describe educational and role influences on ethics. Consider your educational aspirations and career goal when reviewing these sections.

Questions to Ask Yourself

1. What is my comfort level with maintaining an ethical practice as an APN?
2. Will my degree give me the skills necessary to make ethical decisions with the population I wish to serve?
3. Are the professional competencies for ethical practice by my future professional organization applicable to my career goals?
4. What personal and professional challenges will I face in addressing this essential at the MSN or DNP level in my chosen role?

Educational Differentiation

AACN assumes ethical practice is an integral component of all nursing care, and thus, ethics is not specifically addressed within the MSN and DNP *Essentials*. Table 3.16 compares provisions of ANA's Code of Ethics to Essential competencies.

Role Differentiation

The ANA Code of Ethics for nurses is an overarching framework for APN/APRN practice (Epstein & Turner, 2015). A relevant code of ethics supports professional practice so that nurses can practice competently and with integrity. Key elements from the ANA Code of Ethics may explicitly or implicitly work in concert with professional organizations and accrediting body competencies to establish frameworks that guide nursing practice. Table 3.17 demonstrates how ethics is found in the competencies and/or practice standards of APNs/APRNs.

Table 3.16. Translating and Integrating Scholarship Into Practice by Professional Organization

Professional Organization	Competency/Practice Standard	Examples
Nurse Practitioner (NONPF, 2017)	Practice Inquiry Competencies	Provides leadership in the translation of new knowledge into practice; leads practice inquiry; disseminates evidence from inquiry to diverse audiences.
Certified Nurse Midwife (ACNM, 2014)	Hallmarks of Midwifery	Incorporates of scientific evidence into clinical practice; evaluates and utilizes research to provide high-quality, evidence-based healthcare, initiates change, and improves midwifery practice for women and newborns.
Clinical Nurse Specialist (NACNS, 2017)	Nurses/Nursing Practice Sphere	Uses evidence-based knowledge as a foundation for nursing practice to achieve optimal nurse-sensitive outcomes; mentors nurse colleagues in using evidence-based practice principles.
Clinical Nurse Leader (AACN, 2013)	Essential 4: Translating and Integrating Scholarship Into Practice	Facilitates practice change based on best available evidence; disseminates changes in practice and improvements in care outcomes to internal and external audiences.
Certified Nurse Anesthetist (COA, 2018)	Critical Thinking	Provides nurse anesthesia care based on sound principles and research evidence.
Nurse Educator (NLN, 2013)		Uses knowledge of evidence-based practice to facilitate learning; incorporates current research in assessment and evaluation practices.
Nurse Administrator (AONE, 2015)	Knowledge of the Healthcare Environment: Performance Improvement/Metrics	Uses evidence-based metrics to align patient outcomes with the organization's goals and objectives; articulates the organization's performance improvement program and goals.

Table 3.17. Professional Nursing Practice (Ethics) by Professional Organization

Professional Organization	Competency/ Practice Standard	Examples
Nurse Practitioner (NONPF, 2017)	Ethics competencies	Integrates ethical decision-making; evaluates the ethical consequences of decisions; applies ethically sound solutions to complex issues related to individuals, populations, and systems of care.
Certified Nurse Midwife (ACNM, 2014)	Practice in accordance with ACNM Philosophy Standards and Code of Ethics	Develops a professional relationship between a midwife and a woman is to arrive at a plan of care that optimizes the woman's health through informed decision-making, is consistent with professional standards of practice, and is acceptable to both.
Clinical Nurse Specialist (NACNS, 2017)	Patient/Direct Care Sphere Nurses/Nursing Practice Sphere	Facilitates resolution of ethical conflicts in complex patient care situations. Addresses ethical conflict experienced by nurses and the interprofessional team.
Clinical Nurse Leader (AACN, 2013)	AACN Essential 1: Building for Practice From Sciences and Humanities	Applies ethical analysis and clinical reasoning to assess, intervene, and evaluate advanced nursing care delivery.
Certified Nurse Anesthetist (AANA, 2018)	Respect and maintain the basic rights of the patient	Supports and preserves the basic rights of the patient.
Nurse Educator (NLN, 2013)	Pursue systematic self-evaluation and improvement in the nurse educator role	Practices according to legal and ethical standards relevant to higher education and nursing education.
Nurse Administrator (AONE, 2015)	Domain of professionalism	Upholds ethical principles and corporate compliance standards; holds self and staff accountable to comply with ethical standards of practice to discuss, resolve, and learn from ethical dilemmas.

AACN, American Association of Colleges of Nursing; ACNM, American College of Nurse Midwives.

The Move to Competency-Based Standards

Nursing education is in the midst of fundamental changes to how we educate new nurses. Benner and associates (2009) published *Educating Nurses: A Call for Radical Transformation* in which they articulated the strengths and weaknesses of nursing education. The seminal work developed from a national survey of teachers and students and was undertaken as a cooperative study with the National League for Nursing (NLN), the AACN, and the National Student Nurses' Association (NSNA). This work underscored the need for nurse educators to focus on teaching in a way that promoted clinical reasoning skills rather than attainment of knowledge. Simultaneously, a body of evidence began to emerge indicating that competency-based education would better meet the healthcare needs of the public and promote better outcomes through accountability (Calhoun et al., 2011; Carraccio et al., 2002; Frank et al., 2010). In this context, competency may be defined as the measurable mastery of defined knowledge, skills, and attitudes or abilities (KSAs) (Englander et al., 2013; IOM, 2011).

Competency-Based Education

Competency-based education is grounded in a deep understanding of the knowledge, skills, and attitudes needed by professionals working in today's complex healthcare system. Because competencies are measurable, they can be used to ensure attainment of practices that are linked to improved patient outcomes (AACN, 2019). Furthermore, because competency-based education is learner-centered rather than time-centered, this approach requires greater learner accountability while providing for increased flexibility. Competency-based education is well suited to clinical education because of its ability to create clearly measurable expectations and assessment standards (IOM, 2011).

Englander and Associates (2013) conducted an exhaustive review of domains of competence across all health professions. Their goal was to create a robust framework with a standard set of competencies that could be applied to all health disciplines. This seminal work provides a meaningful competency framework across health professional education and creates a common language to assist in understanding differences and commonalities in scope and intent of practice. A competency framework is not intended to dictate educational standards or content; rather, it is used to inform implementation strategies and actions as faculty create curricula that meet measurable practice expectations (Figure 3.8).

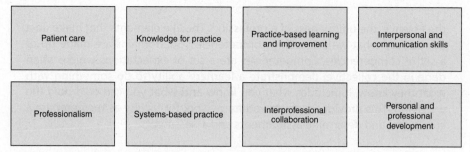

Figure 3.8. Competencies identified by Englander and Associates.

Competency Domains

Englander and Associates' (2013) publication—Toward a common taxonomy of competency domains for the health professions and competencies for physicians—serves as an initial framework for developing competencies. Since publication of this document and medicine's subsequent adoption of competency-based education, other health profession programs have adopted the eight-domain framework including physical therapy, dental, and veterinary education. In particular, the discipline of physical therapy used their competency framework to develop a validated, standardized tool for use by programs in documenting attainment of expected competencies at graduation (Roach et al., 2012). Universal adoption of the eight domains assists in creating a common language between professions and developing an understanding of what the unique contributions each profession adds in meeting individual and community health needs.

In Their Own Words

John McFadden, PhD, CRNA
Professor and Dean, College of Nursing and Health Sciences
Barry University, Miami Shores, Florida

What Are Competencies and Domains?
The term competency is not new. Nurse educators have a long history of engaging in competency-based education. A domain is a grouping of like elements that represent a sphere of knowledge. A group of domains in aggregate capture

(Continued)

the essence, the uniqueness of a profession. The like elements that make up a domain are what we are calling competencies. So, domains are made up of a set of competencies. Competencies are a set of expectations which, when done in the collective, demonstrate a learners' ability to do something with what they know. It includes what you know **and** what you can do. I bold the word and! This provides a structured framework for faculty as they prepare a curriculum and determine assignments and assessments.

Why Make the Change?

I think many practice partners were seeing gaps in nursing education—for example, with respect to population-focused care. They also voiced concern about variabilities among graduates across all degree levels and even among those with the same degrees and credentials. Some employers of our graduates, the public, and even some within our own profession have a difficult time articulating the difference between a graduate of one degree or a higher degree. Fortunately, the AACN leadership determined the time is right to reenvision the *Essentials*, which includes delineating the expected competencies of graduates of baccalaureate, master's, and DNP programs and identifying the necessary curricular elements that must be present in these programs. Development of core domains, domain descriptors, competency statements, and subcompetencies will help define the different expectations of undergraduate- and graduate-level nurses. Competencies can also be used by our practice partners to create standardized expectations of graduates from accredited programs.

What Are Some of the Terms That Need to Be Understood?

We started discussing domains and competencies. Remember, competencies are descriptions of very clear expectations that we make explicit to our learners, their employers, and the public. Competencies need to be objectively demonstrated through a performance that can be replicated in multiple contexts. It is not a check list of tasks that is demonstrated and assessed once. It is not a singular demonstration performed in one setting. Subcompetencies are even more specific, measurable, observable pieces of evidence of competency attainment. Unlike other professions that have one level of practice, nursing has different levels of practice. There needs to be a way to differentiate levels of learners and practice. So, each competency has a set of subcompetencies for the entry into professional nursing practice and another for the advanced professional nursing practice. It might help to think of it going backwards. Try this analogy. A painting (a competency) is made up of individual brushstrokes (subcompetencies). Several paintings put together as a collage (domain) tell a story—or in our case, describe the uniqueness of our profession. The competencies will provide a measurable framework for the expectations of graduates of nursing programs.

(Continued)

How Are Competencies Used Within Curricula?

Competencies can do three things: They provide a framework for what we teach, they set expectations for students, and very importantly, competencies can guide performance assessment. Competencies are designed to be applicable across all care settings and all populations throughout the lifespan. The intent is that any curriculum model can be used to teach competencies and assure that the learner has achieved the competencies.

What Are the Benefits of Moving to Competency-Based Education?

- Currently, nursing struggles with multiple entry points to practice. There is also a great deal of variability in program length, scope, expectations, and quality. We struggle to articulate the uniqueness that nurses bring to healthcare, and we also have difficulty in identifying the differences between the different levels of nursing practice.
- The domains, domain descriptors, competencies, and subcompetencies are being formed with ongoing and robust input from education administrators, faculty, practice partners, and other specialty organizations to promote and affirm their relevancy. This work will facilitate a standard for what graduates KNOW and are able TO DO. The domains articulate nursing knowledge and emphasize nursing's unique disciplinary knowledge.

What Might Be a Few Good References to Learn More About Competency-Based Education?

- Englander, R., Cameron, T., Ballard, A., Dodge, J., Bull, J., & Aschenbrener, C. (2013). Towards a common taxonomy of competency domains for the health professions and competencies for physicians. *Academic Medicine, 888*), 1088–1094.
- AACN's Vision for Academic Nursing. https://www.aacnnursing.org/News-Information/Position-Statements-White-Papers/Vision-for-Nursing-Education
- AACN Board of Directors Approved Common APRN Doctoral Level Competencies. https://www.aacnnursing.org/News-Information/News/View/ArticleId/20950/APRN-Doctoral-Level-Competencies
- Ferrell, B., Malloy, P., Mazanec, P., & Virani, R. (2016). CARES: AACNs new competencies and recommendations for educating undergraduate nursing students to improve palliative care. *Journal of Professional Nursing, 23*(5), 327–333.

Changes in education methodologies and approaches (immersive learning technologies, open-access online courses, microcredentialing, and digital badges) coupled with adoption of competency frameworks in other healthcare disciplines increase the desirability of competency-based education.

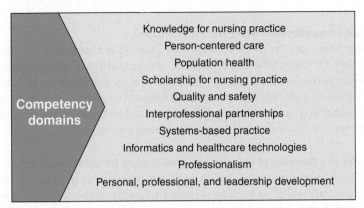

Knowledge for nursing practice
Person-centered care
Population health
Scholarship for nursing practice
Quality and safety
Interprofessional partnerships
Systems-based practice
Informatics and healthcare technologies
Professionalism
Personal, professional, and leadership development

Competency domains

Figure 3.9. American Association of Colleges of Nursing (AACN) draft domains for competency-based education.

In combination with the understanding that nurses need to strengthen their ability to manage patient information, lead teams, and have strong clinical reasoning skills came the movement of other health professions toward competency-based education. Understanding the skills that are needed allows a profession to articulate the services and benefits that they are able to provide (Englander et al., 2013). Figure 3.9 presents the most recent draft of competency domains available at the time of publication. It must be noted that seven concepts are expected to be threaded across and within the ten domains. These concepts include (1) diversity, equity, and inclusion; (2) social justice; (3) determinants of health; (4) communication; (5) ethics; (6) policy and advocacy; and (7) innovation. AACN plans ongoing discussion and work to refine the domains, their descriptors, and the expected competencies for undergraduate and graduate education (AACN, 2019).

Nursing's Journey to Competency-Based Education

Introduced in the latter half of the 1990s, AACN's *Essentials Series* provided the elements and framework for nursing curricula. However, the Essentials focused on content areas as opposed to measurable competency domains that differentiate performance expectations between entry-level nurses, APNs, and other health professionals. As part of licensure requirements, the four APRN roles—nurse practitioner, nurse midwife, nurse anesthetist, and clinical nurse specialist—have competencies as delineated by their respective professional organizations (AACN, 2017). Although they do not sit for a licensing exam, nurse leaders, nurse educators, and CNLs may opt to become certified in their role; these voluntary certifications often carry additional competencies for expected practice. Although nursing has, in some ways, been at the forefront of professional competency development (Englander et al., 2013), no widely accepted definition of nursing competency that is standardized in terms of scope and measurability exists within nursing (AACN, 2017).

In 2018, AACN formed a task force to develop competency domains across entry-level and advanced practice nurses. Thus far, this group has created 10 domains of competence adapted from the original eight identified in Englander et al. (2013) work. These competencies will create a measurable framework to outline performance expectations for nurses at all levels of education. AACN charged The Vision for Nursing Education Task Force (Table 3.18) with clarifying preferred educational pathways for contemporary nursing and outlining

Table 3.18. Future Trends and Needs

Current Trends	Vision
Changing learners • Differences among learners (Baby Boomers, Millennials, Generation Z, Generation X, first-generation learners, second-degree learners) place greater demands on faculty to adapt pedagogical practices to meet student needs **Changing nursing workforce** • Growing demand for an increased number of baccalaureate and higher degree–prepared nurses • Need to educate nurses to practice across settings and populations, addressing the social determinants of health to minimize health disparities • Nurses must be educated to lead primary care teams • The nursing workforce is inequitably distributed across the United States and is particularly acute in rural areas • Diversity within the nursing workforce is necessary, and holistic admission process can help to increase diversity without decreasing workforce preparedness and academic success	**Accelerate diversity and inclusion** • Adopt holistic admission review practices • Support students to ensure success in nursing programs • Foster strategies to increase recruitment and retention of the nursing workforce in all geographic environments • Build a culture of diversity and inclusion in academic nursing

(Continued)

Table 3.18. Future Trends and Needs   (continued)

Current Trends	Vision
Competency-based education movement • This movement reflects current trends in health professions education • Competency-based education models are currently under review for nursing • Impact of competency-based education for nursing must be evaluated in terms of cost, resources, regional accreditation requirements **Changing regulation of nursing practice** • The National Council of State Boards of Nursing (NCSBN) has announced plans for new testing formats and assessment items known as the next generation of NCLEX • Evidence continues to build demonstrating that a higher mix of BSN and higher degree–educated RNs improves healthcare outcomes • Only 16 states have fully adopted the NCSBN *Consensus Model for APN Regulation: Licensure, Accreditation, Certification & Education;* lack of adoption throughout the United States hampers the ability of APRNs to cross state lines and create standardization within the role	**Transition to competency-based education and assessment** • Shift focus from what a learner must know to what a learner must be able to do • AACN should lead development of nationally recognized competencies using a consensus-based process that engages diverse stakeholders • Align competencies with regional accreditation requirements and develop reliable assessment methods
Changing healthcare systems • Critical need to decrease healthcare costs while improving health outcomes • Shift of nurse employment settings from acute care to primary care and community settings • Technology-enabled healthcare services support diagnosis and delivery of care	**Increase collaboration between education and practice** • Develop expanded academic-practice partnerships that include multi-school, multipractice, and regional partnerships • Promote intentional partnerships that cross-engagement across practice and education • Create robust transition-to-practice models

Table 3.18. Future Trends and Needs (continued)	
Current Trends	**Vision**
Changing faculty availability and mix • The critical faculty shortage is largely fueled by an aging faculty workforce, an increased demand for skilled faculty, and an insufficient number of potential faculty in the educational system • Increased concern over the utility of tenure models in the current changing educational climate • Concern in providing a structure that supports nursing faculty workload while allowing for growth and increased practice expertise • Need for increased collaborative efforts between academia and practice	**Increase emphasis of faculty development and career advancement** • Career-long faculty and leadership development opportunities provide for career progression and sustainability of the profession • To become a master teacher in the practice environment or academia, additional preparation in the science of pedagogy is preferable
Changing higher education • Development of awarding microcredentials, digital badges, or stackable credentials • Changes in demands of employers, prospective students, and public • Changing student demographics • Availability of distance learning opportunities and immersive learning technologies **Changing learning technologies** • Increased understanding of evidence-based educational practices is transforming higher education • New models of instruction must engage and challenge the learner • Technology is changing the availability, affordability, and accessibility of learning	**Explore and adopt opportunities for resource efficiencies** • Simulated and practicum experiences should be proportioned to ensure adequate exposure to high-risk, low-volume clinical experiences • Develop regional consortia to collaboratively provide select courses to better utilize scarce resources and expertise • Form simulation learning centers to provide access to new technologies in a more cost-efficient manner

AACN, American Association of Colleges of Nursing; APRNs, advanced practice registered nurse; NCLEX, National Council Licensure Examination.

Compiled from AACN's Vision for Nursing Education Task Force Final Report: *AACN's Vision for Academic Nursing* White Paper, 2019.

broad curricular recommendations for baccalaureate and graduate nursing programs. Table 3.18 presents a summary of the future trends and needs as identified by the task force.

Implications for Nursing Education

As the healthcare system becomes increasingly complex and patient acuities continue to rise, the need for a more highly educated nursing workforce becomes apparent. Because nurses represent the largest healthcare workforce, their ability to impact the health of our nation is unparalleled. In 2010, the Health and Medicine Division (HMD, formerly the Institute of Medicine) of the National Academies of Sciences, Engineering, and Medicine (the National Academies) released the seminal report, the Future of Nursing: Leading change, Advancing Health. Through its deliberations, the committee developed four key messages:

- Nurses should practice to the full extent of their education and training.
- Nurses should achieve higher levels of education and training through an improved education system that promotes seamless academic progression.
- Nurses should be full partners, with physicians and other healthcare professionals, in redesigning healthcare in the United States.
- Effective workforce planning and policy making require better data collection and information infrastructure.

In keeping with HMD's vision for the future of nursing, the Josiah Macy JR. Foundation has emphasized the importance of nursing's role in finding healthcare solutions and advocates for increased preparation that will support nurses in helping to meet primary care needs (2017). Much discussion has ensued related to the best means of preparing nurses to become part of the solution to a fragmented healthcare delivery system.

The American Association of Colleges of Nurses (AACN, 2019) refers to today's nurses as indispensable members of the healthcare team and is currently involved in addressing the educational pathways and changes to transform nursing education. As such, AACN asserts that any solution should be developed within the context of considering academic nursing's role in promoting population health, addressing the social determinants of health, and advancing interprofessional engagement. In 2018, AACN formed the Vision for Nursing Task Force to

BOX 3.1

▶ **AACN'S VISION FOR NURSING EDUCATION ACTION OPPORTUNITIES**

- Increase diversity and inclusion in nursing education and practice

- Transition to competency-based education and assessment

- Increase collaboration between education and practice by expanding formal academic-practice partnerships

- Increase emphasis on faculty development and career advancement

- Explore and adopt opportunities for resource efficiencies

…summarize trends and projected changes in healthcare, higher education, population demographics, learners and learning styles, the nursing workforce, nursing regulation, and patient/population needs…to inform the vision being advanced. To ensure that graduates are ready for contemporary practice required faculty who have an awareness of evolving changes …and a commitment to adapting curricula, teaching strategies, and learning assessment.

(p. 4)

Box 3.1 briefly identifies the resulting recommendations from the task force.

Goals of Competency-Based Education

By adopting standardized competencies based upon a common taxonomy across health professions, communication and coordination among disciplines will improve. Unifying competencies within nursing will also provide direction for standards across nursing education. AACN's vision is one of a collaborative effort among nurse educators, professional organizations, and healthcare organizations and providers that would be ongoing and translated to nursing curricula to ensure that all levels of nursing graduates are better prepared to meet the changing healthcare environment.

This move to a competency-based approach to education is designed to more clearly define expectations to students by providing objective measures of competency mastery (Harden, 2002). Performance-based assessment can then be used to demonstrate a theoretical grasp of learning and the ability to put that learning into practice within clinical or simulated settings. The transition to practice or nurse residency programs could offer an extended opportunity to reinforce and test core competencies in real-world settings that are both safe and monitored.

Web Resources

- AACN Essentials: https://www.aacnnursing.org/Education-Resources/AACN-Essentials
- AACN's Vision for Academic Nursing: https://www.aacnnursing.org/Portals/42/AcademicNursing/pdf/AACN-Vision-for-Academic-Nursing-Memo-White-Paper.pdf?ver=2019-02-15-113532-080
- US Department of Education: Competency-Based Learning: https://www.ed.gov/oii-news/competency-based-learning-or-personalized-learning

---

Summary

APNs are educationally and clinically prepared to lead and advocate for patients and their profession. Their expertise and knowledge are necessary to the development and implementation of health policy. APNs can review policies for the effects on specific patient populations, serving as the voice of patients who need better access and more services in support of their quality of life. They can conduct and analyze research that informs the profession and public about treatment management procedures and methods that improve patient care outcomes. APNs should also advocate for their profession, becoming active members of organizations and associations that focus on health policy; all voices need to be heard on policy issues related to practice, education, and administration of healthcare services. It is crucial that APNs fully implement their roles.

Competency-based education focuses on attainment of objectively defined outcomes. Progression is based on mastery of competencies rather than proficiency of content. This subtle difference pushes the emphasis toward attainment of outcomes independently from time.

Chapter Highlights

- Role competencies of APN/APRNs were discussed and defined by an ethical code of conduct, professional organizations, and accrediting bodies.
- Educational differentiation of competencies between master's vs. doctorally prepared APN/APRNs was explored.
- The competencies of professional organizations were discussed as they impact each of the APN/APRN roles.
- In sync with other professional organizations, AACN is working toward identification of competencies for nurses that will facilitate competency-based standards. This would create a common language to be shared with other healthcare professionals such as physicians, dentists, physical therapists, and veterinarians and better identify the value provided by nurses.

References

Agency for Healthcare Research and Quality (AHRQ). (2018). *Six domains of health care quality*. Content. https://www.ahrq.gov/talkingquality/measures/six-domains.html

Alexander, S., Frith, K. H., & Hoy, H. (2019). *Applied clinical informatics for nurses* (2nd ed.). Jones & Bartlett Learning.

American Association of Colleges of Nursing (AACN). (2006). *The Essentials of doctoral education for advanced nursing practice*. http://www.aacnnursing.org/Portals/42/Publications/DNPEssentials.pdf

American Association of Colleges of Nursing (AACN). (2011). *The Essentials of master's education*. http://www.aacnnursing.org/Portals/42/Publications/MastersEssentials11.pdf

American Association of Colleges of Nursing (AACN). (2013). *Competencies and curricular expectations for clinical nurse leader education and practice*. http://www.aacnnursing.org/Portals/42/AcademicNursing/CurriculumGuidelines/CNL-Competencies-October-2013.pdf

American Association of Colleges of Nursing (AACN). (2019). *AACN's vision for academic nursing white paper, 2019*. https://www.aacnnursing.org/Portals/42/News/White-Papers/Vision-Academic-Nursing.pdf

American Association of Colleges of Nursing (AACN). (2007). *White paper on the education and role of the clinical nurse leader*. http://www.aacnnursing.org/News-Information/Position-Statements-White-Papers/CNL

American Association of Nurse Anesthetists. (2018). *Code of ethics for the certified registered nurse anesthetist*. www.aana.com/docs/default-source/practice-aana-com-web-documents-(all)/code-of-ethics-for-the-crna.pdf

American College of Nurse Midwives (ACNM). (2014). *Competencies for master's level midwifery education*. http://www.midwife.org/ACNM/files/ACNMLibraryData/UPLOADFILENAME/000000000291/Competencies-for-Master's-Level-Midwifery-Education-Dec-2014.pdf

American Nurses Association (ANA). (2015). *Code of ethics for nurses with interpretive statements.*

American Organization of Nurse Executives (AONE). (2015). *Nurse executive competencies.* http://www.aone.org/resources/nec.pdf

American Organization of Nurse Executives (AONE). (2016). *System CNE white paper: The effective system nurse executive in contemporary health systems. Emerging competencies.* http://www.aone.org/resources/aone-system-cne-white-paper.pdf

Anderson, J. E. (2011). *Public policymaking* (7th ed.). Wadsworth.

Arnold, R. D., & Wade, J. P. (2015). *A definition of systems thinking: A systems approach.* https://ac.els-cdn.com/S1877050915002860/1-s2.0-S1877050915002860-main.pdf?_tid=d99b1852-6303-4c09-9d9b-d7435706a9a7&acdnat=1523901683_2bcae0a6c1863d7e8e3ed996164e9bfe

Azar, A. M., Mnuchin, S. T., & Acosta, A., U.S. Department of Health and Human Services, U.S. Department of the Treasury, & U.S. Department of Labor. (2018). *Reforming America's healthcare system through choice and competition.* https://www.hhs.gov/sites/default/files/Reforming-Americas-Healthcare-System-Through-Choice-and-Competition.pdf

Bartol, T. (2018). This medical bill can't be right, can it? *Medscape.* https://www.medscape.com/viewarticle/894850

Brown, M. A. (2012). *The advanced practice registered nurse as a prescriber.* Wiley Blackwell.

Calhoun, G., Wrobel, C. A., & Finnegan, J. R. (2011). Current state in U.S. public health competency-based graduate education. *Public Health Reviews, 33,* 148–167.

Campbell, S. M., Roland, M. O., & Buetow, S. A. (2000). Defining quality of care. *Social Science Medicine Journal, 51,* 1611–1625.

Carraccio, C., Wolfsthal, S. D., Englander, R., Ferentz, K., & Martin, C. (2002). Shifting paradigms: From Flexner to competencies. *Academy of Medicine, 77*(5), 361–367.

Centers for Disease Control (CDC). (2019), *What is health literacy?* https://www.cdc.gov/healthliteracy/learn/index.html

Chilton, L. (2015). *Nurse practitioners have an essential role in health policy.* http://www.npjournal.org/article/S1555-4155(14)00687-4/pdf

CITI Program. (n.d.). *Human subjects research.* https://about.citiprogram.org/en/series/human-subjects-research-hsr/

Colby, S., & Ortman, J. (2015). *Projections of the size and composition of the U.S. Population Reports* (pp. 25–1143). U.S. Census Bureau.

Cordon, C. P. (2013). System theories: An overview of various system theories and its application in healthcare. *American Journal of Systems Science, 2*(1), 13–22. http://article.sapub.org/pdf/10.5923.j.ajss.20130201.03.pdf

Correa-de-Araujo, R. (2016). *Evidence-based practice in the United States: Challenges, progress, and future directions.* https://www.ncbi.nlm.nih.gov/pmc/articles/PMC4804828/

Cosgrove, T. (2016). *Four behaviors that define healthcare leadership: What healthcare leaders need to meet challenge ahead.* https://consultqd.clevelandclinic.org/four-behaviors-define-healthcare-leadership/

Council on Accreditation (COA). (2019). *Standards for accreditation of nurse anesthesia educational programs.* https://home.coa.us.com/accreditation/Documents/Standards%20for%20Accreditation%20of%20Nurse%20Anesthesia%20Programs%20-%20Practice%20Doctorate,%20revised%20October%202019.pdf

D'Eramo, A. L., & Puckett, J. B. (2014). Tools of quality improvement. In P. Kelly, B. A. Vottero, & C. A. Christie-McAuliffe (Eds.), *Introduction to quality and safety education for nurses: Core competencies.* Springer Publishing Company.

D'Eramo, A. L., & Puckett, J. B. (2018). Tools of quality improvement. In Kelly, P., Vottero, B. A., & Christie-McAuliffe, C. A. (Eds.), *Introduction to quality and safety education for nurses: Core competencies* (pp. 417-446). Springer Publishing Company.

Decker, F. (2018). *What is risk management in nursing?* http://smallbusiness.chron.com/risk-management-nursing-69795.html

Elliott, N. (2016). Building leadership capacity in advanced nurse practitioners: The role of organizational management. *Journal of Nursing Management, 23*(1), 77–81.

Englander, R., Cameron, T., Ballard, A., Dodge, J., Bull, J., & Aschenbrener, C. (2013). Towards a common taxonomy of competency domains for the health professions and competencies for physicians. *Academic Medicine, 88*(8), 1088–1094.

Epstein, B., & Turner, M. (2015). The nursing Code of Ethics: Its value, its history. *Online Journal of Issues in Nursing, 20*(2), 4. https://ojin.nursingworld.org/MainMenuCategories/ANAMarketplace/ANAPeriodicals/OJIN/TableofContents/Vol-20-2015/No2-May-2015/The-Nursing-Code-of-Ethics-Its-Value-Its-History.html

Farmer, L., & Lundy, A. (2017). Informed consent: Ethical and legal considerations for advanced practice nurses. *The Journal for Nurse Practitioners, 13*(2), 124–130.

Fawaz, M. A., Hamdan-Mansour, A. M., & Tassi, A. (2018). Challenges facing nursing education in the advanced healthcare environment. *International Journal of Africa Nursing Sciences, 9*, 105–110.

Finkelman, A. (2019). *Professional nursing concepts: Competencies for quality leadership* (4th ed.). Jones & Bartlett Learning.

Frank, J. R., Snell, L. S., Cate, O. T., Holmboe, E. S., Carraccio, C., Swing, S. R., Harris, P., Glasgow, N. J., Campbell, C, Dath, D., Harden, R. M., Iobst, W., Long, D. M., Mungroo, R., Richardson, D. L., Sherbino, J., Silver, I., Taber, S., Talbot, M., & Harris, K. A. (2010). Competency-based medical education: Theory to practice. *Medical Teacher, 32*, 638–645.

Gallup. (2017). *Nurses keep healthy lead as most honest, ethical profession.* http://news.gallup.com/poll/224639/nurses-keep-healthy-lead-honest-ethical-profession.aspx?g_source=CATEGORY_SOCIAL_POLICY_ISSUES&g_medium=topic&g_campaign=tiles

Galvin, H. K. (2019). *Protecting patient privacy rights in EHRs requires thoughtful solutions.* https://www.aappublications.org/news/2019/07/11/hit071119

Goddard, M. (2017). The EU general data protection regulation (GDPR): European regulation that has a global impact. *International Journal of Market Research, 59*(6), 703–705.

Goudreau, K., & Smolenski, M. (2018). *Health policy and advanced practice nursing: Impact and implications* (2nd ed.). Springer Publishing Company.

Grace, P. (2018). *Philosophical foundations of applied and professional ethics.* In *Nursing ethics and professional responsibility in advanced practice.* Jones & Bartlett Learning.

Hanks, R., Starnes-Ott, K, & Stafford, L. (2018). Patient advocacy at the APRN level: A direction for the future. *Nursing Forum, 53*(1), 5–11.

Harden, R. M. (2002). Learning outcomes and instructional objectives: Is there a difference. *Medical Teacher, 24*(2), 151–155.

Haviley, C., Anderson, A. K., & Currier, A. (2014). Overview of patient safety and quality of care. In P. Kelly, B. A. Vottero, & C. A. Christie-McAuliffe (Eds.), *Introduction to quality and safety education for nurses: Core competencies.* Springer Publishing Company.

HealthyPeople.gov. (2020). *What is the Healthy People 2030 framework?* https://www.healthypeople.gov/2020/About-Healthy-People/Development-Healthy-People-2030/Framework

Homeyer, S., Hoffmann, W., Hingst, P., Opperman, R., & Dreier-Wolfgramm, A. (2018). Effects of interprofessional education for medical and nursing students: Enablers, barriers, and expectations for optimizing future interprofessional collaboration – a qualitative study. *BMC Nursing, 17*(13). https://bmcnurs.biomedcentral.com/articles/10.1186/s12912-018-0279-x

Hospitals (2018). *Improving patient care with interprofessional collaboration.* https://www.simula-tioniq.com/blog/content/improving-patient-care-interprofessional-collaboration-0

Huff, R., Kline, M., & Peterson, D. (2015). *Health promotion in multicultural populations: A handbook for practitioners and students* (3rd ed.). Safe Publications, Inc.

Institute of Medicine. (2011). *The Future of Nursing: Leading Change, Advancing Health.* The National Academies Press. http://doi.org/10.17226/12956. http://www.nationalacademies.org/hmd/Reports/2010/The-Future-of-Nursing-Leading-Change-Advancing-Health.aspx

Interprofessional Education Collaborative Expert Panel. (2016). *Core competencies for interprofessional collaborative practice: 2016 update.* Interprofessional Education Collaborative.

Jangland, E., Nyberg, B. & Yngman-Uhlin, P. (2017). "It's a matter of patient safety": Understanding challenges in everyday clinical practice for achieving good care on the surgical ward – a qualitative study. *Scandinavian Journal of Caring Sciences, 31*, 323–331.

Kent, J. (2018). *Population health nurses require changes in education, practices.* https://healthitanalytics.com/news/population-health-nurses-require-changes-in-education-practices

Makary, M. A., & Daniel, M. (2016). Medical error-the third leading cause of death in the US. *British Medical Journal, 353,* i2139. https://www.bmj.com/content/353/bmj.i2139

Mayo, A., & Wooley, A. W. (2016). Teamwork in healthcare: Maximizing collective intelligence via inclusive collaboration and open communication. *AMA Journal of Ethics, 18*(9), 933–940. http://journalofethics.ama-assn.org/2016/09/pdf/stas2-1609.pdf

McGonigle, D., Hunter, K., Sipes, C., & Hebda, T. (2014). Why nurses need to understand nursing informatics. *AORN Journal, 100*(3), 324–327. http://doi.org/10.1016/j.aorn.2014.06.012

McGonigle, D. & Mastrian, K. (2018). *Nursing informatics and the foundation of knowledge* (4th ed.). Jones & Bartlett Learning.

MedPAC. (2019). *Improving Medicare's payment policies for advanced practice registered nurses and physician assistants.* http://medpac.gov/-blog-/the-commission-recommends-aprns-and-pas-bill-medicare-directly-/2019/02/15/improving-medicare's-payment-policies-for-aprns-and-pas

Metzger, R., & Rivers, C. (2014). Advanced practice nursing organizational leadership model. *The Journal for Nurse Practitioners, 10*(5), 337–343. https://doi.org/10.1016/j.nurpra.2014.02.015

National Association of Clinical Nurse Specialists (NACNS). (2017). *Draft core CNS competencies.* http://nacns.org/wp-content/uploads/2017/10/2017-Draft-CNS-Core-Competencies-FINAL.pdf

National League for Nursing (NLN). (2018). *CNE 2018 candidate handbook.* http://www.nln.org/docs/default-source/default-document-library/cne-handbook373ac75c78366c709642ff00005f0421.pdf?sfvrsn=0

National League for Nursing (NLN). (2020). *Nurse educator core competency.* http://www.nln.org/professional-development-programs/competencies-for-nursing-education/nurse-educator-core-competency

National League for Nursing. (2020). *Nurse educator core competency.* http://www.nln.org/professional-development-programs/competencies-for-nursing-education/nurse-educator-core-competency

National Organization of Nurse Practitioner Faculties (NONPF). (2017). *Nurse practitioner core competencies with curriculum content.* https://cdn.ymaws.com/www.nonpf.org/resource/resmgr/competencies/2017_NPCoreComps_with_Curric.pdf

ODPHP. (2018). *Healthy people 2020 leading health indicators.* https://www.healthypeople.gov/2020/leading-health-indicators/2020-LHI-Topics

Ogrinc, G., Davies, L., Goodman, D., Batalden, P., Davidoff, F., & Stevens, D. (2016). Squire 2.0 (Standards for QUality Improvement Reporting Excellence): Revised publication guidelines from a detailed consensus process. *BMJ Quality & Safety, 25*(12), 986-992. https://pubmed. ncbi.nlm.nih.gov/26369893/

Palmer, D. (2018). *What is GDPR? Everything you need to know about the new general data protection regulations.* https://www.zdnet.com/article/gdpr-an-executive-guide-to-what-you-need-to-know/

Pender, N., Murdaugh, C., & Parsons, M. (2015). *Health promotion in nursing practice* (7th ed.). Pearson Education, Inc.

Peters, D.A. (2014). The application of systems thinking in health: Why use systems thinking? *Health Research Policy and Systems, 12*(51), 1–6. https://health-policy-systems.biomedcentral. com/track/pdf/10.1186/1478-4505-12-51

Pestotnik, S., & Lemon, V. (2019). *How to use data to improve quality and patient safety.* https:// www.healthcatalyst.com/insights/use-data-improve-patient-safety/

Petersen, S. W. (2015). Systems thinking, healthcare organizations, global health, and the advance practice nurse leader. In M. E. Zaccagnini & K. W. White (Eds.), *The doctor of nursing practice essentials: A new model for advanced practice nursing* (3rd ed.). Jones & Bartlett Learning.

QSEN. (2020). *QSEN About.* https://qsen.org/about-qsen/

Roach, K. E., Frost, J. S., Francis, N. J., Giles, S., Nordrum, J. T., & Delitto, A. (2012). Validation of the revised physical therapist clinical performance instrument (PT CPI): Version 2006. *Physical Therapy, 92*, 416-426.

Rosen, M. A., DiazGranados, D., Dietz, A. S., Benishek, L. E., Thompson, D., Pronovost, P. J., & Weaver, S. J. (2018). Teamwork in healthcare: Key discoveries enabling safer, high-quality care. *American Psychology, 73*(4), 433-450. https://www.ncbi.nlm.nih.gov/pmc/articles/ PMC6361117/

Rosenbaum, S. (2011). The patient protection and affordable care act: Implications for public health policy and practice. *Public Health Reports, 126*(1), 130-135. https://www.ncbi.nlm.nih. gov/pmc/articles/PMC3001814/

Schub, T. B., & Strayer, D. M. (2016). *Power of nurses to advocate for policy change.* CINAHL Nursing Guide.

Speakman, E., & Arenson, C. (2015). Going back to the future: What is all the buzz about Interprofessional Education and Collaborative Practice. *Nurse Educator, 40*(1), 3–4.

Squires, A., Wade, J., Dominick, P., & Gelosh, D. (2011). *Building a competency taxonomy to guide experience acceleration of lead program systems engineers.* In *9th annual conference on systems engineering research (CSER)* (pp. 1–10). http://www.sercuarc.org/wp-content/ uploads/2014/02/12_Squires_Building-a-Competency-Model1.pdf

Steusse, E. (2014). Clinical nurse leaders and clinical nurse specialists: Harmonious partners. *American Nurse, 9*(4). https://www.myamericannurse.com/clinical-nurse-leaders-and-clinical-nurse-specialists-harmonious-partners/.

Stevens, K. R. (2013). The impact of evidence-based practice in nursing and the next big ideas. *Online Journal of Issues in Nursing, 18*(2). http://ojin.nursingworld.org/MainMenuCategories/ ANAMarketplace/ANAPeriodicals/OJIN/TableofContents/Vol-18-2013/No2-May-2013/ Impact-of-Evidence-Based-Practice.html

Sullivan, M., Kiovsky, R. D., Mason, D. J., Hill, C. D., & Dukes, C. (2015). Interprofessional collaboration and education. *American Journal of Nursing, 115*(3), 47–54.

Tinker, A., & Falk, L. H. (2016). *The top five essentials for outcomes improvement.* https://www. healthcatalyst.com/Outcomes-Improvement-Five-Essentials

Trivedi, A. (2016). *Overview of health care financing.* Merck Manual. https://www.merckmanuals.com/professional/special-subjects/financial-issues-in-health-care/overview-of-health-care-financing

Vanberg, A. D. (2018). The right to data portability and the GDPR: What lessons can be learned from the EU experience? *Journal of Internet Law, 21*(7), 11–19.

Vasuki, R. (2016). The importance and impact of nursing informatics competencies for baccalaureate nursing students and registered nurses. *IOSR Journal of Nursing and Health Sciences, 5*(1), 20–25. http://iosrjournals.org/iosr-jnhs/papers/vol5-issue1/Version-4/D05142025.pdf

Von Bertalanffy, L. (1968). *General system theory.* George Braziller.

Wheatley, M. J. (2006). *Leadership and the new science: Discovering order in a chaotic world.* Berrett-Koehler Publishers.

White, K.M., Dudley-Brown, S. & Terhaar, M.F. (2016). *Translation of evidence into nursing and healthcare.* Springer Publishing Company.

Williams, S. D., Phillips, J. M., & Koyama, K. (2018). Nursing advocacy: Adopting a health in all policies approach. *Online Journal of Issues Nursing, 23.* https://ojin.nursingworld.org/MainMenuCategories/ANAMarketplace/ANAPeriodicals/OJIN/TableofContents/Vol-23-2018/No3-Sept-2018/Policy-Advocacy.html

Williamson, K. (2016). *Evidence-based practice in nursing education: The nuts and bolts of integration (White Paper).* Wolters-Kluwer. http://nursingeducation.lww.com/free-resources/resources/white-papers/evidence-based-practice-in-nursing-education.html

World Health Organization (WHO). (2018). *Constitution of WHO: Principles.* http://www.who.int/about/mission/en/

World Health Organization (WHO). (2016). *What is health promotion?* http://www.who.int/topics/health_promotion/en/

PART TWO

Advanced Nursing Roles

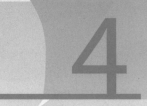

4

Educators

Carolyn Hart • Pegge L. Bell

LEARNING OBJECTIVES

After completing this chapter, you will be able to:

1. Review the history of nurse educators.

2. Define the role and rank expectations of the nurse educator.

3. Discuss differences between pedagogy and andragogy.

4. Delineate the competencies of nurse educators.

5. Explore the certification process for nurse educators.

KEY TERMS

Accreditation: A quality assurance process of evaluating education programs to ensure that specific standards are met.

Andragogy: The methods used to teach adult learners in which the learner is actively involved in knowledge acquisition and the focus is on gaining experience and problem-solving skills.

Boyer's Model of Scholarship: An academic model that provides an expanded definition of scholarship and is used to set expectations for faculty roles.

Clinical track: An academic appointment for faculty whose scholarship is in clinical or advanced practice.

Didactic: The theory or classroom portion of a course (as opposed to clinical or laboratory experiences).

Pedagogy: The methods used to teach learners in which learners rely on educators for acquisition of knowledge.

Rank: The hierarchical structure for academic appointment.

Sabbatical: A period of paid leave for a faculty member to pursue scholarship interests.

Scholarship: The American Association of Colleges of Nursing (AACN) defines scholarship as those activities used to advance the teaching, research, and practice of nursing; this can involve elements of Boyer's Model of Scholarship: discovery, integration, application, and teaching.

Tenure: A permanent academic appointment involving a process of review, usually lasting 6 to 7 years. *Tenure track* is the structure used to indicate an educator is pursuing tenure. Once granted, tenure provides for academic freedom to pursue any academic research without fear of job termination.

Introduction

At all levels of practice, nurses have a role as educators. Nurses, as part of their professional standards, are expected to maintain a primary role in the education of patients and families (Bastable, 2017). This includes teaching across the lifespan, meeting the age and developmental educational needs of diverse populations (Marshall et al., 2015). As nurses increase their expertise, their educational role may expand as they assume responsibilities as preceptors. For nurses who find satisfaction in their role as an educator, multiple career opportunities exist. For example, nurses may assume roles in staff development or as community educators. Although nurses can pursue educator roles in a variety of settings, this chapter will focus on academic nurse educators.

History

Although today's nursing programs are typically located in academic settings and adhere to national accreditation standards, this has not always been the case. Keating (2015) eloquently described nursing education as an "adventure" and the need for systematic nursing education became apparent at the close of the U.S. Civil War. As early as 1893, nurse leaders, including Florence Nightingale, advocated for an educated nursing workforce using standards of practice rather than the hospital apprenticeships that were common in that time where students were viewed as a source of free labor for hospitals (Egenes, 2008). Undeniably, records from the early 1900s indicate that classes were often canceled when students were needed to meet staffing needs. Nursing curriculum focused on character traits and habits, often ignoring Nightingale's principles of education (Keating, 2015).

In the late 1800s, program length was about 1 year and increased to 3 years as time progressed. Nursing education was primarily hospital-based and referred to as "*training*," with predominantly White females earning a diploma rather than a college degree. As scientific and clinical knowledge expanded and care moved from homes to hospitals, administrators and nurse educators realized the need for a more rigorous nursing program (Bacon, 1987). At the same time, practice regulations and standards for nursing education were being developed (Judd & Sitzman, 2014). World War I brought to the forefront the need to have nurses prepared to meet national emergencies. Key changes to nursing education during this era included the founding of the Army School of Nursing and the Vassar Training Camp. In particular, the Vassar initiative helped move nursing education to the academic setting (Bacon, 1987).

Technical institutes began offering course work to nursing students, while education at the university level was only considered for leaders of nursing training schools. As care for patients became increasingly complex due to advances in science and technology, the education of nurses expanded to include 4-year baccalaureate programs at universities. The 1960s and early 1970s saw the emergence of master's programs and the development of increased assessment skills, nurse practitioner programs, and the inclusion of practicum experiences within baccalaureate education (Keating, 2015).

Currently, nurses can enter practice from multiple pathways and degree options: diploma, associate, baccalaureate, or entry-level master's. Although all graduates must pass the NCLEX-RN, hiring practices will differ by institution and area. In locations with multiple nursing programs, supply allows for the demand of higher educational levels. Several changes are underway within nursing education. NCLEX-RN is increasing its use of technology to better determine competency. Additionally, the amount of information that must be mastered by nursing students at all levels requires new ways of teaching as the methods used in previous decades no longer support current demands and content volume (Benner et al., 2010; Christensen & Simmons, 2020). Billings and Halstead (2019) concur, stating this is a "significant time in the history of nursing education—one that requires nurse educators to embrace change and seek opportunities to re-envision the learning environments they co-create with their students" (p. ix). They further postulate that the challenges faced by nursing faculty include (1) closing the education-practice gap, (2) identifying educator competencies for clinical educators and faculty, and (3) translating the science of nursing education into practice. Today's nursing educator faces a very diverse classroom with students who have wide variation in age and life experiences; educators must understand their different learning needs and use teaching strategies that incorporate a respect for students' existing knowledge and build upon their experience (Bradshaw et al., 2019). This is most certainly true and makes the role of nursing educators challenging but imminently rewarding.

Nurse Educator Preparation

Nurse educators work in diverse settings including academe, staff education, communities, insurance companies, schools, and entrepreneurial roles. Educational preparation and degree qualifications are varied and may relate to their practice area rather than knowledge specific to teaching and learning theory. Because of this variety and broad scope of opportunities for nurse educators, content in this chapter will focus on the educational preparation needed to teach in academic settings.

As nursing education has grown and developed higher-level degree programs, nurse educators increasingly are required to obtain higher levels of education.

In Baccalaureate (BSN) programs, educators with doctoral degrees are strongly preferred, and in many cases, this is an expectation. In licensed practical nurse (LPN) programs, movement toward requiring faculty prepared at the master's level has been in progress. In academic settings, faculty with a master's degree are generally hired at the Instructor rank and primarily teach at the undergraduate level; in some cases, they may also be assigned to support Advanced Practice Nurse (APN) courses at the graduate level if they have strong teaching or clinical experience. The faculty shortage has led to many universities posting undergraduate positions with the notation that the terminal degree is preferred, rather than required. For that reason, master's prepared nurse educators are used extensively in undergraduate programs, particularly in clinical rather than classroom instruction. A terminal degree (DNP or PhD) is required for faculty who teach at the graduate levels. Exceptions exist for MSN-prepared faculty with specialized knowledge and skills particularly in advanced practice registered nurse (APRN) programs. Box 4.1 presents expected faculty preparation for different levels of nursing education as identified by the National Council of State Boards of Nursing (NCSBN, 2008).

Rank

Academic **rank** includes instructor, assistant professor, associate professor, and professor and is typically found in programs associated with a 4-year institution. Faculty are assigned rank at the time of hire based on experience in teaching, service, and research or **scholarship**. Progression to a higher rank occurs as a result of a periodic internal review process. This process requires completion of a portfolio as well as peer observation to support and document attainment of the expectations of the next rank. Each institution has guidelines and expectations for rank progression that involve three areas: teaching, service, and scholarship. While some institutions define scholarship as participating or leading research, others use broader interpretations that can include publication or presentation at conferences. Scholarship is discussed in greater detail in Chapter 17. In selecting an institution in which to work, consideration should be given to research expectations. Those who enjoy research may wish to work in an environment where this is an expectation and support is provided to novice researchers. Others may choose to work at institutions where research is not required to meet scholarship expectations.

BOX 4.1

▶ FACULTY PREPARATION EXPECTATIONS

- Full- and part-time faculty for practical and registered nurse programs will have either a master's or doctoral degree in nursing, with graduate preparation in teaching and learning, including curriculum development and implementation.

- In practical nurse programs, BSN-prepared nurses may participate as nursing faculty.

- Clinical preceptors should be educated at or above the level for which the student is preparing.

- When evaluating faculty preparation, boards of nursing should consider the three roles of faculty: collaborator, director of learning, and role model.

- All part-time, adjunct, preceptors, and novice faculty members should be oriented to the nursing program's curriculum and engaged in formal mentorships and faculty development.

- Boards of nursing should collaborate with educators to foster innovation in nursing education.

National Council of State Boards of Nursing. (2008). *Nursing faculty qualifications and roles*. https://www.ncsbn.org/Final_08_Faculty_Qual_Report.pdf.

In institutions with a research focus, instructors may participate in research projects or contribute to an article for publication. Assistant professors are generally building their scholarship and may develop a research trajectory or area of scholarship, depending on the specific focus of their institution. Faculty employed by non–research-focused institutions will build scholarship in other ways that expand their teaching expertise. Faculty can build on their dissertation from their doctoral program or create a new niche for themselves that matches their teaching assignments, clinical areas of interest, or available populations/diseases or opportunities for collaboration. They may seek funding for their endeavors from a number of external sources, and some universities provide "seed money" or a small grant in support of their research activities. The funding levels vary per institute but can provide substantial support for research until experience and reputation have been established. The results of the research activities are published in professional journals and shared at local, state, national, and international conferences depending on their significance and fit with conference objectives. Many universities require that dissemination of research occur in refereed venues, meaning an external individual or panel has reviewed the abstract or draft and accepted it for presentation or publication.

Associate professors and professors have an established research trajectory and therefore may have more opportunities for submitting grants that will provide external funding sources in support of their research. They generally lead teams in research projects and present their findings at national and international conferences and in peer-reviewed journals.

Tenure Track

Nurses contemplating careers as educators frequently have questions about the tenure process. Not all institutions offer tenure, defined as a permanent contract to protect academic freedom. Tenure is a process initiated by the Association of University Professors (AAUP) in the early 1900s (Hunt, 2013) to assure faculty freedom of inquiry, research, and ability to teach different viewpoints in the classroom without reprisal (Figure 4.1). Most institutions expect newly hired faculty to establish themselves as skilled educators within a specific time frame. This may include creating a record of published articles and research, obtaining grant funding, and gaining recognition through service to the community. Faculty who are unable to obtain tenure within the specified period may be expected to leave that institution. Some institutions require promotion to Associate Professor as a condition of tenure. Other institutions may have nontenure track positions although these roles may carry a higher teaching load because of the decreased expectations related to scholarship.

Although the idea of tenure was to promote meaningful classroom discussions that contribute to knowledge development, the basic premise of tenure

Tenure advantages
- Job security is needed to recruit high performing people that might otherwise be paid more in private industry
- Protection from being fired for personal and political reasons
- Freedom to examine controversial topics without censure

Tenure disadvantages
- Faculty with tenure may lack motivation for professional growth
- May be difficult to remove professors with ineffective teaching skills

Figure 4.1. Tenure advantages and disadvantages.

is to promote the common good rather than to further the interests of an individual teacher (AAUP, 2010). Faculty who hold tenure may only be dismissed under extreme circumstances such as closure of a program or financial exigency. While not all institutions offer tenure, it is typically awarded to faculty after at least 6 years of continued engagement, growth, and accomplishment in the three missions: teaching, service, and research or scholarship. Each institution defines the importance of these three missions. While teaching is usually weighted most heavily, the importance of research will vary by institution. Tenure may be followed by periodic reviews to assure faculty are continuing in their professional development. In most cases, faculty who are appointed to a clinical position are not eligible for tenure; however, this practice is changing.

Clinical Track

With the proliferation of APN programs, many universities have established a clinical track for faculty, recognizing that many faculty hold certification in an advanced practice role and need time during the week to practice. The rank system is similar to the traditional ranks discussed above, but with the addition of a clinical designation—clinical instructor, clinical assistant professor, clinical associate professor, and clinical professor. As faculty progress along these levels of rank, so does their involvement with teaching, service, and research. A clinical instructor may assist a senior faculty member with a research project, while a clinical professor could be implementing a new procedure to improve patient care outcomes in a specific population. As universities become more inclusive of faculty who have an active clinical practice, the term *"faculty practice"* has become integral to the nursing educator's role. Faculty in this category generally receive release time from their typical role to engage in direct patient care services. This release time enables APNs, who are also nurse educators, to comply with the recertification requirement that at least 8 hours per week are spent in direct patient care.

Innovative opportunities exist for bedside nurses with advanced degrees to combine clinical practice with education. Joint appointments may be made whereby a specific amount of time is devoted to clinical or bedside practice with the remainder of their workload allotted to teaching for an external educational program. This relationship requires formal agreement between the clinical and educational institutions and may not be available in all areas of the country.

Role Expectations

Nurse educators work at a variety of educational and healthcare settings and in multiple levels of practice. Practice setting and responsibilities will be based upon the educator's academic preparation, type of institution, and rank. The role of nurse educators is to support the mission of the institution. Academic missions are typically focused on three areas: teaching, service, and research or scholarship. The program level and educational setting determines the degree of involvement in the three missions. Nurse educators who teach in non-RN levels of nursing (certified nursing assistant and LPN) have a workload that consists of teaching in the classroom, laboratory, or clinical area with little to no involvement in the other two missions of service and research/scholarship. While nurse educators in associate degree programs have workloads emphasizing the teaching role and service to the institution, they may also have clinical expectations. Faculty with appointments at the baccalaureate (BSN) or higher level programs (MSN, DNP, PhD) engage in the mission areas of teaching and service and have an expectation of scholarship or research.

Questions to Ask Yourself

1. Which level of student would I want to teach? Why?
2. What type of program would I prefer—an online program or a face-to-face? Why?
3. Would a tenure or clinical track be more beneficial to my career goals?
4. How do I feel about being responsible to prepare for a class, develop a syllabus, facilitate learning, and evaluate students? Am I excited? Hesitant?
5. What else do I need to know about this role to assure me that I am a good fit for the role?
6. Do I have a mentor in mind for this role?

Teaching Mission

In support of the teaching mission, accreditation standards require that faculty lead the development, implementation, and evaluation of curricula. Curricular development can be as simple as creation of a new course or as complex and involved as developing an entire degree program. Implementation occurs when nurse educators teach a **didactic** course in face-to-face or online modalities or provide clinical instruction in a variety of settings to achieve the objectives of a clinical course. Faculty are also integral to the evaluation processes of the curriculum—the overall program, individual courses, and student achievement of program or course objectives (Oermann & Gaberson, 2019). Regardless of program, nurse educators must assure that graduates of their program (BSN, MSN, DNP, PhD) can competently practice as outlined by AACN's Essentials (see Chapter 3).

Faculty are charged with preparing course syllabi including course objectives, student learning outcomes, methods of evaluation, and a list of required and recommended textbooks. Most faculty provide a topical outline with separate student learning objectives and references along with a weekly schedule of content and assignments. Nursing programs frequently have a syllabus template to assure that all required areas are included and that across programs and professors, consistent language and formatting is maintained. Additional faculty resources may be available to assist in developing course objectives or student learning outcomes. These resources may include instructional designers and technical support. More information about the role of an instructional designer may be found in Box 4.2.

> BOX 4.2

▶ INSTRUCTIONAL DESIGNERS

Education is not static and information, particularly in healthcare, is constantly evolving. As new information emerges, educational materials must be revised to remain current. Often this is accompanied by the need to deliver content in a more effective manner. Instructional designers (IDs) collaborate with faculty in updating or developing new courses. Their education prepares them to be experts in the theory and practice of design, development, utilization, management, and evaluation of processes and resources for learning. Working with an ID allows faculty to focus on content; the ID, as an expert in technology and education, offers input into how to best use assignments and technology to make sure students are ready for their next challenge.

Faculty workloads at the undergraduate level (Associate degree or BSN) typically include a workload of teaching at least four classes per term or semester. Graduate faculty workloads may be slightly less to reflect their increased involvement with research or scholarship as well as the higher student expectations needed to meet MSN and DNP Essentials. The institution will define how service and scholarship or research expectations affect workload. Universities also may offer a sabbatical to tenured faculty after a number of years of service to concentrate on research for one semester or term.

Student evaluation is a critical part of the teaching mission. Because undergraduate students are preparing for their licensure examination (NCLEX), most of the coursework provides opportunities for multiple choice, NCLEX-format testing. Thus, test-writing can be an important component of undergraduate or graduate clinical education. Licensure and certification examinations rely heavily on application level test items. Different resources exist for educators to develop test-writing skills.

In addition to test-writing skills, nurse educators can expect to be involved in developing expertise in teaching and learning strategies, curriculum development, professional socialization of students, and assessment of outcomes. This expertise is required whether their assigned courses are offered in a face-to-face format or online. Educational preparation will include coursework devoted to these topics. Many programs also require internships or practicums to help develop practical skills. Table 4.1 presents an example of faculty practices within these areas.

With the advent of online nursing programs, nurse educators need to be creative in fostering adult learning principles within the virtual classroom. Special consideration must be given to the ability to share experiences and to learn from others. Challenges exist in building a community of student learners who are engaged. Distance learning techniques for adult learners can be used to ensure students are

Table 4.1. Examples of Faculty Practice

Expected Practice	Examples of Activities
Teaching and learning strategies	• Setting classroom expectations • Maintaining clinical expertise • Using innovative teaching strategies to engage learners
Curriculum development and design	• Updating content to meet national standards • Promoting evidence-based practice • Ensuring that course content meets program goals • Selecting textbooks that meet specific course needs
Professional socialization of students	• Setting clear, professional expectations • Modeling professional behavior • Serving as faculty liaison in student organizations and clubs
Assessment of outcomes and commitment to quality improvement	• Creating tests and assignments that provide a measure of expected outcomes • Using student and peer evaluations to improve course content • Applying objective standards to assess student performance • Participating in the accreditation process and peer evaluations
Improve educational practices	• Using evolving technologies and practices to improve student outcomes • Contributing to evidence-based teaching practices • Disseminating ideas and successful teaching practices

connected and learning appropriate content to achieve their educational and career goals. A number of resources are available to help faculty create a learning environment conducive to adult learners whether in a face-to-face or online environment. For example, the National League for Nursing (NLN) hosts educational conferences with sessions to inspire teaching strategies that engage students at all levels.

In Their Own Words

Barbara J. Patterson, PhD, ANEF, FAAN
Distinguished Professor
Director PhD Program
Associate Dean for Scholarship & Inquiry
School of Nursing
NLN Center of Excellence
Widener University

The key points in understanding my role are… As Director of a PhD program in nursing, I see my role as one who mentors, supports, and facilitates the knowledge and leadership development of the next generation of nurse scholars and leaders. Academic nursing education does not exist as a silo in higher education; nurse academicians are faced with a major challenge in understanding the rapidly changing healthcare context, higher education dynamics, as well as political and global influences. Being a nurse educator requires self-discipline and hard work. Nevertheless, while this may sound cliché, it is extremely rewarding both personally and professionally.

What keeps me coming back every day is… The honor of working with colleagues who are dedicated professionals and have a similar desire to produce the highest quality of practicing nurses and nursing faculty. The stimulation of ideas and excitement of scholarly inquiry, which are crucial components to being a role model for one's students. The moment a student expresses that he/she gets it, links those difficult ideas, that is what is energizing to me.

My greatest challenge is… Learning to say "no" to some of the opportunities that have presented themselves. I am naturally inquisitive and finds numerous opportunities interesting and worth exploring or joining. There are a multitude of possibilities we have as nurses and educators and staying focused and totally engaged in an area of expertise contributes to being recognized

(Continued)

for their personal accomplishments in the nursing profession. Keeping one's focus can be a great challenge. Reaching out for assistance when needed and not being concerned with whether something is the best end product. Nursing and nursing education are processes; they take work and collaboration with others to achieve the best for nursing.

I wish someone had told me... The range of possibilities that were open to me as a novice nurse; while I had a sense of them, I did not appreciate the depth and breadth of opportunities that were open to all nurses. With a wide range of opportunities, comes the risk of saying "YES, let me try that, I can do it" and not always being successful. I wish I had stepped up more in some instances. I wish I had been told to keep a reflective journal of my growth as a scholar so I could revisit it as my professional roles and life circumstances evolve and change.

I need to be a lifelong learner because... It is part of my inherent nature; it is part of me. I love to learn new things; acquiring an understanding of something challenging to me is a highlight of the day. Nursing can no longer accept doing things the way we once did them; whether it is teaching or patient care. The dynamic nature of healthcare and higher education forces us to be current about what is happening in the nation and world. To be a contributing, active player with those making decisions for and about nursing, one has to know the evidence. This requires always reading and searching the literature within nursing and outside of nursing for ideas and data to be able to articulate an argument and advocate for nursing.

Another point to understand is... That one must maintain his/her moral compass. Nurses and nurse educators have a duty to maintain the highest ethical standards in our practices. Students look to us as positive role models and our behaviors can have a long-term impact. To always remain open to a diversity of ideas, it is narrow perspectives that will hinder the growth of the profession. Respectfully engaging in scholarly work is what strengthens us as individuals and professionally.

Service Mission

Departmental and campus-wide committees are organized to ensure the efficient operation of the academic institution, with faculty involvement in determining academic policies. Within nursing programs, faculty will be involved in committees specific to the nursing program. This may involve setting nursing student policies or oversight of nursing curriculum. Service to the institution reflects the larger mission of the university and includes committees focused on promotion and tenure, research (IRB), development (securing funders), student government, faculty affairs, and administration (Deans and Directors). Typically, service will involve some combination of participation at the department and institutional levels. Graduate faculty may additionally be required to serve on thesis or doctoral dissertation or project committees.

Professional growth may be an institutional expectation as a faculty member achieves a higher rank. External service is also a means of establishing a professional reputation beyond the institutional community. Committee service within professional organizations, board membership, or community service are ways of meeting this requirement.

Research or Scholarship Mission

Research and scholarship expectations vary according to a faculty member's rank and institutional policies. Some institutions require that faculty on tenure track participate in and conduct independent research. Other institutions allow the individual to define their own means of meeting scholarship expectations. When investigating potential employment opportunities, this area should be evaluated to ensure that it meets personal expectations and preferences.

All faculty should be fostering development of and ability to maintain an evidence-based practice (EBP) among their students. This is not only one of the AACN's Essentials, but a fundamental role of nurses in the profession: practicing according to the current body of evidence. Faculty at all ranks can make significant contributions to the body of nursing knowledge. Nursing faculty who teach undergraduate clinical courses have opportunities to observe how hospital units are monitoring patient care outcomes, noting when patients are not recovering according to expectations. Nursing faculty can collaborate with hospital-based nurses to address these discrepancies. This process may involve a review of the literature to identify potential interventions, proposal of a change in practice, and evaluation of outcomes. Ultimately, policies can be developed that are more in line with published findings.

Questions to Ask Yourself

1. Which type of teaching assignment is more appealing—classroom/didactic or clinical/laboratory? Why?
2. Is nursing research an area that I would like to explore?
3. In what areas would I like to grow professionally?
4. What nursing organizations would support my professional growth and area of expertise?
5. What service opportunities exist within these organizations?

Dissemination is key to developing as a scholar, regardless of rank. Presentations at local, state, national, and international venues provide validation for research activities and contribute to the science of nursing. Publication is another way that faculty can disseminate findings. Many faculty may first begin presenting at local or regional conferences. One can then develop the skills and confidence to present nationally or internationally. Poster presentations can also be a less intimidating means to disseminate work.

In Their Own Words

Melissa Abreu, MSN-Ed, RN

The key points in understanding my role are… I am a full-time faculty member teaching in an undergraduate Baccalaureate Nursing program in south Florida. My role is to teach didactic courses (Pathophysiology, Medical-Surgical Nursing I, Health Assessment, Maternal and Child Health, Theoretical Foundations, and Business of Healthcare). In addition, I am an advisor for approximately 50 to 60 students with whom I meet each semester in preparation for registration. I review their study habits, goals, and challenges and mentor them throughout the program to ensure they are as successful as possible.

What keeps me coming back every day is… The students! To me it is amazing how I can teach them Pathophysiology or Health Assessment in their first semesters and then have them later in the program for Maternal Child or Business of Healthcare and their thinking, attitude, view on the profession, and

(Continued)

patient care are more developed. I enjoy the challenge of helping the students over the hurdles that try to bring them down. Sometimes it is just being there to listen to them—validate their feelings and encourage them to keep going. But watching them walk across stage and hearing they passed the NCLEX makes every minute worth it!

My greatest challenge is… Fighting for a student's success more than the student fights for themselves. Each student comes to the BSN program for different reasons, but watching a student with the ability to perform who does not take the initiative to perform is the greatest challenge. I can only offer all of the resources, take my time to answer questions, and be available for tutoring, but if they do not bring their best self or choose to not apply themselves, I have to know that at the end I did all that I could to help the student.

I wish someone had told me… Teaching is not as easy as it seems! I knew accepting a faculty role would have different responsibilities compared to a bedside nurse, but having to explain it at the most basic level so the students understand the fundamentals is harder than it seems. It is easy to blurt out lab values and "nurse talk" but when you see 40+ students staring back with that blank stare…I know I went into bedside nurse mode and have to back up to explain it on the students' level. The other thing I wish someone told me was that students will ask the most obscure questions…I'm not a walking medical dictionary! I have had to learn to say "that's a great question, lets look this up with the class so everyone understands." It's hard being put on the spot and not having the answer, I have become very comfortable with saying now "I don't have an answer for that but I will find one for you."

I need to be a lifelong learner because… I need to stay current with best practice at the bedside, healthcare concerns, and funding and stay abreast of new technologies being implemented. I am currently enrolled in a PhD program at Barry University, and I am excited for the opportunity to expand my knowledge so I can share it with my students. When I teach them to evoke change at the bedside and continue to read and research and implement best practices, I want to be sure I am walking the walk as well.

Another point to understand is… While teaching BSN students can be exhausting, challenging, and frustrating, it is more importantly the most amazing experience to see the concepts click…when the students have those "A-HA" moments and share their excitement with you. But more importantly, the hundreds of nursing students I teach will care for thousands of patients. The impact is greater than the four walls of a campus, so installing a strong educational foundation and making the student aware of the impact they will have is why I love teaching.

Role Specifics

Pedagogy is a young learner approach to teaching. At this level, students are not self-directed and depend on their teacher throughout the learning process (Pappas, 2015). Young learners have few personal experiences to contribute to the learning process and rely upon the instructor to focus on content. They are not inquisitive about why they are taking a certain subject and are not able to independently identify what they need to know. Young learners are not so much motivated by intrinsic rewards, but more so by extrinsic factors such as good grades or avoiding failure.

In contrast, andragogy is an adult-focused approach to learning (Pappas, 2015). These students are typically self-directed and, in many cases, have rich experiences that contribute to the learning process. Adult learners are very interested in the knowledge that is perceived to apply to their educational goals. These students have a readiness to learn and typically possess a desire for self-improvement; they may require a rationale for the need for certain courses or in engaging in certain course activities. Adult learners typically view the intrinsic rewards of education as being equally important to extrinsic rewards.

Understanding these concepts can help one develop an approach to teaching that is student-centric (Figure 4.2). As nurses, we develop content expertise with our practice. Understanding how to teach requires a very different set of skills that are very necessary in higher education (Bastable, 2017; Bradshaw et al., 2019). NLN competencies can provide a framework for expectations of a nursing educator. Additionally, while master's degree programs with a specialty in nursing education are available, postgraduate certificates and online courses to develop teaching expertise also exist. Resources include the Nursing Education Speaker Series hosted by Lippincott and the National League for Nursing, NLN OnDemand Courses, Nurse Tim, and others.

Financing Your Education

Because of the national shortage of nurse educators, financial aid options are available. The federal government, through the Health Resources and Services Administration (HRSA) offers a funding opportunity called the

Andragogy
- Based on Knowles' theory of adult learning.
- Emphasizes role of adults as self-directed learners who can be expected to take responsibility for decisions.
- Andragogy makes the following assumptions: (1) Adults need to know why they need to learn something, (2) Adults learn by doing, (3) Adults are more focused on problem-solving skills, and (4) Adults learn best when they value the need to learn specific content.

Pedagogy
- The study of how knowledge and skills are imparted or the method and practice of teaching
- Considers the interactions that must occur for a student to learn
- Involves teaching styles, teaching theory, and assessment
- Four categories of approaches to pedagogy: behaviorism, constructivism, social constructivism, and liberationist

Figure 4.2. Andragogy and pedagogy.

Nurse Faculty Loan Program (NFLP). NFLP is a loan forgiveness program designed to increase the number of qualified nursing faculty teaching in accredited schools of nursing. If accepted into NFLP, qualifying federal student loans can be forgiven in exchange for a set number of years of employment as a full-time faculty member. Some institutions have NFLP funds which they can grant to students in their program while other nurses may apply as an individual when the grant cycle is open, typically in early spring. For those applying on an individual basis, preference is given to those who teach at an institution with a high proportion of underserved students or have a student loan balance that meets or exceeds their yearly income. NFLP information is now accessed through the Nurse Corps Loan Repayment program. Additional sources to secure funding for advanced education include scholarships and grants from professional organizations. Examples include the following:

- Through the American Nurses Association, the Minority Fellowship Program offers doctoral fellowships for minority nurses interested in a career that focuses on behavioral health or substance abuse. More information can be found on their website: https://emfp.org/fellowships.

- Through the National League for Nursing, the **Mary Anne Rizzolo Doctoral Research Award** supports PhD doctoral dissertations related to the use of simulation in nursing education.
- **Sigma Theta Tau International and the National League for Nursing Research Award** is given each year to a nurse researcher or doctoral dissertation student to support the use of technology in nursing education.
- **Sigma Theta Tau International/Rosemary Berkel Crisp Grant** awards up to $5,000 per year for a research project that is ready for implementation in the area of women's health, oncology, or pediatrics.
- **Southern Nursing Research Society (SNRS) Doctoral Dissertation Grant** provides an annual award of $5,000 to a member of the SNRS to complete their dissertation.

Other opportunities include the following:

- The **National Institute of Health's (NIH) Loan Repayment Program** which repays up to $50,000 each year of a researcher's qualified educational debt in return for a commitment to engage in NIH mission-relevant research.
- Check with your institution's Office of Financial Aid for flexible payment options or eligibility to teaching assistant positions.

Populations

Applicants to nursing programs are typically considered adult learners. Wide variation exists among undergraduate nursing students, drawing from high school students, single parents, and those on a second or third career. Students enrolled in accelerated programs (RN-MSN, RN-DNP) may not have an undergraduate degree when they begin taking graduate courses. Nurse faculty are needed at all levels of education, including

- Course and clinical education for LPNs, associate and bachelor's degree nursing programs (ASN, BSN), and graduate education.
- Graduate education including master's and doctoral level education in clinical specialties, administration, education, and research.

Other opportunities for nurse educators that may or may not require a higher level of education include staff development, community education, public health services, and patient or family educators.

While diversity is growing among the applicants to nursing programs, minority populations remain underrepresented and Caucasian females remain the majority. The recent NLN Biennial Survey of Schools of Nursing (2018) found that the percentage of minorities in prelicensure nursing programs was 11.8% Black/non-Hispanic, 9.8% Hispanic, 4.5% Asian or Pacific Islander, 2.6% unknown, and 0.6% Indian. This underrepresentation within undergraduate students results in even less representation of minorities at the graduate levels of nursing. The need to grow a more diverse nursing workforce is necessary to achieve quality healthcare (AACN, 2019). The number of men in nursing is increasing, but still only represents 9.1% of nurses (National Council of State Boards of Nursing's National Nursing Workforce Survey, 2017).

Settings

Just as the populations served by nurse faculty are varied, so too are the settings in which nurse educators are found. In the academic setting, undergraduate programs that prepare students for licensure as a registered nurse are typically conducted in face-to-face settings. However, programs that address postlicensure and graduate education are increasingly offered in the online environment. Advances in technology continue to blur the lines between face-to-face and online environments and may be referred to as hybrid or blended courses. Typically, hybrid courses are those with less than 50% of content offered online. For those roles outside of academics, technology enables the ability to provide education when and where it is needed.

Questions to Ask Yourself

1. How will I finance my education?
2. What kind of a relationship do I want with my peers and students?
3. If I am teaching online, what are the institutional expectations for my presence on campus?
4. What resources are available to help me develop expertise in teaching?
5. What is the promotion and tenure process for my institution of choice?
6. What are the potential logistics of relocating for employment?

Professionalism

The American Nurses Association (2014) writes that "The public has a right to expect registered nurses to demonstrate professional competence." Nurse educators are responsible for providing the means for nursing students to learn those competencies and skills necessary for safe nursing practice (ANA, 2017). As professionals, nurse educators may obtain certification as a nurse educator as an indicator of their expertise. The NLN provides resources for nurses to build their expertise as nurse educators. NLN and Sigma hold conferences with presentations dedicated to nursing education. Other annual conferences of interest to nurse educators include

- Sigma and NLN: Nursing Education Research Conference
- ATI: National Nurse Educator Summit
- AACN Academic Nursing Leadership Conference

Competencies

The NLN defines the competencies of nurse educators as facilitating learning; facilitating learner development and socialization; using assessment and evaluation strategies; participating in curriculum design and evaluation of program outcomes; pursuing continuous quality improvement in the academic nurse educator role; functioning as a change agent and leader; engaging in scholarship of teaching; and functioning effectively within the institutional environment and the academic community. The NLN (Halstead, 2018) promotes competencies for nurse educators designed to foster excellence in this specialty role. Through these competencies, presented in Table 4.2, the NLN seeks to demonstrate the complexity of the faculty role.

The World Health Organization (WHO), recognizing that the education of nurses is a constantly evolving process and one with far-reaching implications for world health, compiled core competencies for nurse educators. With these competencies, it is hoped that improvement of nurse educators will ultimately result in a more effective nursing workforce that is better able to meet world health needs. WHO views these competencies as a means of enhancing the quality of health services; development of these skills within educators is "an essential prerequisite to attaining high standards in nursing practice." Noting

Table 4.2. Nurse Educator Core Competencies

Competency	Task Statement
I: Facilitate learning	Nurse educators are responsible for creating an environment in classroom, laboratory, and clinical settings that facilitates student learning and the achievement of desired cognitive, affective, and psychomotor outcomes.
II: Facilitate learner development and socialization	Nurse educators recognize their responsibility for helping students develop as nurses and integrate the values and behaviors expected of those who fulfill that role.
III: Use assessment and evaluation strategies	Nurse educators use a variety of strategies to assess and evaluate student learning in classroom, laboratory, and clinical settings, as well as in all domains of learning.
IV: Participate in curriculum design and evaluation of program outcomes	Nurse educators are responsible for formulating program outcomes and designing curricula that reflect contemporary healthcare trends and prepare graduates to function effectively in the healthcare environment.
V: Function as a change agent and leader	Nurse educators function as change agents and leaders to create a preferred future for nursing education and nursing practice.
VI: Pursue continuous quality improvement in the nurse educator role	Nurse educators recognize that their role is multidimensional and that an ongoing commitment to develop and maintain competence in the role is essential.
VII: Engage in scholarship	Nurse educators acknowledge that scholarship is an integral component of the faculty role and that teaching itself is a scholarly activity.
VIII: Function within the educational environment	Nurse educators are knowledgeable about the educational environment within which they practice and recognize how political, institutional, social, and economic forces impact their role.

Adapted from National League for Nursing. *Nurse educator core competency.* http://www.nln.org/professional-development-programs/competencies-for-nursing-education/nurse-educator-core-competency.

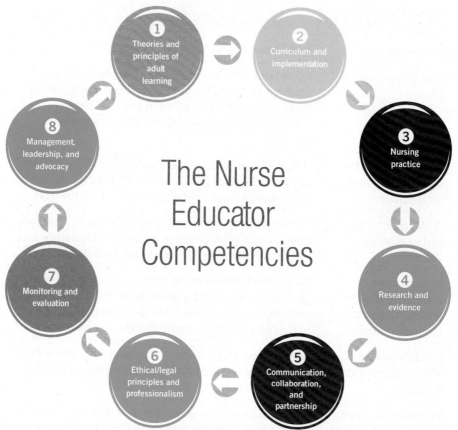

Figure 4.3. World Health Organization's (WHO's) nurse educator competencies. (Based on BMJ Quality & Safety, 25, 986–992. https://qualitysafety.bmj.com/content/qhc/25/12/986.full.pdf)

the domains of the WHO competencies as presented in Figure 4.3, the need for nurse educators to understand diverse topics such as leadership (see Part V), research (see Chapters 12 and 13), and teamwork (see Chapter 16) is evident.

The eight domains of learning and teaching each carry subcompetencies and are further explained through cognitive, affective, and psychomotor domains. These eight domains largely reflect the Essentials developed by AACN (see Chapter 3) but also emphasize the teaching role (Table 4.3). Nursing faculty should possess and model these competencies and are responsible for teaching them to their students.

Table 4.3. Comparison of Professional Competencies

Essentials	WHO	NLN
• Organizational and systems leadership	• Management, leadership, and advocacy	• Function as a change agent and leader
• Quality improvement and safety	• Monitoring and evaluation	• Using assessment and evaluation strategies
• Health policy and advocacy	• Ethical and legal principles and professionalism	• Facilitating learner development and socialization
• Interprofessional collaboration; informatics and healthcare technologies	• Communication, collaboration, and partnership	• Functioning effectively within the institutional environment and the academic community
• Translating and integrating scholarship into practice	• Research and evidence	• Engaging in scholarship of teaching
• Clinical prevention and population health	• Nursing practice	• Pursuing continuous quality improvement in the academic nurse educator role
	• Curriculum and implementation	• Participating in curriculum design and evaluation of program outcomes
	• Theories and principles of adult learning	• Facilitating learning

NLN, National League for Nursing; WHO, World Health Organization.

Certification

As a recognition of the need for highly trained nurse educators, the NLN developed the examination for a Certified Nurse Educator (CNE). With creation of the CNE in 2009, NLN sought to achieve four goals:

- Distinguish academic nursing education as a specialty area of practice and an advanced practice role within professional nursing

- Recognize the academic nurse educator's specialized knowledge, skills, and abilities
- Strengthen the use of core competencies of nurse educator practice
- Contribute to nurse educators' professional development

The CNE is a computer-based examination consisting of approximately 150 multiple-choice questions (NLN, n.d.). Creation of the CNE was a strategic move by the NLN to bring attention to nursing education as a practice discipline. Because nurse educators have a defined practice setting and specific competencies as measure of excellence, development of certification was a logical step. The CNE credential is valid for a period of 5 years at which time renewal through continuing education or reexamination is possible. Attainment of CNE certification is considered a mark of professionalism and is intended to demonstrate expertise in nursing education (Caputi, 2015).

Two options exist for determining eligibility for CNE certification. Both options begin with an active, unencumbered licensure as a registered nurse. In option A, the nurse must have a master's or doctoral degree with a major emphasis in nursing education. If the major emphasis area is not nursing education, then a post-master's certificate in nursing education or completion of nine or more graduate level education courses are acceptable. Option B provides for employment in a nursing program as a substitute for completion of education courses when the major area of emphasis in the master's or doctoral degree in nursing is not in nursing education.

Multiple resources exist to help educators prepare for the CNE. NLN publishes a detailed test blueprint that helps to identify content areas along with the percentage of questions that will pertain to that area. NLN also provides a CNE Handbook, titled *Certified Nurse Educator 2019 Candidate Handbook*. While NLN also maintains the handbook on their website along with a reference list to help with studying for the CNE examination, preparatory webinars are also available from various sources, such as Nurse Tim. Once initial certification is obtained, the nurse educator will need to renew prior to the expiration date. To be eligible for renewal, the educator must meet the required practice requirements and fulfill professional development requirements or retake the CNE examination. The requirements include holding an active, unencumbered license as a registered nurse and two or more years of employment over the past 5 years in an academic faculty role within a university, college, or community college.

Continuing Education

Certified nurse educators have mandated continuing education (CE) hours within specified areas of content for continued certification. Individual state boards of nursing also set requirements for CE hours in order to keep an active nursing license. The number of required hours will vary by state and typically range from 24 to 30 hours every 2 years. Nurses who teach in a clinical capacity may also expect to be required to obtain CEs in that specialty.

When considering continuing education opportunities, nurses should ensure that the offering is recognized by their state board of nursing or by the American Nurses Credentialing Center (ANCC). Most national organizations, such as the NLN or Sigma, are accredited providers of CEs through the ANCC. College courses that are related to nursing practice will generally count as CE credit.

Web Resources

- Educause: https://www.educause.edu/
- IOM Future of Nursing Report: http://nationalacademies.org/hmd/reports/2010/the-future-of-nursing-leading-change-advancing-health.aspx
- Open Educational Resources (OER): https://library.educause.edu/topics/teaching-and-learning/open-educational-resources-oer
- Sigma: https://www.sigmanursing.org/

Blogs

- e-Literate: https://mfeldstein.com/
- The Innovative Educator: https://theinnovativeeducator.blogspot.com/
- Inside Higher Ed: http://insidehighered.com/

Professional Organizations

- American Association of Colleges of Nursing (AACN): http://www.aacnnursing.org/
- American Nurses Association (ANA): https://www.nursingworld.org/ana/
- National League for Nursing (NLN): http://www.nln.org/
- Professional Nurse Educators Group (PNEG): https://pneg.org/
- Quality and Safety Education for Nurses (QSEN): http://qsen.org/

Summary

This chapter provides an overview of the nurse educator role. The historical evolution of the role notes changes to the profession that have influenced expectations and educational preparation of educators. This history demonstrates the drastic change from earlier educator expectations to current roles as scholars in their field of study. Nurse educators are found in multiple settings and, in addition to the education of registered nurses in and outside of academia, can be involved in the education of CNAs and LPNs.

Faculty rank and academic track (tenure and clinical) clarify options for appointment as an educator. While the MSN degree will typically allow nurse educators to teach clinically at the BSN level, prospective nurse educators will need to have more advanced degrees (DNP or PhD) if they plan to teach APN students. Exceptions to policies on faculty appointment exist based upon geographic location and availability of doctorally prepared candidates. This information also prepares nurse educators for decisions about role responsibilities in the three missions of the educator role: teaching, service, and research or scholarship. These variables could influence the type of faculty position and graduate program prospective nurse educators pursue.

Professional competencies of nurse educators as defined by NLN and WHO are contrasted and compared with AACN's Essentials for MSN and DNP graduates. Future nurse educators are encouraged to engage in lifelong learning and to seek certification as a CNE. Resources for professional development and continuing education conferences will foster professional development as an educator.

Chapter Highlights

- Changes to the profession have influenced expectations and educational preparation of educators.
- Nurse educators are found in multiple settings and, in addition to the education of registered nurses in and outside of academia, can be involved in the education of CNAs and LPNs.

- Faculty rank and academic track (tenure and clinical) clarify options for appointment as an educator.
- Prospective nurse educators will need to have more advanced degrees (DNP or PhD) if they plan to teach APN students.
- Role responsibilities for educators include teaching, service, and research or scholarship.
- Professional competencies of nurse educators as defined by NLN and WHO are contrasted with AACN's Essentials for MSN and DNP graduates.
- Future nurse educators are encouraged to engage in lifelong learning and to seek certification as a CNE.
- Resources for professional development and continuing education conferences will foster professional development as an educator.

References

American Association of Colleges of Nursing. (n.d.). *Essentials.* http://www.aacnnursing.org/Education-Resources/AACN-Essentials

American Association of Colleges of Nursing (AACN). (2019). *Enhancing diversity in the workforce.* https://www.aacnnursing.org/News-Information/Fact-Sheets/Enhancing-Diversity

American Association of University Professors. (2010). *Academic integrity.* http://www.aaup.com

American Nurses Association. (2014). *Professional role competences: ANA position statement.* https://www.nursingworld.org/practice-policy/nursing-excellence/official-position-statements/id/professional-role-competence/

American Nurses Association. (2017). *Recognition of a nursing specialty, approval of a specialty nursing scope of practice statement, acknowledgment of specialty nursing standards of practice, and affirmation of focused practice statements.* https://www.nursingworld.org/~4989de/globalassets/practiceandpolicy/scope-of-practice/3sc-booklet-final-2017-08-17.pdf

Bacon, E. (1987). Curriculum development in nursing education, 1890-1952. *Nursing History Review, 2,* 50–66.

Bastable, S. (2017). *Nurse as educator: Principles of teaching and learning for nursing practice* (5th ed.). Jones & Bartlett Learning.

Benner, P., Suphen, M., Leonard, V., & Day, L. (2010). *Educating nurses: A call for radical transformation.* Jossey-Bass.

Billings, D. M., & Halstead, J. (2019). *Teaching in nursing* (6th ed.). Elsevier Saunders.

Bradshaw, M. J., Hultquist, B. L., & Hagler, D. (2019). *Innovative teaching strategies in nursing and related health professions* (8th ed.). Jones & Bartlett Learning.

Caputi, L. (Ed.). (2015). *NLN certified nurse educator review book: The official guide to the CNE exam.* National League for Nursing.

Christensen, L. S., & Simmons, L. E. (2020). *The scope of practice for nurse educators and academic clinical nurse educators* (3rd ed.). Lippincott, Williams, & Wilkins.

Egenes, K. J. (2008). History of nursing. In G. Roux & J. A. Halstead (Eds.), *Issues and trends in nursing: Essential knowledge for today and tomorrow* (pp. 1–26). Jones & Bartlett Learning.

Halstead, J. (2018). *NLN core competencies for nurse educators: A decade of influence.* Wolters Kluwer.

Hunt, D. D. (2013). *The new nurse educator: Mastering academe.* Springer Publishing Company.

Judd, D. J., & Sitzman, K. (2014). *A history of American nursing: Trends and eras.* Jones & Bartlett Learning.

Keating, S. (2015). *Curriculum development and evaluation in nursing* (3rd ed.). Springer Publishing Company.

National Council of State Boards of Nursing. (2008). *Nursing faculty qualifications and roles.* https://www.ncsbn.org/Final_08_Faculty_Qual_Report.pdf

National League for Nursing. (n.d.). *CNE examination: Detailed test blueprint.* http://www.nln.org/docs/default-source/professional-development-programs/detailedblueprint.pdf?sfvrsn=8

Oermann, M. H., & Gaberson, K. (2019). *Evalution and testing in nursing education* (6th ed.). Springer Publishing Company.

Pappas, C. (2015). *5 differences of pedagogy vs andragogy in eLearning.* http://elearningindustry.com/pedagogy-vs-andragogy-in-elearning-can-you-tell-the-difference

World Health Organization. (2016). *Nurse educator core competencies.* World Health Organization. http://who.int/hrh/nursing_midwifery/nurse_educator050416.pdf

5

Administrators

Margaret Norton-Rosko

LEARNING OBJECTIVES

After completing this chapter, you will be able to:

1. Understand the role of senior nurse administrators in leading healthcare entities.

2. Articulate the competencies demonstrated by effective nursing leaders.

3. Demonstrate knowledge of how nurse administrators influence nursing practice and quality patient care.

4. Identify the leadership traits of successful executive nurse leaders.

KEY TERMS

American Organization for Nursing Leadership (AONL): Formerly known as the American Organization of Nurse Executives [AONE]).

Chief Nursing Officer: Responsible for broad services that impact the patient experience and the delivery of care.

Management: Collective body conducting or supervising the business environment.

Nurse executive: Takes an active leadership role with the governing body, senior leadership team, medical staff, management, and other clinical leaders within the organization's decision-making structure and processes.

Nursing leadership: Recognizing nursing as a clinical specialty of its own and the importance of nursing services being led by a highly educated and experienced nurse.

Outcomes: Results or consequences.

Professional development: Supporting nursing education through academic and practice partnership to support teaching and provide clinical sites for learning to ensure a qualified workforce for the future.

Regulatory standards: Standards of care developed by regulatory bodies, the state board of nursing, and specialty organizations that define nursing practice.

Standards and scope of practice: Services those APRNs are deemed competent to perform and permitted to undertake with their advanced professional license.

Transformational leadership: Requires the ability to motivate others to participate in the creation and execution of visionary goals and objectives by exerting their influence not by positional authority.

Value-based care: Focuses on balancing performance in the areas of safety, clinical care, efficiency and cost reduction, and patient-centered experience/coordination.

Introduction

The complexity of healthcare entities requires nurse executives to broaden their knowledge and skills beyond oversight for nursing services. Increasingly Chief Nursing Officers (CNOs) are responsible for broad services that impact the patient experience and the delivery of care. Frequently, CNOs provide executive oversight for pharmacy services, respiratory, patient transport, physical therapy, care management, and various other services. This expanded responsibility and the demand of the current healthcare environment require CNOs to develop a broad range of skills and knowledge including analyzing financial statements, staying abreast of changes in clinical protocols, understanding payers, case mix index (CMI), and population health management while developing and maintaining relationships across the multidisciplinary team. Moving forward, CNOs will be increasingly responsible for a continuum of healthcare that is not restricted to acute care (Haughom, 2017; Vaugh, 2009). This chapter presents insights into the skills and traits needed for nurse leaders at all levels of practice.

History and Evolution

Current senior nursing leadership roles and organizational structures were developed in response to regulatory agencies recognizing nursing as a clinical specialty of its own and the importance of nursing services being led by a highly educated and experienced nurse. Nursing and leadership standards from the Center for Medicare and Medicaid Services (CMS) and the Joint Commission (TJC) dictate that two specific leadership groups are responsible for guiding the activities of caregivers: the medical staff leader(s) and the most senior nurse executive. The nurse executive directs the delivery of nursing care and serves as a member of the hospital leadership team at the senior leadership level. The nurse executive must take an active leadership role with the governing body, senior leadership team, medical staff, management, and other clinical leaders within the organization's decision-making structure and processes. The Joint Commission requires that the most senior nurse executive be included in decisions around the quality and safety of care and in established meetings of the senior clinical management team (Schyve, 2017). The Joint Commission developed a specific standard to delineate the role of the nurse executive in promoting high-quality care. Nursing performance is the foundation for patient care, and the nurse executive develops, manages, and guides improvement for the nursing care team and overall patient care (Woten & Mennella, 2018).

Titles

Nurse leaders function under many titles with varying degrees of responsibilities. Nurse managers and nurse directors may be responsible for one specific area or nursing unit or have oversight of multiple units. As one rises in level of authority, titles may include nurse executive, senior nurse leader, and CNO. Scope of responsibility will reflect the level of authority as well as organizational differences. Generally, managers and directors would report to senior leadership that may include CNOs and nurse executives.

Role Specifics

The role of the CNO on the senior leadership team is to represent nursing as a discipline but more importantly to represent patients (Larkin, 2012) and to facilitate interdisciplinary collaboration. Nurses are experts in care delivery and are well positioned within health systems to identify the inefficiencies in healthcare delivery, risks to patient safety, problems with access to services, barriers to achieving the best patient outcomes, and opportunities to decrease the cost of care (Schub & Strayer, 2016) as presented in Figure 5.1.

An effective leader interprets the importance of this expertise at the most senior level of the organization and influences decisions affecting nursing practice and the patient experience. Historically, physicians have been identified as the highest level experts in healthcare delivery, and they provide important medical expertise, but they are not necessarily positioned well to understand the process issues that are encountered at the level of care delivery. Administrators with business backgrounds possess an in-depth knowledge of financial theories and policies, but they should also trust the expertise of nurses when allocating resources, developing policies, and making decisions related to patient care. Nursing leaders have the responsibility

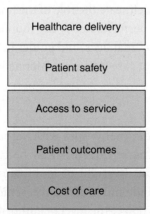

Figure 5.1. Role of a Chief Nursing Officer.

to ensure there is a balanced approach to making decisions that affect nursing practice, patient care, and operations of healthcare entities.

Nurses in executive leadership practice are responsible for creating and setting the vision for patient-centered care, improving healthcare outcomes and population health, and decreasing the cost of healthcare (American Organization of Nurse Executives, 2015). CNOs affect change using a transformational approach to leadership. Transformational leadership requires the ability to motivate others to participate in the creation and execution of visionary goals and objectives by exerting their influence not by positional authority. The relationship developed between leaders and employees transforms the culture and brings value to employees and the organization. The foundation for power in a transformational leadership approach is based on mutual support and a common purpose (Matson, 2014). Executive nursing leaders break down barriers and provide the voice for nurses to have an impact on organizational mission, vision, and goals. This requires an understanding of leadership roles and competencies (Crawford et al., 2017). Transformational leaders have a wide array of skills as presented in Figure 5.2 (Anderson, 2017).

In addition to transformational leadership, nurse executives typically possess other traits that contribute to success. The first of these traits is that of super

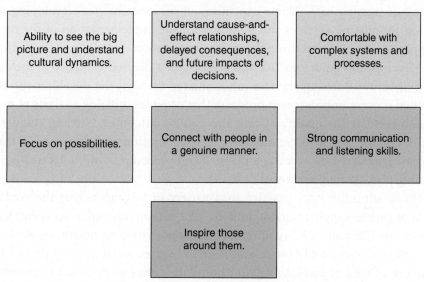

Figure 5.2. Skills of transformational leaders.

integrator. Adept nursing leaders are able to align dissimilar nursing practices, information, and technology into unified systems. Pressures of senior nursing leadership positions require leaders who are savvy negotiators who can exert their influence to transform the care environment and influence culture change. Nurse administrators are also strategic and goal driven as they affect safety practices and create a strong practice environment. Taking a realistic approach to leadership allows leaders to pragmatically manage time, opportunities, and their own need to expand their skills and develop competencies for success. Finally, nurse leaders are well educated and nationally certified, with a proven track record of achieving outcomes (Crawford et al., 2017).

The Joint Commission requires that senior nurse executives demonstrate authority as they function at the most senior level of the organization and coordinate the activities of other nursing leaders, play an active role in the senior leadership team and governing body, and are supported by the organization with written guidance about their responsibilities with a specific job description or contract outlining expectations. Nurse executives should also possess adequate qualifications to function in their position. Minimally, CNOs hold an active nursing license and possess a postgraduate degree. Oversight of nursing services is demonstrated by the ability to direct nursing services, establish guidelines for the delivery of nursing care, and direct the implementation of nursing care. Nurse executives are responsible for developing the vision for nursing services and planning for the implementation of the nursing care delivery model throughout the organization. Policies and procedures are developed to guide practice and are based on the best evidence in the current literature. Nursing services are evaluated through the development of a defined process improvement program that provides ongoing analysis of metrics to evaluate the quality of care and patient outcomes. Nursing standards are developed by the nurse executive in collaboration with the nursing team and are supported by accessible policies and procedures and a defined nurse staffing plan (Woten & Mennella, 2018).

Nurse administrators practice in a variety of settings across the continuum of care to support nursing practice and patient outcomes. As mentioned above, the CMS and TJC require organizations providing healthcare services to name an accountable nurse executive to oversee nursing practice and the delivery of patient care. Acute care hospitals, community-based transitional care, outpatient surgery centers, medical homes, long-term care facilities, and

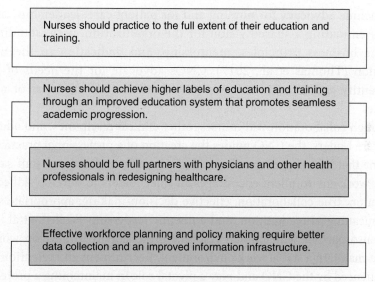

Figure 5.3. Recommendations from *Future of Nursing Report.*

home-care agencies need nursing leaders to evaluate and direct patient care services to ensure quality care. Advanced practice nurse executives practice in a variety of roles within the healthcare system and the advancement of population health multiple settings. They also act as consultants to policy makers, industry, and legislative bodies to promote cost-effective and quality healthcare. The Institute of Medicine (IOM) report on the future of nursing outlined four strategies that should be accomplished to solidify the impact nursing can have on patient care in the future (Robert Wood Johnson Foundation, 2011) as presented in Figure 5.3.

Scope and Standards

The American Nurses Association (ANA) outlines the scope and standards of practice for nursing administration. Nurse administrators are defined as registered nurses who direct and influence the work of others, usually in a healthcare environment. Regardless of the setting, most nursing administration roles include advocacy for nursing and for patient care, leadership, creating and disseminating a shared vision for the organization, understanding and applying business principles, mentorship, and dedication to the nursing profession (Thomas et al., 2017). CNOs advocate for the needs of nurses and identify and monitor metrics to evaluate the effectiveness of nursing practice.

Through collaboration with nurses, other clinical disciplines, and additional healthcare leaders, the CNO guides the creation of a professional practice environment that encourages excellence and promotes patient and staff safety. A healthy work environment encourages all stakeholders to develop skilled communication, true collaboration, effective decision-making, appropriate staffing plans, meaningful recognition, and authentic leadership (Vollers et al., 2009). CNOs also partner with human resource professionals to develop workforce plans to maintain a stable work environment. Recruitment and retention efforts are influenced by the CNO and play a pivotal role in maintaining a professional nursing practice environment.

The American Nurses Credentialing Center (ANCC) offers direction for nursing leaders by providing a framework for nursing practice and research through the Magnet recognition program (Figure 5.4). The Magnet model helps shape the professionalism of nursing, particularly in acute care settings. The framework provides a detailed structure to guide nursing leaders in creating

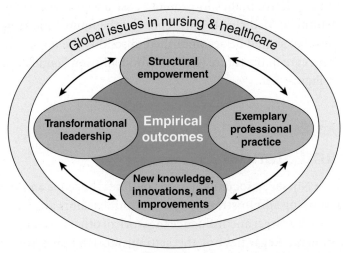

Figure 5.4. American Nurses Credentialing Center (ANCC) Magnet model.

an optimal practice environment while incorporating evidence-based practice and research into nursing structures and processes. Transformational leadership, structural empowerment, exemplary professional practice, new knowledge innovation and improvements, and empirical quality results are the concepts within the Magnet framework that provide guidance for CNOs as they promote professionalism and quality patient care.

Competencies

The American Organization for Nurse Leadership (AONL formerly, American Organization for Nurse Executives [AONE]) in partnership with the Healthcare Leadership Alliance (HLA) has identified competencies that define the skills, knowledge, and abilities intended to guide nurse executive practice. The competency domains within the HLA model reflect multiple dimensions of leadership. Each domain requires mastery of several skills to demonstrate effective leadership practice.

The competency domains for healthcare leadership include communication and relationship management, knowledge of the healthcare environment, leadership, professionalism, and business skills and principles (American Organization of Nurse Executives, 2015). A separate document from the AONL and HLA defines additional expectations for nurses performing the responsibilities of the system CNO role. As healthcare continues to evolve and systems of care merge to create large networks of care, nurses should be represented at the highest level of organizations to guide practice, standardization of care, and allocation of resources; to influence patient-centered decisions to guide population health; and to work with academic and community partners to drive workforce development and education.

An overview of the nurse executive competencies defined by the AONL and HLA are provided in Table 5.1 followed by further detail and an explanation of the skills necessary to effectively practice as a senior nurse executive.

Communication and Relationship Management

Building relationships and communicating at all levels is the foundation for transformational leadership. Motivating and inspiring others is possible when stakeholders believe in the message and in the individual delivering the message.

Table 5.1.   AONL Nurse Executive Competencies

AONL Competencies	Description of Competencies	Examples of Skills
Communication and relationship building	• Effective communication • Relationship management • Ability to work with diversity • Medical staff relationships • Academic relationships	• Build trusting, collaborative relationships • Care about people as individuals; demonstrate empathy while ensuring that organizational goals are met
Knowledge of healthcare environment	• Clinical practice knowledge • Patient care delivery models • Healthcare economics and policy knowledge • Understanding of governance • Knowledge of quality improvement and metrics	• Role model lifelong learning, including clinical subjects such as disease processes, pharmaceuticals, and clinical technology • Articulate federal and state payment systems and regulations which affect organization's finances
Leadership skills	• Foundational thinking skills • The ability to use systems thinking • Succession planning • Change management	• Demonstrate reflective leadership • Consider the impact of nursing decisions on the healthcare organization as a whole
Professionalism	• Personal and professional accountability • Ethics • Advocacy for the clinical enterprise and for nursing practice • Active membership in professional organizations	• Create an environment in which others are setting expectations and holding each other accountable • Create an environment in which professional and personal growth is an expectation
Business skills	• Understanding of healthcare financing • Human resource management and development • Strategic management • Marketing • Information management and technology	• Manage financial resources by developing business plans • Champion a diverse workforce • Provide mentorship to aspiring clinicians and leaders

AONL, American Organization for Nursing Leadership.
Adapted from information obtained from AACN. (2015). *Nurse Executive Competencies*. https://www.aonl.org/system/files/media/file/2019/06/nec.pdf

Top-down leadership is not effective in the current healthcare environment. Every individual should be encouraged to create innovative change, and leaders need to facilitate innovation to improve patient care. Transformational leaders leverage their relationships at every level in the organization to help others enhance their own skill and knowledge to better serve patients and the organization.

In Their Own Words

Margaret Norton-Rosko, DNP, RN, NEA-BC
Chief Nursing Officer

The key points in understanding my role are... Nurse executives first and foremost have an obligation to support the nursing profession and to promote excellence in nursing practice in every setting. Promoting excellence in practice results in quality patient care and encourages goal achievement for the healthcare organizations that employ nurse executives. Nurse executives possess knowledge and skills beyond the clinical scope of practice by demonstrating competency in leadership, management, quality improvement, human resource management, professional development, regulatory guidelines, and healthcare finance. Nurses in executive nursing practice interact with leaders at every level in their practice settings as well as community and government leaders. The role requires flexibility and a passion for continuous learning and developing relationships across the healthcare continuum.

What keeps me coming back every day is... I am passionate about supporting nurses. Nurse executives take care of the people who take care of patients and families requiring care at the most vulnerable points in their lives. Nurses are a generous and caring group who often work beyond their own perceived capacity. Supporting nurses and other clinicians brings me great pride and satisfaction. I feel like I can make a difference for more patients by supporting and encouraging the work of nurses at every level in the healthcare system.

Nursing is one of the greatest professions. It has provided me with a meaningful career and a feeling that I can make a difference every day. Nursing leadership has been more rewarding than I could have ever imagined. Advocating

(Continued)

for nurses and quality patient care is an honor. It allows me to have a positive impact even though I am not working directly with patients. It is also extremely gratifying to make the difference in the life of other nurses. Supporting nurses through professional growth and personal challenges is the most rewarding part of my job. I once sent a note to a new graduate nurse who was struggling through orientation to encourage her to continue her orientation as she was already making a positive impact on patient care. I wanted her to know that I saw several positive qualities in her that would help her to be successful in nursing. She later told me that the note reached her on a day that she had decided she probably was not going to be successful and should leave the profession. The note made an impact, and she decided to show up the next day and keep trying with just a little more confidence than she had the day before. She did successfully complete her orientation and worked for several years in the intensive care unit before moving on to become a Certified Registered Nurse Anesthetist. She reminded me how important it is to be supportive and encouraging to others. Supporting one nurse through a crisis can have an impact on countless patients in the future. The skill, knowledge, and compassion of each nurse touch innumerable lives, and making a difference at that level is very satisfying!

My greatest challenge is… Developing the workforce so the supply of nurses is adequate to meet the needs of patients. Workforce development requires leaders to toil across the healthcare continuum and outside of healthcare to identify a large pool of potential future nurses and to develop creative plans to foster nursing education programs that can accommodate the growing need. The complexity of patient care requires continuous staff development. The ability to adequately and expediently develop nurses to meet patient care needs also impacts the work environment and retention.

I wish someone had told me… To take the first nursing management positions I was offered. I resisted going into an administrative leadership position for several years because I felt I would be abandoning the clinical aspect of nursing. I have learned as much about clinical best practices as a leader as I did at the bedside and feel I can have a bigger impact on the use of best clinical practices within healthcare by becoming proficient at implementing clinical guidelines on a larger scale, not just in my own practice.

I need to be a lifelong learner because… Healthcare changes at a rapid pace! Leaders and clinicians must stay abreast of the changing landscape within healthcare. Leaders need to understand the impact of clinical changes, regulatory guidelines, government requirements, laws impacting healthcare, and the changing reimbursement structures.

> **Another point to understand is...** Nursing is one of the most important con-
> tributors to patient outcomes and organizational success within healthcare
> systems. Nurses make up the largest number of healthcare professionals. It is
> our obligation to be involved and influence changes that affect our profession
> and the care we provide for patients. Every nurse is obligated to act as a leader
> in providing quality patient care and in advocating for the profession.

Effective Communication

Effective communication requires practice and the ability to communicate in
multiple settings, to multiple audiences, using different methods of communication. CNOs make oral presentations to nurses and more diverse audiences.
Nursing leaders must be well versed in nursing and other healthcare topics and
be able to clearly communicate organizational issues to set context for change,
communicate results, and drive innovation. Effective presentations help the
nurse leader gain support for patient care services and effective nursing practice. Nurse leaders need to be comfortable presenting to frontline staff, other
leaders, the multidisciplinary care team, and members of the board and larger
community. Effective communication also includes the ability to clearly convey
a message in writing to similar audiences.

As a senior clinical leader, the CNO is often required to facilitate group discussions at multiple levels within and outside of their organization. Enabling conversations with key stakeholders helps build the trust required within shared governance
structures and healthy work environments. Effective facilitation promotes and supports decision-making by frontline nursing staff and encourages multidisciplinary
efforts to improve the quality of patient care. Facilitation is a foundational element of
quality and process improvement efforts. Creating an environment that encourages
open communication relies on good interpersonal relationships. Effective leaders
work to develop relationships from the board room to the frontline and beyond.
Creating opportunities to interact across the continuum of services enables leaders
to create the relationships necessary to support the work of caregivers.

Relationship Management

Healthcare and nursing services are team sports. They require collaboration and
clear communication to effectively care for patients and improve the quality of
care. The CNO must focus on building collaborative relationships throughout
the organization and should role model several key attributes of collaborative

relationships. Effective conflict resolution starts with creating an environment where leaders and other stakeholders feel safe to disagree and to debate about the most effective solutions to problems. Role modeling effective conflict resolution is an essential skill for leadership within healthcare. Developing a trusting environment takes commitment and attention to details communicating with large teams and multiple stakeholders in a complex environment. The following behaviors will serve leaders well in creating the trust needed to effectively manage relationships:

- Follow up when concerns are raised.
- Keep promises and create processes to consistently follow up on commitments.
- Balance the concerns of individuals with organizational goals and communicating the rationale for decisions when the two are in conflict.
- Encourage staff to be involved in decision-making through formal and informal involvement in shared governance.
- Communicate at all levels with respect to maintaining credibility and relationships.

(AONL, American Organization of Nurse Executives, 2015).

Influencing Behaviors

The goal of demonstrating effective communication and building relationships is to achieve outcomes through engagement of the larger team. Leaders cannot achieve meaningful outcomes unless the team members understand the organizational objectives and are encouraged to participate in creating and communicating this information to others. Promoting a patient-centered vision requires every team member to understand the importance of keeping patients at the center of every action and decision made by the team. When team behaviors are not demonstrated, leaders need to manage the undesired behaviors in a nonjudgmental and nonthreatening manner.

Diversity

Patient-centeredness and safe work environments require leaders and organizations to value inclusion. Organizational values that support cultural competence of the workforce must be supported and developed by nursing leaders. Patient care should include the incorporation of cultural beliefs. Leaders should develop an organizational learning culture that values diversity and demonstrates their respect for the cultural beliefs and norms of their workforce by encouraging opinion sharing and innovation to achieve outcomes.

Questions to Ask Yourself

1. How does a nurse in an administrative role impact quality patient care and nursing practice?
2. What standards guide nursing leadership practice?
3. How do nurse leaders impact organizational governance?
4. What competencies are required for successful nursing leadership practice?
5. What level of education is required for nursing leadership?
6. How do regulatory agencies affect nursing leadership practice?

Community Involvement

Nurse executives have a responsibility to represent nursing outside of their official capacity as a leader in a healthcare organization. The responsibility to the profession requires that nursing leaders represent nursing in a positive fashion to the larger public. This can be accomplished by representing one's organization to constituents within the community, serving on the board of community organizations, representing the community's interests within the larger healthcare system, and by serving as a healthcare resource to community and business leaders.

Medical Staff/Provider Relationships

Two groups are responsible for guiding the activities of caregivers: the medical staff leader(s) and the nurse executive (Schyve, 2017). The partnership between the nurse executive and the medical staff needs to demonstrate a respectful approach to collaboration and conflict resolution. CNOs must understand how to implement the use of medical staff mechanisms to address physician clinical performance and to address disruptive behavior. The AONL competencies suggest that the nurse executive must build credibility with physicians as a champion for patient care, quality, and the profession of nursing. This is accomplished by representing nursing at the medical executive committee and other medical department staff committees. Nurse leaders should collaborate with medical staff leaders to identify metrics to evaluate the effectiveness of care and cooperate to identify evidence-based approaches to improve patient care. Market data should be used by the nurse executive and physician leaders to determine the services needed to serve the needs of the community.

Academic Relationships

The supply and demand for nursing services is one of the biggest challenges that a nurse executive will face. Identifying the current and future workforce needs within an organization requires nursing leaders to partner with others within and outside of the organization to create a workforce development plan that includes professional development and plans for recruitment and retention of the nursing workforce. Ongoing evaluation of current models of care is necessary to create innovative models that will allow for top-of-license practice for every nurse and the creation of supportive roles. Nurse executives should partner with academic programs on many levels to:

- support nursing education through academic and practice partnership to support teaching and provide clinical sites for learning to ensure a qualified workforce for the future;
- evaluate the quality of graduating nurses and develop mechanisms to enhance the quality;
- develop programs for successful transition to practice;
- collaborate in nursing research and translate evidence into practice; and
- collaborate to investigate care delivery models.

Knowledge of the Healthcare Environment

Senior nurse leaders must demonstrate an expert understanding of nursing practice and the responsibilities of all the members of the patient care team. It is important for all practitioners to practice at the top of their license. The CNO facilitates practice by understanding and communicating standards of care developed by regulatory bodies, the state board of nursing, and specialty organizations that define nursing practice. The CNO or designee reviews the credentials of advanced practice registered nurses and ensures that peer review is an element in evaluating practice. Creating a positive work environment also includes the need to leverage the clinical expertise of others in developing evidence-based policies and procedures, and to update them as new evidence becomes available. Incorporating ethical and legal guidelines into clinical and management decision-making further supports patient care and a positive work environment (AONL [formerly AONE], 2015).

Patient Care Delivery Models

The complexity of patient care continues to challenge nursing practice at every level and in every setting. Quality of care is measured and publicly reported, and this allows consumers to compare organizations to determine where they want to receive care. American Organization for Nursing Leadership (formerly AONE) encourages leaders to engage direct care nurses in evaluating the effectiveness of current patient care delivery models and creating more effective models where indicated. Evaluating care requires nurses at every level to understand the metrics used in measuring the effectiveness of care. Nurse-sensitive indicators, such as infection rates, hospital-acquired pressure ulcers, failure to rescue, and falls, provide information about how well nursing teams are structured to prevent patient harm. Other indicators reflect how well structures and processes support care and optimize patient outcomes. These include length of stay, readmission rates, complications, mortality, and patient experience scores. Redesign efforts should include activities that optimize nursing roles, focus on outcomes, and reorganize workflow and resources to improve efficiency and outcomes and decrease the cost of care (Wharton et al., 2016).

Healthcare Economics, Regulations, Policy, and Legislation

Regulatory and financial pressures influence decision-making and resource allocation within the practice environment. It is important that nurse leaders understand regulation and payment issues that affect organizational financial performance. Financial performance is impacted by the CMI, which is a relative value assigned to patients in a diagnosis-related group that reflects the resources required to care for patients within that group. CMI is one factor that should be considered when aligning care delivery models that result in safe and effective care. Value-based purchasing (VBP) focuses on balancing performance in the areas of safety, clinical care, efficiency and cost reduction, and patient-centered experience/coordination of care for Medicare patients. Other payers are also using value-based metrics to benchmark organizational performance. Organizations that perform well are rewarded with financial incentives to continue improvement efforts, while underperforming organizations are penalized.

Professional nurses at every level must lead efforts to collaborate with healthcare organizations—local, state, and federal government; professional associations; certifying organizations; and academic partners—to position the nursing profession as a powerful force to improve healthcare for those we serve. Efforts should focus on improving access to care, patient-centered delivery models, and outcomes as measured by evidence-based metrics that benchmark performance across the industry (Holle & Kornusky, 2018).

 In Their Own Words

Victoria L. Rich, PhD, RN, FAAN
Dean of Nursing, University of South Florida College of Nursing

My role as a college of nursing dean is… To develop clinical and nursing research faculty that transforms nursing students into healthcare professionals who become interprofessional practitioners, clinical leaders, educators, and researchers. To successfully accomplish this outcome, I must focus on the four FAST initiatives: (F) Fundraising for scholarships and research, (A) Accreditation from state and national professional bodies, (S) Strategic visioning, and (T) Teaching and retaining faculty and staff talent.

What keeps me coming back every day is… Realizing that individual healthcare professionals can no longer practice in silos. Each healthcare professional *must* appreciate and respect one another's knowledge basis and create wholesome, individualistic plans of care for patients, families, populations, and society. As an International Patient Safety Consultant for the last 20 years, I experienced numerous systems' failures in healthcare that resulted in harm or the death of patients. Over and over again, the error occurred because of a lack of communication, care integration, and interprofessional partners not understanding scopes of practice nor accountability. Medical errors also have a second victim: the nurse, doctor, or pharmacist who caused the harm is usually the victim of poor system processes. Often they leave the profession with a sense of guilt and moral distress.

My greatest challenge is… Twofold. The first challenge is to foster and develop meaningful academic-service partnerships. The two cultures remain islands, and collaborative outcomes remain scant.

I spent over 30 years in the service part of healthcare as a COO, CNE, and Consultant. I understand the knowledge gaps of all healthcare practitioners. It was easy to evaluate the pros and cons of academia. I frequently remarked:

(Continued)

"Why aren't the nurses prepared to take on patients? Why do I have to create the nurse practitioner? What do I need a nurse researcher for? Why do I have to teach nurses to be good teachers?" Now, as the Dean of Nursing, I have experienced challenges in academics, program structure, and the time it takes to address standards and handle student and family genomics.

My second challenge is a philosophical one. As the profession of nursing evolves into a highly educated discipline of clinicians, researchers, and leaders, we cannot forget that we truly are the profession "Who cares for others when they cannot care for themselves." How will we balance our sophistication within the basic needs of patients from cradle to grave?

My work now as a Senior Professional of both service and academia is to assist in defining meaning and purpose that result in performance outcomes.

I wish someone had told me... To practice being patient and humble and to initiate a new program or idea *only* after all stakeholders involved have had a voice in the discussion. This includes more than the nursing profession. We learn from each other, and a major leadership skill is to "model the way without pride or expectation, but because it is the right thing to do."

I need to be a lifelong learner because... Human genomic nursing science and research has exploded. Big data and practice-based evidence for populations have revolutionized the care of humans. Due to scientific knowledge and discoveries constantly updating, the lifelong learner must be proficient in triple loop learning. Triple-loop learning requires (1) learning a new concept, (2) applying the new learning, and (3) changing direction and system outcomes. Lifelong learning implies accountability and leadership in change as master skills.

The sustainability of the human race relies on communication, evidence, and respect for diversity. The profession and discipline of nursing are postured to lead with other interprofessional healthcare mavens.

Organizational Governance

Many healthcare organizations are governed by a board that consists predominantly of lay people not experienced or knowledgeable about clinical practice. Very often, physicians also sit on governing boards as voting members. The CNO is in a unique position to act as a resource to governing board members who have the responsibility to set the direction of the organization, ensure effective management, enhance assets, achieve quality goals, and act as a stakeholder on behalf of the community

(Harder, 2006). The governing body has ultimate authority to oversee fiduciary responsibilities, credentialing, and performance management. The CNO should be comfortable representing patient care concerns to the board and should actively participate in strategic planning and quality initiatives. Collaborating with physicians on the governing board will help provided adequate representation of clinical disciplines and concerns as the board exerts its authority in decision-making.

Patient Safety

Senior leaders in healthcare organizations are responsible for creating a work environment that values patient safety. This requires developing an organization-wide patient safety program that defines patient safety goals, creates a system to reliably monitor risks to patient safety, quickly responds to patient safety concerns and events, and has a commitment to zero patient harm. Nurse executives play a key role in developing and communicating the patient safety message and allocating staffing and equipment resources required to deliver safe care (Disch et al., 2011). Healthy work environments encourage direct caregivers and all employees to speak up when they identify a concern to patient safety. Just cultures support a nonpunitive approach to investigating safety events and reward staff members for identifying and reporting unsafe conditions. Investigating safety concerns requires focus on inadequate systems and processes, not on individual errors committed by people. Familiarity with high-reliability concepts and human factors analysis are important elements of administering an effective safety program. Monitoring the culture of safety using a nationally benchmarked survey is an important effort often led by nursing and patient safety leaders.

Performance Improvement and Metrics

The Institute for Healthcare Improvement defines the focus of improvement efforts for the healthcare industry as the Triple Aim. This strategy encourages healthcare organizations to focus on improving population health, improving the patient care experience (quality, safety, and satisfaction), and reducing cost (Institute for Healthcare Improvement, 2020). Application of high-reliability principles can help drive necessary improvement efforts. Integrating these principles into an organization's quality and safety programs reduces clinical variation, improves the use of evidence-based practices, and enhances nurse-sensitive patient outcomes (Oster & Deakins, 2018). The five characteristics of high-reliability organizations are those that possess a sensitivity to operations, are preoccupied with failure, readily defer to expertise, are reluctant to simplify, and are committed to resilience (Patient Safety Network, 2017). Sensitivity to operations means that work groups understand processes and functions beyond their own department. This improves unit-to-unit collaboration and engagement of everyone in the organization. Preoccupation with failure means that individuals are watching for the next possible event and are ready to intervene to prevent the error from reaching a patient. Deferring to expertise requires humility from every member of the team and a shared vision for the goal of zero harm to patients. This requires the ability to recognize that rank and title are not synonymous with expert knowledge in every situation. Reluctance to simplify discourages healthcare workers from developing workarounds, encourages event analysis to determine the root cause of issues, and focuses on the development of solutions to fix the root cause. Transparency is required as high-reliability organizations commit to resilience. Leaders must be comfortable admitting when errors occur, engage in effective management of errors, and nurture organizational learning from events (Oster & Deakins, 2018).

Nursing usually constitutes the largest cost center in most healthcare organizations. It is imperative that nursing can demonstrate the value it brings to the organization by positively affecting patient outcomes and managing cost (Oster & Deakins, 2018). Effective nurse leaders can articulate the organization's performance improvement program and goals. They use evidence-based metrics to align patient outcomes with the organization's goals toward the Triple Aim. Quality metrics are determined by identifying process problems, measuring success at improving specific outcomes, analyzing root causes or variation from standards, managing implementation, and sustaining success (AONL). Several process improvement methodologies can be employed as a framework for process improvement including PDCA (plan, do, check, act), DMAIC (define, measure, analyze, improve, control) Lean, and Six Sigma. Nurse leaders should become familiar with these methods and develop expertise in the method used within the organization. Competency in process improvement drives the ability for nurse leaders to be effective in meeting the needs of patients, staff, and the organization.

Risk Management

An effective risk management system helps organizations identify areas of risk for potential liability and patient harm. Risk management often works closely with the quality and safety programs within organizations to identify trends that might affect patient safety and organizational outcomes. Nurse executives should ensure that systems are in place to allow prompt reporting of potential liability and that staff at every level is educated about risk reporting and compliance issues (American Organization of Nurse Executives, 2015). Improvement efforts to correct areas of liability are often led and sustained by nurse leaders using some of the skills and competencies discussed under performance improvement.

Leadership

Senior nursing leaders are pivotal to the success of the interdisciplinary leadership team in healthcare organizations. They establish the vision for patient care and nursing practice by focusing on efforts to improve the overall patient experience and population health while reducing costs. These efforts require transformational leadership. Transformational leadership focuses on the dynamic between leaders and their followers and encourages exchange of ideas at every level. This engagement encourages leaders and followers to challenge each other's thinking to attain a higher level of achievement. Transformational leaders guide others to where they need to be to meet the requirements of the future by facilitating growth and development of team members (Jones et al., 2017). Transformational leaders understand the importance of every member of their team practicing and contributing to their fullest potential to drive improvement in patient outcomes.

Foundational Thinking Skills and Personal Growth

Authentic leadership begins with an understanding of what drives individuals to want to influence the behaviors and performance of a team. Demonstrating the ability to reflect on one's own practice and understand internal motivation are important attributes for nurse leaders. Personal values and beliefs help create a consistent method of decision-making and guide the development of a creative vision for nursing practice and patient care. Willingness to explore new knowledge leads to the ability to critically analyze issues and consider the viewpoints of others to improve outcomes and create a healthy work environment (American Organization of Nurse Executives, 2015).

Systems Thinking

Systems thinking encompasses four primary attributes: a dynamic system, holistic perspective, pattern identification, and transformation. It allows individuals to impact cause and effect through collaboration with others using one's individual ability to influence the greater whole (Statler et al., 2017). Systems thinking forces leaders to think beyond the immediate impact of issues and decisions to understand the complexity of interacting parts within the healthcare system. This helps create a broader vision for patient care and nursing practice. CNOs and other senior nurse leaders must be able to comprehend the complexity of the healthcare system and view it from a holistic perspective to evaluate the impact of their decisions on the entire healthcare enterprise. Coaching nurses to understand systems thinking while caring for patients will improve care by pushing nurses to understand that each care decision and intervention may result in a dynamic patient response that affects multiple systems.

Succession Planning

Effective succession planning creates conditions for sustained organizational performance and superior patient outcomes regardless of the presence of an individual leader. Transformational leaders need to focus on developing future leaders, so they are ready for the demands that an evolving healthcare environment will require. Each leader in the nursing hierarchy of an organization should identify at least one successor for their role so the organization can anticipate sustained outcomes and a more stable future. The CNO should take the lead on developing a workforce analysis plan and identify strategies to ensure a qualified workforce. The CNO should create criteria to identify the best candidates for development. Exposing future leaders to a variety of environments and perspectives will broaden their ability to apply systems thinking to create a vision for the future. Including mentoring and role modeling in succession planning will help future leaders develop relationships and observe how effective leaders drive organizational outcomes (Robinson-Walker, 2013). Senior leaders should establish mechanisms to identify potential leaders and support them through formal mentoring and educational programs (American Organization of Nurse Executives, 2015).

Change Management

Acting as a change agent begins with being able to identify that change is necessary. The need for change is often triggered because an organization is not meeting expected goals or because a patient experienced an unexpected outcome. Nurse leaders need to develop the skills necessary to act as effective change agents. Kotter's (1995) change theory demonstrates components of effective change management as presented in Figure 5.5.

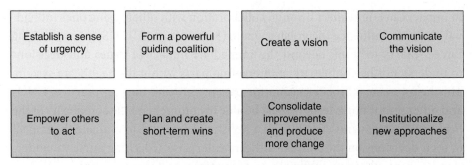

Figure 5.5. Components of effective change management.

Regardless of the change theory used, leaders must be open to change and adapt their leadership style to situational needs and role model a willingness to consider new approaches.

Professionalism

Nurse executives act as role models for the profession by demonstrating the highest level of knowledge, competence, and skill to guide nursing practice. Advocating for the profession includes promoting the clinical perspective in organizational decision-making and involving nurses in decisions about their practice and work environment. They hold themselves accountable for communicating professional expectations and guiding their teams to strive for excellence. They demonstrate the importance of lifelong learning and work within healthcare organizations to create structures that support ongoing formal education and certification for nurses. They actively participate in professional organizations and create opportunities for nurses at every level to do the same. Career planning is an important component of a nurse leader's role. They focus on their own career path by seeking input and mentorship from others to propel their own development. Recognizing the importance of succession planning, they actively look for future leaders and encourage them to explore career development opportunities (American Organization of Nurse Executives, 2015).

Representing the interests of patients and families and advocating for population health are linked to the nursing profession's obligation to society. The Code of Ethics for Nursing is a set of provisions that describe the goals, values, and obligations of the nursing profession and express its values and commitments to society (Epstein & Turner, 2015). Nurse leaders must fully grasp the code of ethics to guide professional practice. It is necessary to evaluate ethical dilemmas through the eyes of these standards and hold others accountable to fulfilling the commitment the profession has to society:

- The nurse practices with compassion and respect for the inherent dignity, worth, and unique attributes of every person.
- The nurse's primary commitment is to the patient, whether an individual, family, group, community, or population.
- The nurse promotes, advocates for, and protects the rights, health, and safety of the patient.
- The nurse has authority, accountability, and responsibility for nursing practice; makes decisions; and takes actions consistent with the obligation to promote health and to provide optimal care.
- The nurse owes the same to duties to self as to others, including the responsibility to promote health and safety, preserve wholeness of character and integrity, maintain competence, and continue personal and professional growth.
- The nurse, through individual and collective effort, establishes, maintains, and improves the ethical environment of the work setting and conditions of employment that are conducive to safe, quality healthcare.
- The nurse, in all roles and settings, advances the profession through research and scholarly inquiry, professional standards development, and the generation of both nursing and health policy.
- The nurse collaborates with other health professionals and the public to protect human rights, promote health diplomacy, and reduce health disparities.
- The profession of nursing through its professional organizations must articulate nursing values, maintain the integrity of the profession, and integrate principles of social justice into nursing and health policy.

(American Nurses Association, 2015)

Business Skills and Principles

The final competency for nurse executives described by AONL and HLA is the development of business skills necessary to successfully operate patient care services within an organization. It is not enough to maintain clinical knowledge and skills to be an effective leader. Nursing is often the largest part of the workforce, and to effectively advocate for resources, leaders need to understand and execute financial strategies.

Financial Management

Patient care decisions have a financial impact on healthcare organizations. It is necessary for leaders to educate their teams about the impact of their decisions and to seek input from their teams about the resources they need as annual operating budgets are developed. Review of routine financial statements is necessary for appropriate management of financial resources. Becoming proficient in negotiation is necessary when competing for scarce resources and when developing and monitoring contracts with physicians and other service providers.

Human Resource Management

Nursing represents a large segment of the workforce in most healthcare settings. Managing human resources includes workforce planning and employment decisions. Learning how to identify organizational needs and the right talent to form a highly functioning team require collaboration with human resource professionals and an understanding of the culture of an organization. Understanding market data that describe the supply and demand of eligible candidates and compensation principles is necessary in developing a solid recruitment plan in a competitive environment. Once a team has been created, it is necessary to focus on retention through the implementation of professional development programs, reward and recognition, and the creation of safe and healthy work environments. Contributing to the development of behavioral standards and holding staff accountable to those standards require both compassion and tenacity. Workplace harassment and bullying are concerns in healthcare settings, and accomplished nurse leaders implement programs to address these issues to keep workers safe.

Strategic Management

Creating a successful strategic plan for nursing that aligns with the organizational strategic plan can be an effective way to achieve success. Different frameworks can be used when creating a strategic plan. The SWOT (strengths, weaknesses, opportunities, and threats) methodology is used in many settings and focuses on the current state to identify tactics to support the strategic direction of an organization. The SOAR (strengths, opportunities, aspirations, and results) helps focus strategic planning exercises on what the organization wants to become as it provides a future-oriented perspective (Wadsworth et al., 2016). Whichever method is used, the result should contribute to the creation of operational objectives, goals, and tactics required to achieve strategic objectives.

The nursing strategic plan should support the dialogue by the nurse executive to defend the business case for nursing. The strategic plan should include promoting the image and influence of nursing.

Information Management and Technology

The final set of skills related to developing competency in the business arena for nurse executives is understanding the importance of information management and technology. The CNO or a designee often provides leadership for the adoption and implementation of information systems. Information management goes beyond the implementation of a functional medical record for the entry of patient data. It requires creating systems that allow organizations to aggregate patient-level data into population-level statistics to inform decision-making around process improvement, resource allocation, program development, workforce planning, and meeting regulatory reporting requirements. These data can also be used to help determine what technology should be implemented to improve patient care. Nurses need to provide input for choosing technology and evaluating its efficacy related to patient safety and workflow implications.

Certification

Like other nursing specialties, nursing leadership practice requires specialized knowledge and competencies. CNOs should encourage certification by leading by example. Knowledge and competency can be validated through national certification. Certification provides validation by a nongovernmental agency that a professional has met predetermined standards that qualify the individual for practice in a specialty area of nursing with recertification signifying ongoing high achievement (Garrison et al., 2018). CNOs and other nurses in formal leadership positions should consider certification in nursing leadership. Many professional nursing organizations offer certification in clinical and leadership specialties. The most recognized and accessible leadership certifications within nursing are supported by the ANCC and AONL. These certifications require a minimum number of practice hours as a nursing leader and successful completion of a certification examination. Once certification has been achieved, it is maintained through ongoing nursing leadership practice and continuing education credits.

The American Academy of Nursing recognizes excellence in nursing leadership by distinguishing leaders as a Fellow in the American Academy of Nursing

(FAAN). Fellows are recognized for their outstanding careers and are highly educated, with more than 90% of fellows holding a doctoral degree and the remaining fellows holding a master's degree. Academy fellows have an ongoing obligation to contribute to the nursing profession, to the academy, and to improving healthcare for the nation. Specifically, fellows focus on enhancing the quality of health and nursing care, promoting healthy aging and human development across the continuum of care, reducing health disparities, shaping healthy behaviors and environments, integrating mental and physical health, and strengthening the nursing and health delivery system on a national and global scale (American Academy of Nursing, 2015).

The American College of Healthcare Executives (ACHE) also supports a fellowship program. The Fellow of the American College of Healthcare Executives (FACHE) program is open to healthcare executives with clinical and nonclinical backgrounds and requires membership in the ACHE, academic preparation, healthcare management experience, continuing education credits, and community and civic involvement. The Board of Governors Examination is also required to achieve FACHE.

Education

General agreement exists that CNOs and other senior nursing leaders should hold an advanced degree. Applicable degree options include DNP, PhD, MSN, MBA, and MHA. Regardless of the degree, nursing leaders gain credibility by connecting with clinicians, staff, and patients to understand patient care requirements and to assess the effectiveness of the care delivery model and nursing practice. Learning through immersion in the patient care environment is supported by the knowledge gained through formal education that supports systems thinking, implementation science, data-driven decisions, experiential knowledge, understanding of evidence-based practice, and business acumen.

Professional Organizations

- Fellow American College of Healthcare Executives (FACHE): https://www.ache.org/
- American Organization for Nursing Leadership (AONL): https://www.aonl.org/
- American College of Healthcare Executives: https://www.ache.org/

Web Resources

- American Nurses Association (ANA): https://www.nursingworld.org/
- American Nurses Credentialing Center (ANCC): https://www.nursingworld.org/ancc/
- Nurse Executive-Board Certified (NE-BC): https://www.nursingworld.org/our-certifications/nurse-executive/
- Nurse Executive Advanced-Board Certified (NEA-BC): https://www.nursingworld.org/our-certifications/nurse-executive/
- Certified in Executive Nursing Practice (CENP): https://www.aonl.org/

Summary

Nursing administrators carry a heavy burden within the larger healthcare system. They carry accountability to ensure top-of-license practice for the largest group of healthcare providers within the healthcare system while ensuring quality patient care, stabilization of the nursing workforce, and support for advancing the nursing profession by incorporating the recommendations from the IOM's future of nursing report and practice guidelines defined by the ANA and specialty nursing organizations. An advanced level of education coupled with experience is necessary to achieve competency in five key areas of practice: communication and relationship management, knowledge of the healthcare environment, leadership, professionalism, and business skills and principles.

Chapter Highlights

- Senior nurse leadership roles were developed in response to regulatory agencies' recognition the role is a clinical specialty with responsibilities over guiding caregiver activities. The role of the CNO on the senior leadership team is to represent nursing as a discipline, but more importantly to represent patients.
- Nursing leaders have the responsibility to ensure there is a balanced approach to making decisions that affect nursing practice, patient care, and operations of healthcare entities.
- AONL developed senior leadership roles and competency domains that support a transformational leadership style.

- Adept nursing leaders are able to align dissimilar nursing practices, information, and technology into unified systems.
- Nurse administrators are also strategic and goal-driven as they affect safety practices and create a strong practice environment.
- The competency domains for healthcare leadership include communication and relationship management, knowledge of the healthcare environment, leadership, professionalism, and business skills and principles.
- Building relationships and communicating at all levels is the foundation for transformational leadership.
- Senior leaders in healthcare organizations are responsible for creating a work environment that values patient safety. This requires developing an organization-wide patient safety program that defines patient safety goals, creates a system to reliably monitor risks to patient safety, quick response to patient safety concerns and events, and a commitment to zero patient harm.
- Effective succession planning creates conditions for sustained organizational performance and superior patient outcomes regardless of the presence of an individual leader.

References

American Academy of Nursing. (2015). *Academy fellows.* https://www.aannet.org/about/fellows

American Nurses Association. (2015). *Code of ethics for nurses with interpretive statements.* http://www.nursingworld.org/code-ofethics

American Organization for Nursing Leadership. (2015). *AONL nurse executive competencies.* https://www.aonl.org/system/files/media/file/2019/06/nec.pdf

Anderson, D. (2017). *Self-mastery: The foundation of co-creating and great transformational leadership.* https://blog.beingfirst.com/self-mastery-the-foundation-of-co-creating-and-great-transformational-leadership

Crawford, C., Omery, A., & Spicer, J. (2017). An integrative review of 21st-century roles, responsibilities, characteristics, and competencies of chief nurse executives. A blueprint for the next generation. *Nursing Administration Quarterly, 41*(4), 297–309.

Disch, J., Dreher, M., & Davidson, P. (2011). The role of the chief nursing officer in ensuring patient safety and quality. *The Journal of Nursing Administration, 41*(4), 177–185.

Epstein, B., & Turner, M. (2015). The nursing code of ethics: Its value, its history. *The Online Journal of Issues in Nursing, 20(2).* http://ojin.nursingworld.org/MainMenuCategories/ANAMarketplace/ANAPeriodicals/OJIN/TableofContents/Vol-20-2015/No2-May-2015/The-Nursing-Code-of-Ethics-Its-Value-Its-History.html

Garrison, E., Schulz, C., Nelson, C., & Lindquist, C. (2018). Specialty certification: Nurses perceived value and barriers. *Nursing Management, 49*(5), 42–47.

Hader, R. (2006). Board Governance: What's your CNO's role? *Nursing Management, 37*(3), 32–34.

Haughom, J. (2017). *Healthcare decision support helps CFOs achieve their top goal: Timely, accurate, agile decision making.* https://www.healthcatalyst.com/healthcare-decision-support-helps-CFOs-achieve-top-goal

Holle, M., & Kornusky, J. (2018). *Evidence-based care sheet: Nursing leadership and the future of nursing.* CINAHL Information Systems.

Institute for Healthcare Improvement. (2020). *The IHI triple aim.* http://www.ihi.org/Engage/Initiatives/TripleAim/Pages/default.aspx

Institute of Medicine (US) Committee on the Robert Wood Johnson Foundation Initiative on the Future of Nursing, at the Institute of Medicine. (2011). *The future of nursing: Leading change, advancing health.* National Academies Press. https://www.ncbi.nlm.nih.gov/books/NBK209880/. https://doi.org/10.17226/12956

Jones, O., Polancich, S., Steaban, R., Feistritzer, N., & Poe, T. (2017). Transformational leadership. *Journal of Healthcare Quality, 39*(3), 186–190.

Kotter, J. (1995). Leading change: Why transformational efforts fail. *Harvard Business Review,* 59–65. https://hbr.org/1995/05/leading-change-why-transformation-efforts-fail-2

Larkin, H. (2012). Focus on the C-suite frontliner in chief. *Hospitals and Health Networks, 86*(5), 33–36.

Matson, K. (2014). Revisiting the past, revamping the future: The leadership edition. *Nursing Management, 45*(8), 47–51. https://www.researchgate.net/publication/264291973_Revisiting_the_past_revamping_the_future_The_leadership_edition

Oster, C., & Deakins, S. (2018). Practical applications of high reliability in healthcare to optimize quality and safety outcomes. *The Journal of Nursing Administration, 48*(1), 50–55.

Patient Safety Network. (2017). *High reliability.* https://psnet.ahrq.gov/primer/high-reliability.

Robinson-Walker, C. (2013). Succession planning: Moving the dial from should to must. *Nurse Administration Quarterly, 37*(1), 37–43.

Schub, T. B., & Strayer, D. M. (2016). *Power of nurses to advocate for policy change.* CINAHL Nursing Guide.

Schyve, P. (2017). *Leadership in healthcare organizations: A guide to the Joint commission leadership standards* (2nd ed.). The Government Institute. https://nrchealth.com/wp-content/uploads/2017/06/WP_JC_Leadership-in-Healthcare-Organizations_Second_Schyve_Carr.pdf

Statler, A. M., Phillips, J. M., Ruggiero, J. S., Scardaville, D. L., Merriam, D., Dolansky, M. A., Goldschmidt, K. A., Wiggs, C. M., & Winegardner, S. (2017). A concept analysis of systems thinking. *Nursing Forum, 54*(4), 323–330.

Thomas, T. W., Seifert, P. C., & Joyner, J. C. (2017). Registered nurses leading innovative changes. *The Online Journal of Issues in Nursing, 21*(3). https://ojin.nursingworld.org/MainMenuCategories/ANAMarketplace/ANAPeriodicals/OJIN/TableofContents/Vol-21-2016/No3-Sept-2016/Registered-Nurses-Leading-Innovative-Changes.html

Vaughn, C. (2009). *Reinventing the CNO.* http://www.hcpro.com/HOM-227787-3749/Reinventing-the-CNO.html?page=2

Vollers, D., Hill, E, Roberts, C., Dambaugh, L. & Brenner, Z. R. (2009). AACN's healthy work environment standards and an empowering nurse advancement system. *Critical Care Nurse, 29*(6), 20–27.

Wadsworth, B., Felton, F., & Linus, R. (2016). Soaring into strategic planning engaging nurses to achieve significant outcomes. *Nursing Administration Quarterly, 40*(4), 299–306.

Wharton, G., Berger, J., & Williams, T. (2016). A tale of two units: Lessons in changing the care delivery model. *The Journal of Nursing Administration, 46*(4), 176–180.

Woten, M., & Mennella, H. (2018). *Nurse executive role, the Joint commission.* CINAHL Information Systems.

6

Clinical Nurse Leaders

Grace Buttriss

LEARNING OBJECTIVES

After completing this chapter, you will be able to:

1. Review the history of clinical nurse leaders.

2. Define the role and expectations of the clinical nurse leader.

3. Discuss the benefits of the clinical nurse leader role.

4. Differentiate the competencies and expectations of clinical nurse leaders.

5. Examine the certification process for clinical nurse leaders.

KEY TERMS

Care Coordination: The deliberate organization of patient care activities among two or more participants, including the patient and/or the family to facilitate the appropriate delivery of healthcare services.

Care Transitions: The movement of patients between healthcare locations, providers, or different levels of care within the same location as their conditions and care need change.

Certification: A mark of distinction that highlights professional accomplishments.

Clinical Macrosystem: Systems or organizations that contain clinical microsystems.

Clinical Mesosystem: Links microsystems together to support patients along the continuum of care.

Clinical Microsystem: Frontline units where patients and healthcare providers interact.

Clinical Nurse Leader: A master's-educated nurse, prepared for practice across the continuum of care within any healthcare setting in today's changing healthcare environment.

Evidence-Based Practice: The conscientious, explicit, and judicious use of current best evidence in making decisions about the care of the individual patient.

Skill Set: Defined nursing skills specific to a role.

History and Evolution

The role of the clinical nurse leader (CNL) evolved from the information provided in a 1999 Institute of Medicine report, *To Err Is Human: Building a Safer Healthcare System* (IOM; now the National Academies of Sciences, Engineering and Medicine). The IOM report concluded that healthcare in the United States was not as safe as it should have been and preventable medical errors exceeded attributable deaths due to motor vehicle accidents, breast cancer, and AIDS. These three causes of death have received more public attention than all preventable medical errors combined (Kohn et al., 2000).

These medical errors have contributed to a loss of trust in the entire healthcare system and compromised patient safety. Secondarily healthcare workers' satisfaction, morale, and productivity have decreased. These combined factors have altered patients' lives and significantly affected their healthcare outcomes in terms of extended length of hospital stays, near misses, disability, and in some cases death.

The Quality of Healthcare in America Committee of the IOM determined that the avoidable harm caused by healthcare employees was at an unacceptable level (IOM, 2000). The committee convened to develop a plan to reduce future patient harm caused by the significant number of avoidable medical errors caused by healthcare workers and unsafe conditions (Kohn et al., 2000).

The IOM's Quality and Safety Report (1999) led to a joint meeting between the Council on Graduate Medical Education (COGME) and the National Advisory Council on Nursing Education (NACNEP). This meeting was held to assess all issues that affect the relationships between physicians and nurses related to patient safety, systems, and collaborations in order to promote the concept of patient safety (Kohn et al., 2000).

Contemporary healthcare systems entered the new millennium fraught with challenges to provide the safe environments for those trusted to their care (IOM, 2003). According to Reid and Dennison (2011), over the last two decades, healthcare's quality-safety-performance-improvement infrastructure has burgeoned, but the provision of safe, quality care for both patients and families has remained challenging. Decisions related to safety were not being made within patient care areas, but rather in facility administrative offices (O'Grady et al., 2010). A substantial disconnect was noted between patient care providers and the quality data collected to guide patient safety efforts and the achievement of sustainable outcomes (Reid & Dennison, 2011).

As changes in the complexity of the healthcare system continued to evolve, the American Association of Colleges of Nursing (AACN) began the process of reviewing the literature on practice and regulation, initiating discussions and forums, and consulting with and eliciting feedback from representative nursing organizations. These organizations included American Organization for Nursing Leadership (AONL), National Council of State Boards of Nursing (NCSBN), Advanced Practice Registered Nursing (APRN) groups, and health system nurse leaders. From these discussions, the AACN generated recommendations from the Task Force on Education and Regulation beginning to initiate the process of developing and creating a new nursing role (AACN, 2013).

AACN (2003) held an invitational meeting that included nursing practice and educational partners who were committed to the development and advancement of a new role. This meeting led to an assembly of the AACN Board of Directors from which the White Paper draft on the *Role of The Clinical Nurse Leader* was developed. The CNL was designated as an advanced generalist prepared at the master's level to enhance patient care delivery and outcomes. The educational requirements for the CNL were designed to bring a higher level of clinical competence and knowledge directly to the patient at the point of care. These efforts aimed to equip the CNL to address the critical need to improve patient care outcomes (AACN, 2013) while serving as a professional clinical resource for both nursing and interdisciplinary healthcare teams (Harris et al., 2018).

The AACN Board of Directors made policy and educational preparation decisions based on the recommendations set forth by the Task Force on Education and Regulation for Professional Nursing Practice 1 and 2 (TFER1 and TFER 2). These recommendations were adopted to guide AACN's process in assuring patients and families that they were being provided with a premier nursing workforce. These recommendations took into consideration the present-day and ongoing healthcare needs of the nation and the educational preparation of nurses (AACN, 2004).

The AACN accepted leadership for the CNL role and engaged stakeholders to create a legal scope of practice, credentialing process, and educational requirements and curricula (AACN, 2004). CNL curricula included 77 registered education-practice partnerships committed to piloting the new CNL role by the development of a CNL educational and collaborating practice program. These partnerships involved university deans and healthcare system chief nurse executives dedicated to supporting the development and implementation of this new graduate level nursing role.

The CNL curriculum and competencies were based on AACN's *The Essentials of Master's Education in Nursing* (AACN, 2011). The CNL competencies reflected a national, consensus-based process, which included a national expert panel and an external validation panel that represented both CNL nursing education and clinical practice. The expert panel included representation from both the Commission on Nurse Certification (CNC) and the Clinical Nurse Leader Association (CNLA). These members replicated the process utilized for the development of previous nationally recognized nursing competencies, such as those developed for clinical nurse specialist and nurse practitioner roles (AACN, 2013a, 2013b).

The CNL curricula were based on these guidelines, and programs were charged with including a minimum of 400 clinical/practice hours during the educational process with 300 of these hours designated for the final clinical immersion experience.

- Five different educational pathways support the educational process of the CNL role. An explanation of these CNL model programs is provided in Figure 6.1 (AACN, 2018b).

Model A

Master's degree program designed for Bachelor of Science in Nursing graduates

Model B

Master's degree program for Bachelor of Science in Nursing graduates that includes a post-BSN residency that awards master's credit

Model C

Master's degree program designed for individuals with a baccalaureate degree in another discipline

Model D

Master's degree program designed for Associate Degree in Nursing graduates (RN-MSN)

Model E

Postmaster's certificate program designed for individuals with a master's degree in nursing in another area of study

Figure 6.1. Models of clinical nurse leader (CNL) competencies.

Role Specifics

CNLs provide evidence-based care that effects positive patient outcomes in all clinical settings. According to AACN (2013a, 2013b), the primary qualities of a CNL include clinical leadership, risk anticipation, lateral integration of care, information manager, patent advocate, and information manager.

Populations Served

Certified CNLs practice in many different clinical settings across the lifespan. The CNL role seeks to improve patient care while working collaboratively to bridge any gaps between interdisciplinary teams and patients. These clinical areas include acute care hospitals as the highest area of practice, healthcare systems, home healthcare, homeless shelters, community outpatient centers, institutions of higher education, nonprofit organizations, rehabilitation centers, private practice, and student health centers among others (AACN, 2018b).

In Their Own Words

Mary Stachowiak, DNP, RN, CNL
Assistant Professor and Director of the MSN in Clinical Leadership Program Rutgers School of Nursing, Newark, NJ (as founding president of the Clinical Nurse Leader Association).

How did CNL programs get started?
Two of the early adapter Universities in Portland Maine and Portland Oregon held a meeting at the 2008 AACN-CNL Summit to discuss the potential of creating a professional organization for the CNLs. We were supported by two advisers: James Harris DSN, APRN-BC, MBA, CNL, and Michael Bleich PhD, RN, NEA-BC, FAAN. I was one of the 12 individuals who volunteered to put forward a proposal to the AACN. The first proposal was rejected and a second group of 12 CNLs (a couple from the original group, a few new members) formed a Steering Committee which contained the same advisers. The new proposal included a business plan, and the results of a survey sent to all CNLs to determine interest in a professional organization. The second proposal was accepted.

I unofficially chaired the Steering Committee, and we worked with a lawyer (contacted through the AACN) to become a 501c3 (charitable institution), spoke to NONPF (and anyone else we could), and received mentoring from individuals at the AACN. We wrote the mission, vision, and bylaws and formed the structure of the board of directors (BOD). We voted on the name (Clinical Nurse Leader Association), designed the logo, and purchased a URL. We established membership dues and membership benefits.

A good friend of my son's set up our first website. We hired managerial support from the AACN. We voted on the first officers (President, VP, Treasurer, and Secretary) and presented a working organization at the 2009 AACN-CNL Summit and began developing membership.

What Was Accomplished During Your Presidency?
After the formation of the organization, I remained president for 2 years. We set up a board of directors which included a practice partner, educational partner, a representative from AACN, and the CNC. We held our first annual CNL

(Continued)

conference at the Maine Medical Center in partnership with the VA (at the time, the VA was the largest employer of the CNL). We started a monthly CE program that I hosted in partnership with UMDNJ (my alma mater). We negotiated a discount for our members at the AACN-CNL Summit and for CNC merchandise. We developed a quarterly newsletter that was available on the CNLA and CNC websites. We changed our managerial support from the AACN to the CNC. We created an annual membership experience and expectations survey used to guide the 1-year and 5-year strategic plans. We had a member of the CNLA on the AACN-CNL planning committee each year. We gained independence from the AACN within 3 years. We were able to sponsor a snack at the annual summit.

What Are Future Goals for the Organization?
This changes a bit with each president. We are now the International CNLA with members in Japan. A partnership was created with a nursing journal (Bobbie Shirley, MS, RN, CNL did that). There are awards to recognize outstanding members. The goal is to grow and sustain membership and to support CNLs, as practitioners, students, or educators.

What is the Current Relationship With the AACN?
The CNLA continues to sponsor a snack at the AACN-CNL Summit, and our annual meeting is during the conference.

What Are Your Thoughts on the Competencies Adhering to the Essentials?
The AACN gathered a group to look at CNL competencies and published them in 2013. The group did a beautiful job crosswalking the MSN Essentials to the CNL competencies. There are two main paths to become a CNL. One is a post-BSN to MSN, the other is for second degree (bachelor's degree not in nursing) to MSN. Both sit for the same CNL certification. The second-degree student graduates as an entry to practice (generalist) nurse and is considered a novice nurse. Many of these graduates remain at the bedside. The post-BSN student graduates with advanced nursing practice skills. The current research on the CNL does not differentiate the outcomes of the two programs. CNL programs are accredited as part of their university accreditation. There is not, as of yet, a CNL-specific accreditation. Any accreditation must indicate adherence to the MSN Essentials. The CNC certification process does require an attestation from the university stating that at least 300 clinical hours were dedicated to a CNL practicum.

Services Provided

AACN (2013a, 2013b) defines the CNL role as "a master's educated nurse, prepared for practice across the continuum of care within any healthcare setting in today's changing healthcare environment" (p 4). The CNL oversees care coordination, provides direct patient care in complex situations, applies evidence-based practice into patient care, ensures patients benefit from the latest innovations within healthcare, evaluates patient outcomes, and assesses the risk for individual patients and cohorts. The CNL has the decision-making authority to change care planning as necessary, based on patient need. CNLs provide management of care across healthcare settings while implementing cost-saving measures, augmenting process improvement and standards of care based on evidence-based practice and nationally recognized standards (AACN, 2018b). The CNL is a generalist clinician whose role was created to augment the roles of both clinical nurse specialists and nurse practitioners whose nursing focus is more specialized. A graduate nursing education is essential due to the higher level of clinical competence needed and the knowledge required at the point of patient care and within the healthcare team.

AACN (2018a) identifies the CNL as a leader in the healthcare delivery system in all settings in which healthcare is delivered. The CNL is educationally prepared for their direct clinical leadership role at the point of patient care (**microsystem**) to ensure that care is safe, evidence-based, of high quality, and targeted toward outcomes for the specific population the CNL serves. The CNL is "not one of nursing administration or management and assumes responsibility for outcomes through the assimilation and application of evidence-based information" (*Competencies and Curricular Expectations for Clinical Nurse Leader Education and Practice* para. 4). The role of the CNL, as identified by AACN (2018a), is presented in Box 6.1.

The CNL also focuses on specific areas to improve clinical outcomes at the point of patient care. These areas are considered to be clinical leadership competencies as presented in Figure 6.2 (AACN, 2004).

AACN (2004) noted that the CNL role was established to "oversee the care coordination of a distinct group of patients and actively provides direct patient care in complex situations" (Talking Points, para. 8). The CNL collects and evaluates patient care outcomes, assesses risk, and has the ability and authority to modify patient plans of care as needed. The CNL clinician also functions

BOX 6.1

▶ FUNDAMENTAL ASPECTS OF CNL PRACTICE

- Clinical leadership for patient care practices and delivery, including the design, coordination, and evaluation of care for individuals, families, groups, and populations;

- Participation in identification and collection of care outcomes;

- Accountability for evaluation and improvement of point of care outcomes, including the synthesis of data and other evidence to evaluate and achieve optimal outcomes;

- Risk anticipation for individuals and cohorts of patients;

- Lateral integration of care for individuals and cohorts of patients;

- Design and implementation of evidence-based practice(s);

- Team leadership, management and collaboration with other health professional team members;

- Information management or the use of information systems and technologies to improve healthcare outcomes;

- Stewardship and leveraging of human, environmental, and material resources; and

- Advocacy for patients, communities, and the health professional team.

as a vital member of interdisciplinary teams by communicating, planning, and implementing care in conjunction with team members, patients, and families. This coordination fills potential patient care gaps and maintains consistent communication between teams, patients, and families in specific microsystems and upon transfer between units where lapses of care are common (Reid & Dennison, 2011). CNLs collaborate with interdisciplinary teams to identify risk analysis strategies to prevent errors or breaks in processes and the resources necessary for optimal patient care outcomes.

The CNL is a frontline patient care provider, leader, and coordinator for the entire healthcare team. The CNL applies the nursing process through the use of

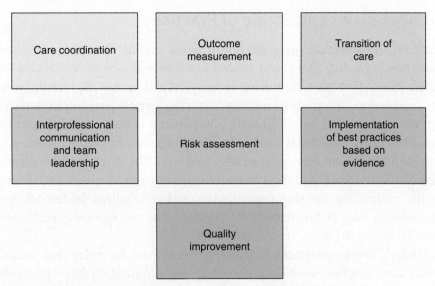

Figure 6.2. Clinical nurse leader (CNL) competencies.

strategic assessments, diagnosis, intervention, and the evaluation of the clinical area in order to guide team efforts for systematic, quality, and safety improvements (O'Grady et al., 2010).

The CNL manages individual microsystems by augmenting the roles of administration, manager, clinical nurse, provider, and case manager to decrease fragmented patient care. Metrics such as clinical nurse turnover rates, hospital-acquired conditions, patient satisfaction scores, and length of stay and readmission rates are select focal points of both CNL curricula and the role (Rankin, 2017).

Professionalism

The role of the CNL is distinctive in evaluating patient care outcomes, assessing patient risk, evaluating patient care plans, and providing input and modifications as deemed necessary. The CNL functions within the interdisciplinary healthcare team by communicating, planning, implementing, and evaluating patient care with other professional members of the healthcare team (AACN 2004).

Competencies and Scope of Practice

The CNL competencies were developed based on the *Essentials of Masters Education in Nursing (2011)* and created in collaboration with AACN and two expert panels. The master's nursing core, as defined by AACN, includes three key components. The graduate nursing core is the foundational curriculum content deemed essential for all students who pursue a master's degree in nursing regardless of the functional focus. The direct care core is essential content to provide direct patient services at an advanced level. The functional area content includes those clinical and didactic learning experiences identified and defined by the professional nursing organizations and certification bodies for specific nursing roles or functions (CNL competencies and clinical expectations) (AACN, 2013a, 2013b).

Master's degree programs that prepare graduates for roles that include direct care practice, including the CNL, are required to have graduate-level content in physiology/pathophysiology, health assessment, and pharmacology. AACN recommends that CNL curricula include three separate graduate-level courses in these content areas. From a practice perspective, it is imperative that CNLs practicing at the point of patient care have a background in these three areas (see Figure 6.3), which also facilitates

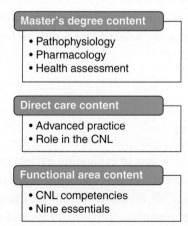

Figure 6.3. Clinical nurse leader (CNL) educational content areas.

the transition of CNL graduates into Doctor of Nursing practice programs (AACN, 2013a, 2013b).

The CNL competencies include nine essentials that were created to reflect and mirror the Master of Science in Nursing Essentials (AACN, 2013a, 2013b) (Table 6.1).

Essential 1: Background for Practice From Science and Humanities

1. Interpret patterns and trends in quantitative and qualitative data to evaluate outcomes of care within a microsystem and compare to other recognized benchmarks or outcomes, e.g., national, regional, state, or institutional data.
2. Articulate delivery process, outcomes, and care trends using a variety of media and other communication methods to the healthcare team and others.
3. Incorporate values of social justice to address healthcare disparities and bridge cultural and linguistic barriers to improve quality outcomes.
4. Integrate knowledge about social, political, economic, environmental, and historical issues into the analysis of and potential solutions to professional and healthcare issues.
5. Apply concepts of improvement science and systems theory.

Essential 2: Organizational and Systems Leadership

1. Demonstrate working knowledge of the healthcare system and its component parts, including sites of care, delivery models, payment models, and the roles of healthcare professionals, patients, caregivers, and unlicensed professionals.
2. Assume a leadership role of an interprofessional healthcare team with a focus on the delivery of patient-centered care and the evaluation of quality and cost-effectiveness across the healthcare continuum.
3. Use systems theory in the assessment, design, delivery, and evaluation of healthcare within complex organizations.
4. Demonstrate business and economic principles and practices, including cost-benefit analysis, budgeting, strategic planning, human and other resource management, marketing, and value-based purchasing.
5. Contribute to budget development at the microsystem level.

Table 6.1. CNL Competencies and Examples

Essential	Examples
Background for practice from science and humanities	Evaluates patient care outcomes of a specific cultural group to determine the bio/psycho/social influences Solves a problem by considering the social, political, environmental, and historical issues
Organizational and systems leadership	Uses systems theory to assess, design, and deliver healthcare Uses business and economic principles and practices to realign budgets
Quality improvement and safety	Assesses a population older than 65 years for their fall risk Introduces a new medication plan with educational training to minimize drug errors
Translating and integrating scholarship into practice	Leads an initiative that changes how patient education is delivered to young adults who rely heavily on technology for learning Applies evidence-based practices to a quality improvement plan
Informatics and healthcare technologies	Access state and national databases to determine the incidence of communicable diseases in their area Creates a phone app that allows nursing staff to track their patients' laboratory results
Health policy and advocacy	Provides testimony to a senate committee on the effects of the Affordable Care Act on patient's ability to afford healthcare Advocates for the creation of a CNL position on the medical-surgical unit
Interprofessional collaborating for improving patient and population health outcomes	Coordinates an interdisciplinary team of nurses, pharmacists, and home health aides to facilitate discharge plans for elderly patients Consult with a statistician to assure the priority health risks for the unit being addressed
Clinical prevention and population health for improving health	Develops a plan for health promotion that will engage the seniors in the community Proposes an afternoon program for kids in the neighborhood that will provide mental health services
Master's-level nursing practice	Leads the implementation and evaluation of educational programs offered to improve clients' nutrition and physical activity Assesses the staff's cultural competence

CNL, clinical nurse leader.

6. Evaluate the efficacy and utility of evidence-based care delivery approaches and their outcomes at the microsystem level.

7. Collaborate with healthcare professionals, including physicians, advanced practice nurses, nurse managers, and others, to plan, implement, and evaluate an improvement opportunity.

8. Participate in a shared leadership team to make recommendations for improvement at the **micro-, meso, or macrosystem** level.

Essential 3: Quality Improvement and Safety

1. Use performance measures to assess and improve the delivery of evidence-based practices and promote outcomes that demonstrate delivery of higher value care.

2. Perform a comprehensive microsystem assessment to provide the context for problem identification and action.

3. Use evidence to design and direct system improvements that address trends in safety and quality.

4. Implement quality improvement strategies based on current evidence, analytics, and risk anticipation.

5. Promote a culture of continuous quality improvement within a system.

6. Apply just culture principles and the use of safety tools, such as failure modes and effects analysis (FMEA) and root cause analysis (RCA), to anticipate, intervene, and decrease risk.

7. Demonstrate professional and effective communication skills, including verbal, nonverbal, written, and virtual abilities.

8. Evaluate patient handoffs and transitions of care to improve outcomes.

9. Evaluate medication reconciliation and administration processes to enhance the safe use of medications across the continuum of care.

10. Demonstrate the ability to develop and present a business plan, including a budget, for the implementation of a quality improvement project/initiative.

11. Use a variety of datasets, such as Hospital Consumer Assessment of Healthcare Providers and Systems (HCAHPS), nurse-sensitive indicators, National Data Nursing Quality Improvement (NDNQI), and population registries, appropriate for the patient population, setting, and organization to assess individual and population risks and care outcome.

Essential 4: Translating and Integrating Scholarship Into Practice

1. Facilitate practice change based on best available evidence that results in quality, safety, and fiscally responsible outcomes.
2. Ensure the inclusion of an ethical decision-making framework for quality improvement.
3. Implement strategies for encouraging a culture of inquiry within the healthcare delivery team.
4. Facilitate the process of retrieval, appraisal, and synthesis of evidence in collaboration with healthcare team members, including patients, to improve care outcomes.
5. Communicate to the interprofessional healthcare team, patients, and caregivers current quality and safety guidelines and nurse-sensitive indicators, including the endorsement and validation processes.
6. Apply improvement science theory and methods in performance measurement and quality improvement processes.
7. Lead change initiatives to decrease or eliminate discrepancies between actual practices and identified standards of care.
8. Disseminate changes in practice and improvements in care outcomes to internal and external audiences.
9. Design care based on outcome analysis and evidence to promote safe, timely, effective, efficient, equitable, and patient-centered care.

Essential 5: Informatics and Healthcare Technologies

1. Use information technology, analytics, and evaluation methods to
   a. Collect or access appropriate and accurate data to generate evidence for nursing practice.
   b. Provide input in the design of databases that generate meaningful evidence for practice.
   c. Collaborate to analyze data from practice and system performance.
   d. Design evidence-based interventions in collaboration with the health professional team.
   e. Examine patterns of behavior and outcomes.
   f. Identify gaps in evidence for practice.
2. Implement the use of technologies to coordinate and laterally integrate patient care within and across care settings and among healthcare providers.

3. Analyze current and proposed use of patient-care technologies, including their cost-effectiveness and appropriateness in the design and delivery of care in diverse care settings.
4. Use technologies and information systems to facilitate the collection, analysis, and dissemination of data including clinical, financial, and operational outcomes.
5. Use information and communication technologies to document patient care, advance patient education, and enhance accessibility of care.
6. Participate in ongoing evaluation, implementation, and integration of healthcare technologies, including the electronic health record (EHR).
7. Use a variety of technology modalities and media to disseminate healthcare information and communicate effectively with diverse audiences.

Essential 6: Health Policy and Advocacy

1. Describe the interaction between regulatory agency requirements (such as The Joint Commission [TJC], Centers for Medicare and Medicaid Services [CMS], or Healthcare Facilities Accreditation Program [HFAP]), quality, fiscal, and value-based indicators.
2. Articulate the contributions and synergies of the CNL with other nursing and interprofessional team member roles to policy makers, employers, healthcare providers, consumers, and other healthcare stakeholders.
3. Advocate for policies that leverage social change, promote wellness, improve care outcomes, and reduce costs.
4. Advocate for the integration of the CNL within care delivery systems, including new and evolving models of care.

Essential 7: Interprofessional Collaboration for Improving Patient and Population Health Outcomes

1. Create an understanding and appreciation among healthcare team members of similarities and differences in role characteristics and contributions of nursing and other team members.
2. Advocate for the value and role of the CNL as a leader and member of interprofessional healthcare teams.
3. Facilitate collaborative, interprofessional approaches and strategies in the design, coordination, and evaluation of patient-centered care.
4. Facilitate the lateral integration of healthcare services across the continuum of care with the overall objective of influencing, achieving, and sustaining high-quality care.

5. Demonstrate a leadership role in enhancing group dynamics and managing group conflicts.
6. Facilitate team decision-making through the use of decision tools and convergent and divergent group process skills, such as SWOT, Pareto, and brainstorming.
7. Assume a leadership role, in collaboration with other interprofessional team members, to facilitate transitions across care settings to support patients and families and reduce avoidable recidivism to improve care outcomes.

Essential 8: Clinical Prevention and Population Health for Improving Health

1. Demonstrate the ability to engage the community and social service delivery systems that recognize new models of care and health services delivery.
2. Participate in the design, delivery, and evaluation of clinical prevention and health promotion services that are patient centered and culturally appropriate.
3. Monitor the outcomes of comprehensive plans of care that address the health promotion and disease prevention needs of patient populations.
4. Apply public health concepts to advance equitable and efficient preventive services and policies that promote population health.
5. Engage in partnerships at multiple levels of the health system to ensure effective coordination, delivery, and evaluation of clinical prevention and health promotion interventions and services across care environments.
6. Use epidemiological, social, ecological, and environmental data from local, state, regional, and national sources to draw inferences regarding the health risks and status of populations to promote and preserve health and healthy lifestyles.
7. Use evidence in developing and implementing teaching and coaching strategies to promote and preserve health and healthy lifestyles in patient populations.
8. Provide leadership to the healthcare team to promote health, facilitate self-care management, optimize patient engagement, and prevent future decline including progression to higher levels of care and readmissions.
9. Assess organization-wide emergency preparedness plans and the coordination with the local, regional, and National Incident Management System (NIMS).

Essential 9: Master's-Level Nursing Practice

1. Conduct a holistic assessment and comprehensive physical examination of individuals across the lifespan.
2. Assess actual and anticipated health risks to individuals and populations.
3. Demonstrate effective communication, collaboration, and interpersonal relationships with members of the care delivery team across the continuum of care.
4. Facilitate modification of nursing interventions based on risk anticipation and other evidence to improve healthcare outcomes.
5. Demonstrate the ability to coach, delegate, and supervise healthcare team members in the performance of nursing procedures and processes with a focus on safety and competence.
6. Demonstrate stewardship, including an awareness of global environmental, health, political, and geo-economic factors, in the design of patient care.
7. Facilitate the lateral integration of evidence-based care across settings and among care providers to promote quality, safe, and coordinated care.
8. Facilitate transitions of care and safe handoffs between healthcare settings and providers.
9. Evaluate the effectiveness of health teaching by self and others.
10. Facilitate the implementation of evidence-based and innovative interventions and care strategies for diverse populations.
11. Design appropriate interventions using surveillance data and infection control principles to limit healthcare–acquired infections (HAI) at all points of care
12. Advocate for patients within the healthcare delivery system to effect quality, safe, and value-based outcomes.
13. Collaborate in the development of community partnerships to establish health promotion goals and implement strategies to address those needs.
14. Evaluate the care of at-risk populations across the lifespan by identifying and implementing programs that address specialized needs.
15. Engage individuals and families to make quality of life decisions, including palliative and end-of-life decisions.

16. Assess an individual's and group's readiness and ability to make decisions and develop, comprehend, and follow a plan of care.
17. Assess the level of cultural awareness and sensitivity of healthcare providers as a component of the evaluation of care delivery.
18. Demonstrate coaching skills, including self-reflection, to support new and experienced interdisciplinary team members in exploring opportunities for improving care processes and outcomes.
19. Use coaching techniques to assist individuals in developing insights and skills to improve their current health status and function.

Certification

Certification as a CNL is provided through the Commission on Nurse Certification (CNC), which was established in 2007 as a certifying autonomous arm of the AACN. CNC oversees initial and renewal certification to ensure those pursuing certification have met the accepted standards of practice as a CNL. The CNC is responsible for the validity, reliability, and legal defensibility of the CNL certification program (AACN, 2018b).

CNC (2018) asserts that the CNL certification is based upon a national standard of requisite knowledge and experiences, thereby assisting employers, the public, and healthcare professionals in the assessment of the CNL role. Earning a CNL certification validates a high level of professional achievement and exhibits commitment to the profession, demonstrates proficiency and a broad base of knowledge beyond RN licensure, proves that the CNL has set standards and knowledge of the profession, assures the public that the CNL is well prepared for safe practice, and promotes lifelong learning and professional development (AACN, 2018b).

CNL-certified professionals demonstrate proficiency in the CNL content and are committed to ongoing professional development to maintain the certification. The designation as a CNL demonstrates that board-certified nurses convey graduate-level clinical knowledge and competencies to the patient's point of care while serving as an important resource for the entire interdisciplinary healthcare team.

In Their Own Words

Veronica Rankin, MSN, NP-C, CNL, RN-BC, CMSRN

The key points in understanding my role are… My role as the Clinical Nurse Leader Coordinator at Carolinas Medical Center is to ensure that the practice of the Clinical Nurse Leader (CNL) is aligned with the White Paper created by the AACN concerning the role. I ensure that while our group of CNLs serve as the master's-prepared advanced generalist of healthcare, ensuring that care is evidence based and effective in improving patient outcomes, that we also stay true to the purpose of the role. It can be difficult at times to be a pioneer in a new role designed to serve as the troubleshooter in an area saturated with silo-work, variability, and pressure to work to the highest level of efficiency despite the availability of resources. This role requires assertiveness and a tenacious attitude toward rejecting the status quo of mediocre care quality. The key points in understanding my role is to grasp the fact that the CNL is the change agent of healthcare, serving as the guardian of the nursing profession, coaching and mentoring at the point of care to ensure the best outcome for the patient population.

What keeps me coming back every day is… There are a few aspects that keep me coming back every day to this role. The first aspect is the fact that I know that patients depend on nursing to holistically nourish their spirit as well as their physical body. As a nurse, I believe that we are blessed with the opportunity to be there for someone who is experiencing the most frightening, vulnerable moments in their lives that they may or may not live through. I know that our ministry is one of the most important with the highest level of responsibility, trust despite the unknown. The addiction of being there for my patient so that they will not feel or die alone is indescribable, and despite my worst day, it keeps me coming back for more. The second aspect that keeps me coming back for more is my faith in the profession of nursing. I sincerely believe that without nurses, healthcare would fail. I take pride in knowing that I serve beside the strongest care providers in the world who provide top quality care despite the lack of resources, time, and oftentimes the energy to do so. I serve with those who routinely put the needs of their patients or coworkers before their own simply because of their human responsibility. I serve with those who give their all during their work shift and then go home to continue to give to their family, friends, and community without a second thought. I am extremely proud to say that I am a nurse and that keeps me coming back every day for more.

(Continued)

My greatest challenge is… My greatest challenge is knowing that despite our best effort, we cannot fix everyone and we cannot solve every problem for our patients. In more than 14 years of nursing, there have been many times that I have walked out of patient's rooms praying for them and hoping for a cure for their situation. Unfortunately, in some situations, our best efforts cannot change the inevitable. This challenge is probably the hardest for any healthcare provider. What amazes me throughout this challenge is the patient who never gives up faith that things will get better or those determined to enjoy the life they are dealt. That always makes this challenge easier to deal with and I try to share that perspective with everyone I encounter.

I wish someone had told me… I wish someone had told me prior to nursing school that nurses give the most with the least. I wish someone would have told me that nursing will teach you the communication skills that you never knew you had. I wish someone would have told me that there will be days that you will depend on your nursing colleagues to get you through. I wish someone would have told me that there will be days that you will feel that you have nothing else to give but one patient will refill your cup in a matter of seconds. I wish someone would have told me that nursing is much like parenthood, a lot of hard work and deep-seeded satisfaction resulting in a legacy of ripples that reach farther than the mind can imagine. Had someone told me these things, I would have run even faster toward this profession than I did.

I need to be a lifelong learner because… I am the healthcare provider that will touch the patients of today and tomorrow. My patients depend on me to remain up-to-date on research and evidence-based practice to save their lives and/or expedite their recovery. My less experienced colleagues depend on me to help coach and mentor them to become better clinicians. My equally or more experienced colleagues depend on me to hone all facets of my nursing experience and knowledge base to carry the load in providing top quality care to an aging, higher acuity patient population. My quality of life depends on my continued learning and developing both professionally and personally. I believe that when you stop learning, you become obsolete. That is not the path I have chosen for myself or any colleague I encounter.

Another point to understand is… Nursing is truly a calling. Although many take on the job role, everyone cannot truly be a nurse within their hearts. Nursing is a ministry that is felt from within. It drives individuals to put themselves second in order to ensure the well-being of another. Recognition of these points will help bridge the gap in our imperfect healthcare world with the hope that we are progressing toward perfection every day for the sake of those that depend on us.

Upon successful completion of a CNL master's or post-master's in a nursing program with a CNL curriculum from an accredited university, potential candidates or faculty members teaching in a CNL curriculum are qualified to take the CNL examination. Successful completion of the examination provides the examinee with the opportunity to use the CNL credential and become certified as a CNL for a 5-year time period.

The CNL certification examination is a computer-based, three-hour examination that reflects the CNL job analysis study guided by the CNC and Schroeder Measurement Technologies, Inc (SMT). The National Commission for Certifying Agencies (NCAA) accredits the CNC CNL certification program (AACN, 2018b).

A scientific research-based job analysis study is conducted every 2 years by both CNC and SMT and includes a literature review to develop a listing of the knowledge, skills, and abilities essential to CNL nursing practice (CNC, 2017). The research-based job analysis also explores and profiles the role of the CNL, the core skills for the role, and competencies prevalent among CNLs across a variety of experiences. The core skills are established based on information related to training, frequency, and importance of practice, education level, practice settings, and clinical locations. Job analysis advisory committee members are then chosen to create a list of knowledge, skills, and abilities representative of the CNL role.

Beta testing is conducted to ensure analysis of responses is reflective of CNL practice across clinical settings, geographical locations, and responsibilities of the role. A content examination outline is then established based on the responses from the beta testing to provide future examinees with a certification blueprint for individual examination preparation.

The examination-testing period is open four times per year and coincides with the completion of academic semesters. The examination may be administered at registered schools of nursing or at designated testing centers upon receipt of approval from CNL program directors. Notification of examination results occurs immediately after completion of the examination and is reported as a pass or fail result. Candidates who are unsuccessful receive a diagnostic breakdown of the examination to identify content area for future studying for subsequent examinations. Candidates who are unsuccessful are required to test in future testing cycles to allow additional study time of weak content areas (Box 6.2).

BOX 6.2

▶ THE CNL CONTENT OUTLINE AS IDENTIFIED BY THE CNC (2017)

I. Nursing leadership (32% of examination)

A. Horizontal leadership (7% of examination)

1. Apply leadership change and complexity theories.

2. Apply strategies to guide the collaborative team to use clinical judgment to make safe patient care decisions.

3. Facilitate delegation of patient care coordination activities.

4. Appraise and evaluate coordinated care activities.

5. Demonstrate accountability for microsystems healthcare outcomes.

6. Practice as a role model for other healthcare providers; including coaching and mentoring the healthcare team.

7. Coordinate evaluation and update plans of care at an advanced level collaboratively with the interprofessional team and the patient.

8. Organize a framework for systematic collaborative team practices to address the complexity of patient care issues.

9. Serve as a partner and leader in the interprofessional health team.

10. Manage and lead group processes to meet care objectives and complete healthcare team responsibilities.

11. Develop effective working relationships within an interprofessional team to influence microsystem outcomes.

12. Demonstrate higher order critical thinking and problem-solving skills.

B. Healthcare advocacy (6% of examination)

1. Initiate partnerships to identify health disparities, establish health promotion goals, and implement strategies to address those concerns.

2. Interface between the patient and the healthcare delivery system to protect the rights of patients and to affect quality outcomes; knowledge of patient rights and responsibilities.

3. Ensure that patients, families, and communities are well informed in creating a patient-centered plan of care.

4. Negotiate and advocate for the nursing profession, the CNL role, and the interprofessional team to healthcare providers, policy makers, and consumers.

5. Identify and propose microsystem resources to meet the needs of target populations.

6. Explain healthcare issues and concerns to key stakeholders including elected and appointed officials, policy organizations, and healthcare consumers.

7. Translate appropriate healthcare information to advocate for informed healthcare decision-making.

8. Recommend improvements in the institution or healthcare system and the nursing profession.

9. Advocate for patients, particularly the most vulnerable.

C. Implementation of the CNL role (7% of examination)

1. Demonstrate professional identity and practice in developing the CNL role.

2. Explain the capacity of CNL practice to improve healthcare processes and outcomes.

3. Exhibit qualities of a microsystem leader within and across interprofessional teams.

4. Appraise and apply current and new CNL evidence, competence, and practice.

(Continued)

5. Synthesize CNL practice outcomes for dissemination at system, regional, national, or international level.

6. Collaborate with a network of CNL professionals at the system, regional, national, or international level.

7. Coordinate the healthcare of patients across the care continuum.

8. Integrate an interprofessional approach to discuss strategies to identify and acquire resources for patient populations. Coordinate and perform risk analysis using appropriate evidence-based tools to predict patient risk and safety issues within and across microsystems.

9. Apply care management skills and principles to provide and coordinate patient care within and across specific episodes of illness and throughout the care continuum.

10: Manage, monitor, and influence the microsystem environment to foster health and quality of care across the care continuum.

11. Apply systems and organization theory in the design, delivery, and evaluation of healthcare delivery across the care continuum.

D. Patient assessment (3% of examination)

1. Perform an advanced comprehensive assessment of the patient across the lifespan (e.g., health history, culture, socioeconomic status, spirituality, health literacy).

2. Perform an advanced assessment of microsystems across the care continuum to determine patient population care needs.

E. Ethics (2% of examination)

1. Apply patient-centered ethical decision-making frameworks to clinical situations that incorporate moral concepts, professional ethics, and law.

2. Apply legal and ethical guidelines to advocate for patient well-being and preferences.

3. Identify and analyze common ethical dilemmas including the impact on patient care and outcomes.

4. Evaluate ethical decision-making from both a personal and organizational perspective and analyze how these two perspectives may create conflicts of interest.

5. Collaborate with the ethics committee and recognize their role in healthcare delivery.

II. Clinical outcomes management (23% of examination)

A. Illness/disease management (9% of examination)

1. Coordinate the provision and management of care at the microsystem level and across the care continuum.

2. Evaluate care for patients across the lifespan with particular emphasis on health promotion and risk reduction services.

3. Identify patient problems that require intervention, with special focus on those problems amenable to nursing intervention.

4. Evaluate and determine readiness, needs, and interventions for safe transition of care.

5. Design and modify patient care based on analysis of outcomes, evidence-based knowledge, and patient's goals of care.

6. Analyze microsystems of care and outcome datasets to anticipate patient risk and improve quality of care delivery.

7. Apply theories of chronic illness care and population health management to patient and families.

8. Integrate community resources, social networks, and decision support mechanisms into care management.

9. Recognize differences in responses to illness and therapies based on patient's cultural, ethnic, socioeconomic, linguistic, religious, and lifestyle preferences.

10. Identify disease patterns and their implications on patient's activation for self-care and on-going care.

(Continued)

11. Use advanced knowledge of pathophysiology, assessment, and pharmacology to anticipate illness progression and response to therapy and to guide, teach, and engage patients and families regarding care.

12. Use knowledge of cost and affordability issues in managing patient illness/disease across the care continuum.

13. Synthesize literature and research findings as the foundation for the design of interventions for illness and disease management.

14. Coordinate and implement education programs for patients and health professionals.

15. Identify and interpret epidemiological patterns in order to manage illness and disease.

B. Health promotion and disease prevention and injury reduction/prevention management (9% of examination)

1. Collaborate with interprofessional team members to promote health and/or prevent disease.

2. Employ strategies to engage patients in therapeutic partnerships with interprofessional team members for disease management and self-care activation.

3. Identify and/or modify interventions based on evidence to meet specific patient needs for health promotion and disease prevention.

4. Design and implement interventions to modify risk factors and promote engagement in healthy lifestyles for diverse populations.

5. Assess protective, predictive, and genetic factors that influence the health of patients.

6. Develop clinical and health promotion programs for patient populations to reduce risk, prevent disease, and prevent disease sequelae, particularly related to chronic illness.

7. Recognize the need for and develop community partnerships to establish risk reduction strategies to address social and public health issues.

8. Incorporate cultural definitions of health into health promotion and disease prevention strategies.

9. Incorporate theories and research in creating patient engagement strategies to promote and preserve health and healthy lifestyles.

C. Healthcare policy (5% of examination)

1. Recognize the effect of healthcare policy on health promotion, risk reduction, and disease and injury prevention with emphasis on vulnerable populations.

2. Recognize the interactive effect of economics on national/global health policy related to health outcomes.

3. Analyze the effect of local, state, and/or national healthcare policy as they apply to the standards of care and scope of practice in the microsystem.

4. Identify the influence of regulatory guidelines and quality controls within the healthcare delivery system.

III. Care environment management (45% of examination)

A. Knowledge management

1. Collect data that document the characteristics, conditions, and outcomes for various patient groups.

2. Apply knowledge of technology, equipment, treatment regimens, or medication therapies to anticipate risk.

3. Compare and evaluate trends of institutional and unit data to national benchmarks.

4. Identify variations in clinical outcomes among various groups to determine where nurses have the greatest impact at the microsystem level.

5. Synthesize data, information, and knowledge to evaluate and achieve optimal patient outcomes.

6. Integrate assessment data into information management systems for decision support.

(Continued)

7. Analyze and disseminate microsystem data that impact health outcomes.

8. Employ strategies to engage the interprofessional team to impact healthcare outcomes.

9. Distinguish the impact of health literacy of patient engagement and activation for self-care.

B. Healthcare systems/organization

1. Apply knowledge of teamwork to manage change and disseminate information at the systems level.

2. Critique and/or modify existing policies and procedures based on current evidence.

3. Implement system-based strategies that decrease healthcare disparities.

4. Apply theories of systems thinking to address problems and develop solutions.

5. Distinguish how healthcare delivery systems are organized and their effect on patient care.

6. Identify the economic, legal, and political factors that influence healthcare delivery.

C. Interprofessional communication and collaboration skills

1. Analyze patterns of communication and chain of command that impact care within the interprofessional team and across settings.

2. Apply concepts of communication skills including critical listening during assessment, intervention, evaluation, and education of patients, families, and the healthcare team.

3. Employ effective negotiation skills.

4. Employ appropriate communication techniques and strategies that address social, political, economic, environmental, technological, and historical issues.

5. Utilize interprofessional communication, collaboration, and group process concepts to meet care objectives and complete healthcare responsibilities.

6. Translate and interpret data for the patients, families, and the healthcare team.

7. Communicate effectively in a variety of written and spoken formats.

8. Construct relationships with interprofessional team including management and administration.

9. Incorporate knowledge of cultural differences to bridge cultural and linguistic barrier.

10. Integrate emotional intelligence in communication and collaboration with patients, families, and the healthcare team.

IV. Recognize and utilize the roles and responsibilities of the interprofessional team

A. Team coordination

1. Perform, teach, delegate, and manage skilled nursing procedures in the context of safety.

2. Demonstrate effectiveness in group interactions, particularly in skills necessary to interact and collaborate with other members of the interprofessional team.

3. Evaluate underlying assumptions and relevant evidence that influence patient and interprofessional team behavior.

4. Establish and maintain effective working relationships within an interprofessional, multicultural team to make ethical decisions

5. Facilitate group processes to meet care objectives to ensure completion of interprofessional team responsibilities.

6. Identify areas in which a conflict of interest may arise and propose resolutions or actions to resolve/prevent the conflict.

7. Promote a positive and healthy work environment and a culture of retention.

(Continued)

8. Incorporate patient/family/interprofessional team input to design, coordinate, and evaluate plans of care.

B. Quality improvement and safety

1. Employ quality improvement methods in evaluating individual and aggregate patient care.

2. Evaluate healthcare outcomes through the acquisition of data and the questioning of inconsistencies.

3. Develop and implement the redesign of patient care utilizing assessment methodologies including but not limited to gap analysis, FMEA, RCA, plan-do-study-act (PDSA) cycles, and microsystem assessment.

4. Gather, analyze, and synthesize data related to risk anticipation to reduce risk and maintain patient safety.

5. Employ strategies to guide the interprofessional team in quality improvement activities within the microsystem to impact the meso- and macrosystems.

C. Evidence-based practice

1. Create framework within the microsystem to integrate patient and family preferences, interprofessional clinical expertise, and best evidence into clinical decisions.

2. Develop foundations for assessment and clinical decisions by applying evidence-based practice.

3. Synthesize quantitative or qualitative evidence for critical thinking and decision-making to achieve optimal patient outcomes.

4. Select relevant sources of evidence to meet specific needs of patients, microsystems, or communities when planning care.

5. Use current evidence to improve patient care.

6. Identify relevant outcomes and measurement strategies that will improve patient outcomes and promote cost-effective care.

D. Healthcare finance and economics

1. Propose cost-effective strategies and/or interventions to the interprofessional team that improve efficiency and patient care outcomes.

2. Serve as a steward for the environmental, human, and material resources while coordinating patient care.

3. Evaluate the fiscal context in which practice occurs.

4. Identify high-cost/high-volume activities to benchmark costs nationally and across care settings.

5. Apply ethical principles in regard to healthcare delivery relating to healthcare financing and economics.

6. Identify the impact of financial policies on healthcare delivery and patient outcomes.

7. Interpret the impact of both public and private reimbursement policies that may affect patient care decisions.

8. Evaluate the effect of healthcare financing on access to care and patient outcomes.

9. Examine current healthcare economic concepts including but not limited to return on investment (ROI), value-based purchasing (VBP), bundled payments, and basic marketing strategies.

E. Healthcare informatics

1. Assess, critique, and analyze information sources.

2. Design care utilizing informatics and patient care technology.

3. Apply multiple sources of systems data in designing processes for care delivery.

4. Evaluate clinical information systems in order to provide feedback related to efficient and accurate documentation.

5. Apply ethical principles in the use of information systems.

6. Evaluate the impact of new technologies on patients, families, and healthcare delivery.

(Continued)

7. Identify and assess the relationships between information systems, accurate communication, error reduction, and healthcare system operation.

8. Analyze and disseminate healthcare information among the interprofessional team and across the care continuum.

9. Validate accuracy of consumer-provided information regarding culturally relevant health issues from multiple sources.

10. Utilize technology for health promotion and disease prevention.

11. Collaborate with quality improvement and information technology teams to design and implement processes for improving patient outcomes.

12. Utilize current technology to anticipate patient risk.

13. Demonstrate to other healthcare providers the efficient and appropriate use of healthcare technologies to maximize healthcare outcomes.

14. Access, critique, and analyze information from multiple sources (CNC, 2017).

Continuing Education

CNL certification renewals occur after 5 years, and according to CNC (2018), recertification ensures the public that the certified CNL continues to maintain current and relevant knowledge of the CNL role. Requirements for renewal include current RN licensure; professional practice attestation of a minimum of 2000 hr in the prior 5-year certification period; a minimum of 50 contact hours that supports the CNL role, job analysis, and competencies (hours earned to renew RN license accepted); completion of a survey about current role responsibilities; and individual preparation for random audits of records and continuing education records by electronic or hard copy format (AACN, 2018b).

In Their Own Words

Bobbi Shirley, MS, RN, CNL, OCN

The key points in understanding my role are... I graduated from a post-BSN master's degree and became certified as a CNL in 2009 (first certification offered in 2007). As a post-BSN CNL, I entered the workforce with expertise in my specialty. Over the years I continued to gain expertise in oncology and advanced nursing skills that have allowed me to clinically manage the patients on my unit to improve their quality of care. As part of my role within the microsystem, I follow the complex oncology patients throughout the hospital. For example, I administer all chemotherapy desensitizations in the ICU and I am appraised of all clinical trials/protocols. Most often, complex patients are referred to me by their provider. Although I primarily follow the complex oncology patient, nononcology providers often request that I follow their complex patients too, and when I am able, I do. I have an excellent relationship with the providers who often call me for a clinical update, a review of the consultant's input, and any suggestions that I have. I bring in other healthcare team members as needed. I coach providers in comprehensive documentation of the diagnosis, diagnostics, patient status, and the clinical plan. I am involved in the discharge plan of the complex patient and complete postdischarge phone calls to improve transitions of care.

I work closely with the staff to model and mentor best practice. I continuously review and compare our current practice to best standards of practice to maintain the highest levels of quality for the oncology population. The staff rely on my clinical knowledge, and they now search the literature for best practices independently, which is something that I am most proud of. I am there to advocate for the patient and to meet with the healthcare team.

My role as a CNL is amazing; staff come to me with issues, and using my advanced skill set, I resolve them. I make sure that I regroup with the staff with the good, or the bad, to close any communication gaps. The patients rely on me to manage their care, see the big picture, and assure accurate communication within (and beyond) the healthcare team.

The patients are grateful for my presence. I speak to them to improve their healthcare literacy and help them understand their plan of care. They know that I will not only evaluate their understanding, but their clinical status and their medical plan. This is well beyond the typical oncology navigator. I initiate difficult conversations with healthcare providers/team member's and families regarding the overall plan of care and the patient's goals. Bottom line, I keep patients safe. I have the opportunity to sit with patients and families to explain

(Continued)

their plan of care, their goals, and their disease process. I am able to connect the patient to internal and external resources. For example, one recent patient had their electricity cut off, I called the electric company and had it turned back on. It was a small thing to do, but for a patient who was struggling with a difficult diagnosis, it made a huge difference.

Beyond the management of the individual patient, I also complete a risk assessment for the patient population. This allows me to keep an eye on trends in quality and risk.

I proudly take responsibility for quality outcomes and find that my skill set is often appreciated by the macrosystem, as I am often pulled into committees to provide loop closure.

Quality is my passion, as it is with all of the CNLs at Maine Medical Center (MMC). All CNLs at MMC are heavily involved in quality not only on a unit level but also hospital wide. My day begins with reviewing all quality risk factors for my unit. I review all central lines, Foley catheters, pressure ulcers, skin assessment scales, falls, bowel movements, and trend blood sugars greater than 180 and readmissions within the month. I then go out to the nurses and follow up to ensure precaution standards are in place. I take a deeper dive into each of these single data points. For example, if a patient is going to a nursing facility, they must have had a bowel movement within the last 24 hours. Falling short of this quality standard results in a delay in discharge affecting the organization's bed flow. I complete a root cause analysis on all areas of quality, for example, I am currently working on an RCA for a catheter-associated urinary tract infection (CAUTI). This will include discussions with nurses and CNAs for their input. During the RCA process, I take the opportunity to educate staff on the standards of practice for catheter care, including the importance of removing them ASAP. I then present to the hospital quality interprofessional council my findings and actions. They have indicated that they were impressed with the thoroughness of my process. I love presenting my work to others because it stimulates conversations and produces changes in hospital policies. I enjoy challenging hospital policies because I feel they should be reviewed frequently by the latest literature.

What keeps me coming back every day is… I work closely with the complex patients and staff. I check in daily with patients; seeing them move seamlessly through the healthcare system just makes my day. I answer all their questions and hold providers and healthcare professionals accountable for their actions and for the care that my patients receive. Everyone (nurse and provider) are juggling many patients and many responsibilities. Despite doing their best, care remains fragmented. I help the staff and providers to keep the patients from falling through the cracks. I have had both patients and providers tell me

(Continued)

that every patient should have a CNL. I have to agree—the CNL is the thread that binds the patients to the rest of the healthcare team. We see the patient holistically, as well as part of a community that they will return to. It has been my observation that without CNL support, patients return to the hospital within 30 days (often much sooner). This indicates poorly coordinated care and an inadequate discharge plan and impacts the patients' quality of life. It also results in insurance reimbursement issues.

My greatest challenge is… I love my job, but often work beyond my 40 hours per week (Monday through Friday) resulting in a work-life balance challenge.

I wish someone had told me… The challenge, of course, is that as a salaried employee, I am not reimbursed for the extra hours. It would be beneficial if CNLs could bill insurance companies for the care coordination they provide, but unfortunately, that is not the case (but I can always hope).

I need to be a lifelong learner because… It keeps me honest and up-to-date with my practice. I am forward thinking, which is a by-product of past experiences and previous education. I need to maintain my clinical expertise to assure that my patients receive the absolute best care, which is, of course, a major motivator. I am always thinking ahead for my patients and staff, looking to see what comes next.

As a previous president of the Clinical Nurse Leader Association (CNLA), I had the opportunity to see the "big picture" at the national level. Without a doubt, that experience has assured that I should stay abreast of factors (internal and external) that will impact my patients and my institution.

Another point to understand is… Knowing the structure of your organization, microsystem versus macrosystem, is key. Many CNLs are great in their microsystem, but it is vital for success to have macrosystem understanding and interaction. You know you have succeeded when you are asked to be on several macrosystem projects. A CNL has the full picture of the overall design of the healthcare system and can move the institutional goals to microsystem practice. The support of the executive team is tied to the success of the position.

"The CNL assumes accountability for patient care outcomes through the assimilation and application of evidence-based information to design, implement, and evaluate patient plan of care" (Harris et al., 2018). This is my elevator speech.

Summary

The CNL role and unique skill set have been found to positively impact patient and family satisfaction, clinical performance, and financial and safety outcomes. The research demonstrates that the CNL has the knowledge and skill set to sustain these positive performance metrics over time with a significant decrease in near misses, medical errors, infection rates, medication errors, length of stay, infection rates, and cost. The CNL is committed to ongoing clinical improvements to maintain positive nursing practice outcomes by supporting advocacy, education, and the implementation of competent patient care.

Chapter Highlights

This chapter provides an overview of the following:

- The CNL role was created by an interprofessional team led by AACN to address the issues with patient safety.
- The CNL role functions at the microsystem level to assist nursing staff and patients to improve health outcomes.
- The competencies of the CNL are aligned with the AACN Essentials.
- Upon graduation, CNLs are qualified to sit for national certification.
- CNLs do not need a second RN license to practice to their full capacity.

References

American Association of Colleges of Nursing (AACN). (2011). *The essentials of master's education.* http://www.aacnnursing.org/Portals/42/Publications/MastersEssentials11.pdf

American Association of Colleges of Nursing. (2013a). *Competencies and curricular expectations for clinical nurse leader education and practice. White paper on the education and role of the clinical nurse leader.* www.aacnnursing.org/News-Information/Position-Statements-White-Papers/CNL

American Association of Colleges of Nursing. (2017). *CNC publications & resources.* http://www.aacnnursing.org/CNL-Certification/CNC-Publications-Resources

American Association of Colleges of Nursing. (2018). *Commission of nurse certification (CNC).* https://www.aacnnursing.org/CNL-Certification/Commission-of-Nurse-Certification

American Association of Colleges of Nursing. (2018a). *Clinical nurse leader.* http://www.aacnnursing.org/CNL

American Association of Colleges of Nursing. (2018b). *CNL certification*. http://www.aacnnursing.org/CNL-Certification

American Association of Colleges of Nursing. (2013b). *Competencies and curricular expectations for clinical nurse leader education and practice*. http://www.aacnnursing.org/Portals/42/AcademicNursing/CurriculumGuidelines/CNL-Competencies-October-2013.pdf

Harris, J. L., Roussel, L. A., & Thomas, P. L. (2018). *Initiating and sustaining the clinical nurse leader role: A practical guide* (3rd ed.). Jones and Bartlett Learning.

Institute of Medicine Committee on Quality Health Care in America. (2000). *To err is human: Building a safer health system*. National Academy Press. https://doi.org/10.17226/9728

Institute of Medicine (US) Committee on the Health Professions Education Summit. (2003). *Health professions education: A bridge to quality*. National Academies Press.

Kohn, L. T., Corrigan, J. M., & Donaldson, M. S. (Eds). (2000). Institute of Medicine (US) Committee on Quality of Health Care in America. *Errors in health care: A leading cause of death and injury*. National Academies Press.

O'Grady, T. P., Clark, J. S., & Wiggins, M. S. (2010). The case for clinical nurse leaders: Guiding practice into the 21st century. *Nurse Leader, 8*(1), 37–41. https://www.nurseleader.com/article/S1541-4612(09)00291-2/abstract

Rankin, G. S. V. (2017). Clinical nurse leaders: Fulfilling the promise of the role. *Medsurg Nursing, 26*(1), 21–24, 32.

Reid, K. B., & Dennison, P. (2011). The clinical nurse leader (CNL)(R): Point-of-care safety clinician. *Online Journal of Issues in Nursing, 16*(3), 4. https://doi.org/10.3912/OJIN.Vol16No03Man04

PART THREE

Advanced Practice Registered Nurse Roles

7

Overview of Clinicians

Cindy Weston

LEARNING OBJECTIVES

After completing this chapter, you will be able to:

1. Provide a historical overview of the four APRN roles.

2. Compare and contrast core competences of the four APRN roles.

3. Describe the impact of prescriptive authority on APRN roles.

4. Review the principles of reimbursement with an overview of billing and coding.

KEY TERMS

Billing: Submission of a claim to a third-party payer to receive reimbursement for treatment and services.

Coding: A standardized process of assigning alphanumeric codes that represent healthcare diagnoses, procedures, services, and equipment.

Collaboration: Professional partnership in a team that utilizes the strengths of each person to work toward a common goal. May be a legal definition of a physician-nurse practitioner relationship in some states.

Controlled substance: Medication or substance considered to have abuse or dependency potential.

Delegation: Permission granted from a physician to a nurse practitioner for the performance of certain professional activities, such as the prescription of medication. May be a legal definition of a physician-nurse practitioner relationship in some states.

Full-practice authority: The allowance of a nurse practitioner to evaluate, diagnose, initiate treatment, and prescribe pharmacotherapy under the exclusive licensure of the state board of nursing.

Legend drugs: Medications and substances that require a prescription for dispensing.

Population focus: The particular area of concentration in a nurse practitioner's educational program and practice.

Prescriptive authority: Independent prescribing of medications, equipment, supplies, devices, treatments, and services.

Reimbursement: Compensation after healthcare services are rendered.

Introduction

This chapter provides an overview of the four advanced practice registered nurse (APRN) clinician roles: nurse practitioner (NP; see Chapter 8), certified nurse midwife (CNM; see Chapter 9), certified registered nurse anesthetist (CRNA; see Chapter 10), and clinical nurse specialist (CNS; see Chapter 11). Topics covered include a brief history of the different roles, educational preparation, core competencies, prescriptive authority, and reimbursement. Beginning with Lillian Wald and the Henry Street Settlement in the late 1890s, individuals have advanced nursing practice to meet the needs of the patients they serve. Over time, the nursing profession has distinguished itself with four roles of APRNs (Figure 7.1).

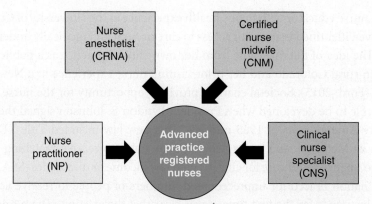

Figure 7.1. Advanced practice registered nurse (APRN) roles.

Nurse Practitioner

The strength of a nurse practitioner (NP) is a focus on health, wellness, and holistic care. The nurse practitioner blends the foundations of nursing practice and theory, which include health promotion and disease prevention, with advanced training to diagnose, prescribe, and manage acute and chronic health conditions to meet the needs of patients and populations. In 2019, there were approximately 270,000 nurse practitioners delivering care across the United States in a variety of settings (AANP, 2019). Nurse practitioners are increasing access to affordable, quality healthcare with a reported 1 billion patient visits annually in the United States (AANP, 2018). According to Loretta Ford, recognized as a creator of the role, the nurse practitioner role did not develop in response to a physician shortage but in order to increase access to care (Ford, 1979). "The nurse practitioner model of professional practice was originally designed to meet the needs of ambulatory populations to maintain health, yet there remain tremendous unmet needs in acute and long-term care settings for which nurses have the potential, opportunity, and accountability to respond" (Ford, 1979, p. 521). Indeed, the nurse practitioner role has developed with population foci to improve health and access to primary care, acute care, long-term care, mental health, specialty care, and other areas.

History and Evolution

Attempts to expand nursing practice faltered prior to the era of change in 1965 that enabled the creation of the nurse practitioner role (Collins, 2015). Dr. Loretta

Ford, a nurse educator with public health experience at the University of Colorado in Denver, identified issues with access to care in rural and medically underserved areas. The idea of the role came from her own clinical practice as a public health nurse in rural Colorado and her prior visiting nurse experience in a New Jersey ghetto (Ford, 2015). Societal changes provided opportunity for the nurse practitioner role to be developed when President Lyndon B. Johnson signed the Social Security Amendments of 1965 into law. This new law included Title XIX, later known as Medicaid, and was a provision for states to receive matching federal funds to finance healthcare for citizens with low income or disabilities (SSA, 1965). As the nation braced for unprecedented numbers of people to receive access to health insurance for the first time, it was clear that the existing system might not withstand the increased need, particularly in rural and underserved areas.

Dr. Ford, in **collaboration** with Dr. Henry Silver, a pediatrician from the University of Colorado, studied data indicating that 50% of a pediatrician's time was spent in well-child checks and 20% in minor problems (Silver & Ford, 1967). It made sense that an expanded nursing role might be able to address routine and minor issues, freeing the physician to care for patients with more complex needs. An intense 4-month program was developed with both theoretical and clinical components in the primary care of children (Silver & Ford, 1967; Silver et al., 1967). Registered nurses with a master's degree in Public Health were selected to receive advanced training and were initially called pediatric public health nurse practitioners (Ford, 1975; Silver & Ford, 1967; Time, 1966). The title was thought to be too long, so "public health" was dropped for easier use; yet, Dr. Ford felt that public health and primary care was an essential focus for the role (Ford, 1975).

Early Years

Although trained in pediatrics with a focus on health and prevention, the new nurse practitioners delivered total family-centered care (Silver et al., 1967). Two of the most important aspects of care were careful assessment and prompt referral. Dr. Silver noted, "[The nurse practitioner] doesn't have to know the specific difficulty. She simply has to know enough to say to herself, 'Oh-oh, I've listened to 3,000 hearts, and this one isn't right. This one is for the doctor'" (Time, 1966, para. 3). As graduates emerged from the program, they located their practice to areas with known barriers to care. The pediatric nurse practitioners (PNPs) were deployed to field stations, schools, and clinics in rural areas of Colorado where they maintained office hours and performed home visits (Casey, 2015; Silver et al., 1967). Time magazine (1966) called the students "a new breed of nurse."

The PNP role later expanded to include both rural and urban settings. With their strong background in public health, they focused on disease prevention and health promotion.

Among the first graduates and bilingual herself, Susan Stearly settled in the Hispanic community of Trinidad, Colorado, where only seven physicians served the region (*Time*, 1966). Her first task was to gain the trust of children and adults in the community. Within 3 months, she had 45 patients (*Time*, 1966). As she began to identify problems requiring a physician's care, she promptly referred and gained the trust of the medical community (*Time*, 1966). Like nurses before and after her, she took a holistic perspective on healthcare. The patient was treated in the context of family and community with an understanding of the broader landscape of socioeconomic stressors and social determinates of health. Then, as now, these pioneer nurse practitioners understood their work to be grounded in nursing theory, with the goal of collaborating with medical providers.

In Their Own Words

Loretta Ford, EdD, NP, FAAN
The "Mother" of the Nurse Practitioner Movement (Ligenza, 2015)

How did the nurse practitioner role begin?
The nurse practitioner role spread because the agencies had health needs for the patients they were serving. The agencies, such as the Veteran Affairs (VA), Planned Parenthood, and others took it upon themselves to prepare nurses in advance training for their particular population. This became an asset and a liability. The asset was the agencies had very good nurses familiar with the needs of the particular population, but the liability was the agencies were not choosy about academic credentials. These first nurse practitioners were high performers but because they did not have professional degrees, they were eventually exploited because they could not get into the academic programs without first obtaining a baccalaureate degree. But that group of nurses and the original agencies that prepared them deserve a tremendous amount of credit for keeping the nurse practitioner movement alive while the educators grew up. The educators eventually moved because the students demanded the nurse practitioner preparation. Early on, academia could see the applicability of nurse practitioners in various populations. The nurse practitioner role developed in response to community health needs.

(Continued)

How did the nurse practitioner role spread?

One strategy of strength Dr. Henry Silver and I developed that led to our success was communication. We were committed to writing about the role and success. When news of the nurse practitioner role got into *Time* magazine (1966), the public became aware. Public and professional communication of the nurse practitioners was important. The stories of how nurse practitioners were influencing communities helped drive the movement. These early nurse practitioners were influential and came from good programs; they were pioneers and deserve a tremendous amount of credit.

Why was the nurse practitioner role so successful?

The success (of nurse practitioners) was predicated on the emphasis of the nursing aspects of health promotion and wellness. The strength of the nurse practitioner is in the way we practice through the culture of health and wellness. We must maintain innovative nurse practitioner leaders committed to the nursing role of holistic healthcare, population and community health needs, and attention to social determinates of health. The nurse practitioner role came out of public health nursing, and it should never lose that focus of orientation toward health and wellness or self-care and empowerment with an educated populous (Figure 7.2). Health and wellness is valuable to the country. A healthy population is human capital and should be invested in with health services and education. A healthy population is creative, innovative, and productive. Health is of great economic value to our country. Healthcare is a human right and just as important as all of our rights in this country.

What opportunities are available to nurse practitioners?

Nurse practitioners have great opportunities to move out of traditional roles in entrepreneurship to meet health needs of populations creatively through technology, digitalization, and new ways of healthcare delivery. Nurse practitioners should never try to become miniphysicians or practice under a medical model focused on disease and illness. The nurse practitioners' strength is the nursing foundation. Patients must be given hope and attention with the nurse practitioner listening to what the patient determines is the problem. Although the current payment system is disease focused and mitigates against self-care, the nurse practitioner should maintain focus on health promotion and disease prevention. Nurse practitioners are not a substitute for physicians; they have some of the same skills, but practice under a nursing model focused on helping a patient's behavior change toward health. We must watch our language and not call everything "medicine" in healthcare. Adversity is not a bad thing. In adversity, you learn a lot about yourself. One of the greatest threats to the nurse practitioner role is apathy. We must stay engaged and we must always remember the most important word in nurse practitioner is *nurse*.

Written by Cindy Weston based on a personal interview with Dr. Loretta Ford.

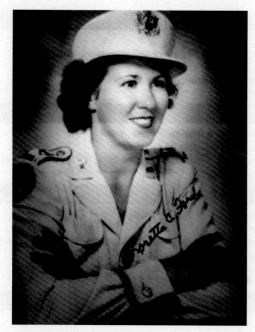

Figure 7.2. Dr. Loretta Ford, circa 1943 Army Air Corps.

Evolving Roles for Nurses

The nurse practitioner role eventually gave rise to other specializations, and the four APRN roles are presented in Figure 7.1. Among nurse practitioners (Chapter 8), much variety exists with recognized specialties in roles such as family, pediatrics (acute and primary care), adult acute, and others. Other areas also developed including CNMs (Chapter 9), CRNAs (Chapter 10), and CNSs (Chapter 11) (Figure 7.3).

Certified Nurse Midwife

Midwifery is a role that has existed since ancient times; however, nurse midwifery reports origins in Europe when nurses gained specialized training in childbearing and delivery. The role was introduced in the United States as an expansion of public health nursing through the Frontier Nursing Service in 1925 (Keeling, 2015) when public health nurses provided care in the rural Appalachian Mountain territory. The role now includes wellness care of women, family planning, and

Strengths

- Our nursing foundation
- Our culture of health and patient self-empowerment
- Our holistic approach
- Transparent communication

Weaknesses

- Movement towards a medical/illness model
- NPs who desire to practice as physicians
- Reimbursement not focused on patient behavior change toward health

Opportunities

- A healthy population as human capitol
- Focus on wellness
- Entrepreneurship: technology, aging populous, community needs and values, digitalization of patients
- Interprofessional team-based care

Threats

- Apathy
- A view that NPs are a substitute for physicians
- A view of healthcare as a privilege versus a right
- Risk aversion

Figure 7.3. A SWOT analysis of the nurse practitioner (NP) role by Loretta Ford.

gynecological care. As of February 2019, there were more than 12,000 CNMs licensed in the United States (ACNM, 2019). CNMs are defined as primary care providers and have prescriptive authority in all 50 states. The professional organization for CNMs is the American College of Nurse Midwives, and they receive national board certification through the American Midwifery Certification Board.

Certified Registered Nurse Anesthetist

CRNAs report their beginning during the Civil War era when a nurse administered anesthesia to wounded soldiers (Matsusaki & Sakai, 2011). As the 20th century approached, nurses and physicians were working collaboratively to provide anesthesia during surgical procedures (Matsusaki & Sakai, 2011). In 2019, there were more than 40,000 CRNAs, and they are among the highest earners of all APRNs (BLS, 2019). They also have prescriptive authority in all 50 states, and like all APRNs, CRNAs contribute to increased access and reduced costs of healthcare. The American

Association of Nurse Anesthetists (AANA) serves as the professional organization for CRNAs, and they may seek national board certification from the National Board of Certification and Recertification for Nurse Anesthetists (NBCRNA).

Clinical Nurse Specialist

The CNS emerged after World War II as nurses received higher education and training as clinical experts who would bridge the gap between theory and practice (Montemuro, 1987). CNSs training leverages clinical expertise, leadership, educational programs, and research to improve health outcomes and direct patient care practices. Population, setting of practice, medical subspecialty, type of care, and type of problem define specialties within the CNS role (NACNS, 2019). By 2019, 41 states in the United States include CNSs within the definition of APRNs, but 11 states still had no provision of prescriptive authority for CNSs. There are approximately 72,000 CNSs in the United States with the majority working in hospital settings (NACNS, 2017). The CNSs professional organization is the National Association of Clinical Nurse Specialists, and CNSs may receive national board certification through the American Nurses Credentialing Center (ANCC) or other organizations depending on the educational tract.

Questions to Ask Yourself

1. How has the history of APRN role development affected current practices?
2. In reviewing core competencies for the four APRN roles, are you confident in your ability to pursue your career choice?
3. How confident are you in assuming a collaborative practice?
4. As an APRN, how can I advance the health of my community?

Consensus Model

Population foci have changed and revised in dynamic response to identified needs in healthcare. With new population foci and growth in all APRN roles, the APRN Consensus Model (2008) was developed by the National Council of State Boards of Nursing (NCSBN) to facilitate continuity in licensing, accreditation, credentialing, and education across the United States. As a result of the Consensus Model, APRNs have seen increasing consistency in requirement nationwide improving mobility and enabling APRNs to seek licensure more easily in other states. The Consensus Model has also clearly differentiated the APRN roles (NCSBN, 2020a). The APRN Consensus Model can be found online at https://ncsbn.org/aprn-consensus.htm. An interactive map of implementation status provides a score for each state with increasing points for the degree of independence, prescriptive authority, and consensus in titles, roles, license, education, and certification. The NCSBN APRN Consensus Implementation Status Map is a dynamic document that changes as states progress toward consensus (NCSBN, 2020b). Viewers can interact with the table at the website by clicking to see what points have been achieved and which ones are still lacking. The APRN Consensus Work Group uses a pyramid to describe the education and preparation for APRN roles, including that of the nurse practitioner (NCSBN, 2020b). The base or foundation is the APRN core courses, including the "3 Ps," advanced pathophysiology, advanced pharmacology, and advanced physical assessment. Building on the "3 Ps" foundational base is differentiation into a specific role, the CNP, CRNA, CNM, or CNS (AACN, 2011; NCSBN, 2020b). The **population focus** describes the way that basic training will be applied to a specific group and differentiates those within the role. Examples within the CNP role include family/across the lifespan, women's health or pediatrics, and other population foci. These elements determine licensure and scope of practice. Beyond that level, the APRN Consensus Work Group describes specialty certification identified through affiliation with professional organizations, continuing education, and additional training. The top of the pyramid reflects a small number of APRNs, who will seek differentiation, subspecialty, or additional training foci, within the context of the chosen population.

 In Their Own Words

Anne Thomas, PhD, RN, AGNP, FAANP

The impetus for developing a consensus model… The impetus for developing the Advanced Practice Registered Nurse (APRN) Consensus Model related to the significant growth in what is now known as the four APRN roles: certified nurse anesthetists, certified nurse-wives, certified nurse practitioners, and clinical nurse specialists. The national growth of APRNs provided increased access

(Continued)

to care particularly for underserved or uninsured individuals in those living in rural and underserved areas. This growth also provided consumers with new options when choosing a healthcare provider. Favorable outcomes were demonstrated by numerous studies that examined the quality, effectiveness, safety, outcomes and cost of care, patient satisfaction, and access as it related to APRN practice. Clearly, the role of APRNs and their integral role in answering the need for expanding access to cost-effective and quality healthcare was appreciated.

However, there was no uniform model that regulated practice and there was inconsistency regarding the expectations for education, certification, and licensure. Specifically, each state independently determined the necessary entry-level certifications and regulations to obtain recognition and/or licensure for APRN practice. This resulted in APRNs experiencing difficulty in interstate mobility as it related to scope of practice and ability to obtain recognition or licensure. The first APRN Consensus conference was held in June 2004 and its outcome was the formation of a national, multiorganizational workgroup to focus on APRN practice. In 2008, the collaborative work of representatives from more than 60 stakeholder organizations resulted in the future model of all APRN regulation known as the Consensus Model for APRN Regulation: Licensure, Accreditation, Certification, and Education.

The initial challenges to implementation of the consensus model... Many of the initial challenges of implementing the APRN Consensus Model still exist today. The ongoing and most impactful issue is the challenge to fully align the model with individual state practice acts, which subsequently allows APRNs to function at their full scope of practice as independent practitioners. Another immediate concern was the ability to provide transparent communication regarding the components of APRN regulation. The communication network known as LACE, for the four pillars of the model, was recommended in the Consensus Model to facilitate communication about APRN regulation and the Consensus Model to APRN stakeholders. Members of LACE include key regulatory agencies that represent licensure, accreditation, certification, and education.

Within each of the essential components of the Consensus Model, significant changes were described that required national stakeholders to create and implement systems to provide uniformity in nursing regulation. After 10 years following implementation of the model, challenges still exist. Curriculum development, which required alignment of the new accreditation standards using new competencies with specific population foci, needed to be created. Institutions of higher education needed to comply with the recommendation

(Continued)

that new APRN programs obtain accreditation or preapproval prior to enrolling students. Certification challenges involved interpretation of acute and primary care as related to population foci and the role of APRN specialties. The acute and primary care conundrum was initially confusing for employers and remains an issue because of ambiguous job descriptions that may blend acute and primary care responsibilities, which result in APRNs needing to obtain dual certifications. Finally, in the absence of a single certifying agency, the Consensus Model required that certification examinations were held to new standards because of their routine use in meeting regulatory requirements. This included that the examinations evaluated the APRN core, role, and population focus of the practice and explicated that the applicant could only sit for the certification in which they were educated.

The consensus model is important to nursing practice because... APRNs are an integral provider in today's healthcare system. Promoting patient safety, cost-efficient care, quality outcomes, accessibility, continuity of service, and consumer trust in APRN care management are inherent in the APRN role. The Consensus Model provides significant benefits to nursing practice because it provides the framework for uniformity in the regulation of APRNs and eliminates the inconsistencies in licensure, accreditation, certification, and education. Standardization promotes consistent expectations for consumers, policy makers, healthcare professionals, as well as the organizations representing the four pillars of the Consensus Model. National consistency and quality promote research related to the effectiveness of APRN practice, which demonstrates the contribution of advanced practice nursing to evolving and complex healthcare system. As noted previously, standardization has also increased interstate mobility for APRNs regarding congruency in licensure and certification.

My advice to nurse practitioner students... Students are well advised to review and use the Consensus Model when determining their role and scope of their practice. Licensure and scope of practice are defined at the level of the role and population focus. If primary care is chosen and the APRN chooses to expand their role to acute care, more formal education may be needed to obtain additional certification. Likewise, if a new population focus is selected, it is likely that additional formal education and certification is required. All states are not fully aligned with the Consensus Model, and APRN students should understand the regulations regarding prescriptive authority, required collaboration with physicians, required postgraduate residency, certification, and educational requirements among others. An APRN's ability to practice at the full extent of their education and training cannot be taken for granted and must be evaluated carefully in the state in which they practice.

(Continued)

> **The future of the consensus model is…** The Consensus Model is now over a decade old, and the healthcare system that existed when it was created has changed significantly. Similarly, APRN roles have evolved, specialty certifications for APRNs are more common, new nursing accreditation organizations have been instituted, state regulatory agencies have made progress in moving APRN practice to full scope authority, the Doctor of Nursing Practice as entry in APRN practice has gained momentum through the endorsement of major APRN organizations, and discussion about opening up the Consensus Model to revisit the population foci has occurred. LACE, the organization created to promote transparency of communication regarding the Consensus Model, is updating its organizational structure and work processes to provide more efficient and effective services. Is it time to revisit or revise the original intent and implementation of the Consensus Model to address the changes that have occurred since its inception, or have the changes occurred because the model provided the framework and we are just at the beginning of optimizing its foundational underpinnings? The new generation of APRNs that were educated and employed after the model was implemented and are now answering the call to improve and lead our healthcare system are key to understanding the future of the model.

Core Competencies

In 1990, the National Organization of Nurse Practitioner Faculties (NONPF) published the first competencies expected of all nurse practitioners (Price et al., 1992). This was a landmark decision, with the result of standardizing approaches to APRN education. As more specialties emerged within the APRN roles, there was a demonstrated need to define and organize specialties. In 2008, NCSBN published a Consensus Model that recognized the specialty areas as a "population focus." Competencies for population foci were refined in 2013 by a multiorganizational task force and for nurse practitioners included family/lifespan; neonatal; acute care pediatric; primary care pediatric; psychiatric-mental health; women's health/gender related; and adult-gerontology (NONPF, 2013).

In a similar fashion, all APRN roles have developed core competencies appropriate to their specialty. The table below depicts an overview of the core competencies for NP, CNM, CNS, and CRNA roles. Core competency details for these roles are provided in their respective chapters (Table 7.1).

Table 7.1. APRN Core Competencies

NP	CNM	CRNA	CNS
Scientific foundation competencies	Hallmarks of midwifery	Perform and document a thorough paresthesia assessment and evaluation	Direct care competency
Leadership competencies	Professional responsibilities	Obtain and document informed consent	Consultation competency
Quality competencies	Midwifery management process	Formulate a patient-specific plan for anesthesia care; participate in the ongoing review and evaluation of anesthesia care to assess quality and appropriateness	
Practice inquiry competencies	Midwifery management fundamentals	Implement and adjust the anesthesia care plan	Collaboration competency
Technology and information literacy competencies	Midwifery care of women	Monitor, evaluate, and document the patient's physiologic condition	Coaching competency
Policy competencies	Midwifery care of the newborn	Document pertinent anesthesia-related information	Research competency
Health delivery system competencies	Knowledge of issues and trends in health care policy and systems	Evaluate the patient's status; verify infection control policies and procedures	Systems leadership competency
Ethics competencies	Advocacy for health equity, social justice, and ethical policies in health care	Adhere to appropriate safety precautions as established within the practice; respect and maintain the basic rights of patients	Ethical decision-making moral

APRN, advanced practice registered nurse; CNM, certified nurse midwife; CRNA, certified registered nurse anesthetist; CNS, clinical nurse specialist.

Prescriptive Authority

As the APRN role evolved and expanded during the late 1960s to early 1980s, the need to prescribe medications became apparent. APRN students must learn about the different types of medications and then study the pharmacological principles of prescribing, in concert with diagnosing. Legend drugs, also called "dangerous drugs," refer to any substance that requires a prescription for dispensing. Typically, "over-the-counter medications" is the term that describes drugs that someone may obtain without a prescription, though these may still be used as part of the APRN's treatment plan. The term controlled substances refers to medications with potential for abuse and dependency (DEA, 2018). Controlled substances are divided into five categories or schedules, referred to as Schedules I-V (DEA, 2018). The Durham-Humphrey Amendment of 1951 required a written prescription from a physician or dentist for the sale of medications considered unsafe for use without medical supervision (FDA, 2018). The term prescriptive authority refers to the legal ability to write prescriptions for noncontrolled and controlled medications (Perry, 2009). In some states, APRNs prescribed under delegation beginning in the 1970s, meaning that they were granted or delegated authority by a physician. It was not until the 1980s that APRNs gained legislated prescriptive authority in some states. By 2006, almost all states authorized nurse practitioners to prescribe medications including controlled substances (Bullough, 1983; Perry, 2009). Alaska, Arizona, Idaho, New Hampshire, Oregon, and Washington were among the first states to expand practice for APRNs, including the ability to prescribe without delegation from a physician, with the goal of filling the primary care provider gap in rural and medically underserved areas (Bullough, 1983; Hartz, 2014; Vestal, 2013). Prescriptive authority was an essential component of meeting the needs of patients, and these states recognized that research indicated APRN prescribing was safe and effective.

Rather than a national standard of prescriptive authority for APRNs, prescriptive authority varies by state. Currently, all states permit CNPs and CNMs to prescribe legend drugs and controlled substances but with varying degrees of regulation. Some require oversight by a physician, described by different states as collaboration, delegation, or supervision. Many states permit APRNs to practice and prescribe medications to the full extent of their education and training without supervision. In all 50 states, the State Board of Nursing regulates APRN practice, and in a few states, APRN practice involves additional regulation through the State Board of Medicine. Some states still require a prescriptive authority agreement or collaborative agreement with a physician that includes established protocols for prescribing, oversite, and chart review or discussion of one or more cases. The APRN must abide by the scope of practice guidelines and legislative requirements for prescriptive authority within the state of practice. It is the APRN's responsibility to stay informed of state law and regulation. In order to prescribe controlled substances, the APRN must register with the federal Drug Enforcement Agency (DEA, 2018). States vary in the limitations of APRNs to prescribe schedule II/IIN controlled substances, but all states allow CNPs prescriptive authority for schedule III, IV, and V controlled substances (Table 7.2).

The delegation of prescriptive authority can pose some special challenges to APRNs in states with a restricted scope of practice. In some states, should the delegating physician leave the country, become incapacitated, die, or simply decide not to delegate any more, the APRN must immediately stop working unless a new delegating physician can be found. Circumstances such as these have occurred, abruptly leaving patients without anyone to attend to their needs, even though the APRN may still be available. This can have an immediate detrimental effect on the income of both the APRN and the delegating physician and may cause closure of a practice. In some states, geographical boundary requirements for delegation have been removed, but the fact that face-to-face meetings are still required places a burden on APRNs who serve in a region where no physicians wish to delegate. Delegation or supervision often incurs a fee paid directly from the APRN to the physician. Since this is not regulated, APRNs in a geographical area or specialty with few willing physicians to delegate may pay considerably more. Lucrative economic gain for physicians is one reason that some are so reluctant to give APRNs **full-practice authority**.

Collaborative Agreement

For APRNs living in states without full-practice authority, medical aspects of care such as the ability to diagnose, prescribe, and perform certain procedures are delegated through a collaborative practice or prescriptive authority agreement

Table 7.2. Prescriptive Authority by State

State	Who May Prescribe	Schedule Drugs Allowed	Collaborative Practice Agreement Required
AK, CO, HI, ND	CNP, CNM, CNS, CRNA	II-V	No
AL	CRNP, CNM	III-IV, limited II	Yes
AZ, ME	CNP, CNM	II-V	No
CA	NP, CNM	II-V	Yes
CT	APRN, CRNA, CNM	II-V	Yes
DC	NP, CNS, CNM, CRNA	II-V	No
DE	NP, CNS, CRNA, CNM	II-V	Yes
FL	ARNP, CNM, CRNA	III-V	Yes
GE, AR	CNP, CNM, CRNA, CNS	III-V	Yes
ID	NP, CNM, RNA, CNS	II-V	No
IL	CNP, CNM, CRNA, CCNS	III-V	Yes
IN, KS, OH	NP, CNM, CNS	II-V	Yes
IO	CNP, CCNS, CNM, CRNA	II-V	No
KY, LA	CNP, CNS, CNM, CRNA	II-V	Yes
MA	CNP, CNM, CRNA, PCNS	II-V	Yes (but not CNM)
MD	CRNP, CNM	II-V	No
MI	NP, NM, NA	III-V	Yes
MN	CNP, CNM, CNS, CRNA	II-V	No with limits
MO, WV	CNP, CNM, CNS, CRNA	III-V	Yes
MS, NJ	CNP, CNM, CRNA	II-V	Yes
MT, OR, WI, WY	CNP, CNS, CNM, CRNA	II-V	No

(continued)

Table 7.2. Prescriptive Authority by State (continued)

State	Who May Prescribe	Schedule Drugs Allowed	Collaborative Practice Agreement Required
NC	CNP, CNM	II-V	Yes
NE	CNP, CNM, CRNA	II-V	Yes for CNP, CNM
NH	CNP, CNM, CRNA, CNS(MH)	II-V	No
NM, RI	CNP, CNS, CRNA	II-V	No
NV	CNP, CNS, CNM	III-V	No with limits
NY	NP, CNM (limits)	II-V	No with limits
OK, SC	CNP, CNS, CNM	III-V	Yes
PA	CRNP	II-IV	Yes with exceptions
SD	CNP, CNM (limits)	II-V	No
TN	CNP, CNS, CNM, CRNA (limits)	II-V	Yes
TX	NP, CNS, CNSM, NA	III-V	Yes with exceptions
UT	APRN, APRN-CRNA, CNM	III-V	Yes for schedule II
VA	LNP, CNM, CNS	II-V	Yes
VT	CNP, CNM, CNS, CRNA	II-V	Yes with exceptions
WA	NP, CNM, CRNA	II-V	No

Adapted from Stokowski, L. A. (2018). *APRN prescribing law: A state by state summary*. https://www.medscape.com/viewarticle/440315. (For the most up-to-date information, check with your state board of nursing)

APRN, advanced practice registered nurse; ARNP, advanced registered nurse practitioner; CNM, certified nurse midwife; CRNA, certified registered nurse anesthetist; CNS, clinical nurse specialist; CNP, certified nurse practitioner; NP, nurse practitioner.

signed by another licensed healthcare provider, typically a physician but in some states may be a dentist or podiatrist. Some states require this delegated relationship for a set number of hours following the initial APRN licensure referred to as a *transition of practice period*; others require the agreement indefinitely with annual review and renewal (Phillips, 2018). Some states require monthly or periodic chart review meetings with the delegating physician to share information relating to patient treatment and care and discuss patient care improvements. APRNs should check the state board of nursing's nurse practice act to identify the required terms and elements of collaborative practice agreements. Each type of APRN (nurse practitioner, CNM, CNA, or CNS) can access their professional organizations for information on collaborative practice agreements and discover sample templates. The American Association of Nurse Practitioners (AANP) provides a color-coded map of the United States to identify states that allow full practice by nurse practitioners and those states with reduced or restricted practice (https://storage.aanp.org/www/documents/state-leg-reg/stateregulatorymap.pdf). Reduced practice indicates at least one element of APRN practice (such as prescribing scheduled medications) is not allowed. Restricted practice indicates the APRN can engage in practice but in a restricted manner (for example, prescribing certain scheduled medications only under delegation of a physician).

CNMs can access the midwife-schooling website for a list of state regulations for CNMs (https://mana.org/about-midwives/state-by-state). CNMs can identify states that allow practice and independent prescribing and compare with those states that require a collaborative agreement. The website can be accessed at https://www.midwifeschooling.com/independent-practice-and-collaborative-agreement-states/.

CRNAs can also access websites and identify states that allow full-practice authority or restricted practice with required supervision of a physician anesthesiologist. One such website provided by Verywell Health can be accessed at https://www.verywellhealth.com/which-states-allow-crnas-to-practice-independently-1736102.

CNSs may also find state differences in full-practice authority vs. required supervision, with full or no prescribing authority. The delegation requirement indicates the state requires a written collaborative practice agreement specifying scope of practice and medical acts allowed with or without medical supervision. No prescribing authority indicates the CNS is not authorized to prescribe pharmacologic and nonpharmacologic therapies. The National Association of

Clinical Nurse Specialists has a color-coded map on their website indicating in which states CNSs can fully practice or have restrictions. Access to this map is found at http://nacns.org/advocacy-policy/policies-affecting-cnss/scope-of-practice/. Sample collaborative practice or prescriptive authority agreements can be found in the state professional APRN organizations.

Consultation

Regardless of state requirements of a formal collaborative practice agreement or prescriptive authority agreement, all APRNs should engage in collegial practice that may require referral and engagement in consultation with other members of the healthcare team. APNs by virtue of advanced education will hold leadership positions that provide opportunities to serve as consultants. CNSs' knowledge is sought by RNs when caring for complex patients. The CNS, who has knowledge and clinical expertise in a specific disease or population, can serve as consultant and collaborator. One of the four primary roles of the CNS is consultant, as they serve the nurse who is providing the patient care services (Proehl, 2016). As a consultant the CNS can assist the RN to reduce patient complaints of pain, disease symptoms, or drug side effects by exploring evidence-based practices that could ameliorate aggravating these symptoms. This form of consultation does not require a formal written request by the RN to appreciate the expertise of the CNS.

In contrast, there will be occasional situations when the APRN will need the consultative services of another healthcare provider. According to Current Procedural Terminology (CPT) guidelines, the APRN can request a consultation of physicians and nonphysicians such as APRNs, physician assistants, physical therapists, occupational therapists, speech pathologists, and social workers (Dowling, 2019). Consultation occurs when the APRN requests advice from another healthcare provider on diagnosis, treatment, or a failure in standard treatment for a specific patient. Consultation by nonphysicians can be provided if the service is within the scope of practice and licensure requirement in the state where the nonphysician practices—and the requirements for physician collaboration and supervision—are met.

The referring APRN should make a request of a qualified physician/nonphysician to initiate the consultation process. A consultation is an evaluation and management (E/M) service provided by the consulting physician/nonphysician to either recommend care for a specific condition or problem, determine whether to accept responsibility of the ongoing management of the patient's entire care, or for the care of a specific condition or problem (Dowling, 2019). The APRN should document in the patient's chart the request for consultation and the specific reason for the consultation. When coding for a consultation, all three elements of history, examination, and medical decision-making should be present.

The rendering consultant can focus their visit with the patient, if the referring APRN has provided adequate documentation about the patient. The consultant will use this documentation to focus the patient's visit, complete their examination and assessments of the patient, and provide a written report regarding their opinion on the patient's condition, their findings, and recommendations or follow-up activities on which the APRN may act (Dowling, 2019).

Referral

A referral involves the transfer of all or certain aspects of care to another provider. APRNs will consult with and refer to a physician specialist or other member of the healthcare team when patient conditions indicate. Examples of referral include enlarged thyroid, palpable breast mass, and loss of hearing in one or both ears. The APRN should be aware of the referral process at their employment site, as gaps in following up on referrals can result in missed or delayed diagnoses and delayed treatment (Ghandi, 2017). Malpractice claims can be costly and time consuming, emphasizing the need for a systematic approach to referrals.

Key to the success of a referral is communication and a systematic approach. The APRN should provide written details of the patient to the specialist and to the patient so they will know what to expect. The patient should receive an appointment with the specialist, where they will receive a treatment plan. This can require either the APRN's office calling for an appointment or the patient receiving the contact information and making their own appointment. The APRN should consider the level of commitment and compliance before asking the patient to make their own appointment. The specialist should then examine and document their findings in order to create a treatment plan. This treatment plan should be shared with the APRN, who should acknowledge receipt of the plan and communicate the plan to patient and their family. Closing the loop of communication is paramount in the cases of consultation and referral (Ghandi, 2017).

Signature Authority

Signature authority refers to the APRN's ability, through state authorization, to certify and sign documents related to healthcare of their patients within their scope of practice. Some states permit APRNs to sign death certificates, handicap-parking certificates, and worker's compensation forms, whereas other states require a physician to sign these documents (Phillips, 2018). Advocacy for signature authority continues on a national level to permit APRNs to sign home healthcare orders and prescribe therapeutic shoes for diabetes.

Reimbursement

Prior to the 1920s, individuals paid reimbursement for healthcare services directly to a physician or dentist. By the 1930s, prepaid medical plans were becoming available and evolved into the modern-day third-party payer system (Kongstvet, 2009). By 1965, Medicaid was established to provide reimbursement for healthcare delivered to low-income families with children, elderly, and disabled population. As discussed earlier, Medicaid services expanded access to healthcare and served as the impetus to the development of the APRN role. In the early years of the APRN role, APRN compensation data were hidden within grant funding, global reimbursement, or physician provider numbers. As the APRN roles developed and expanded, legislation was enacted to decrease healthcare costs while increasing healthcare coverage and access. The Omnibus Budget Reconciliation Act of 1990 allowed direct reimbursement to nurse practitioners practicing in rural areas; despite this, many nurse practitioners experienced delays in processing claims and received letters of denial for services from the Health Care Financing Administration (HCFA) (Brandon, 1998; OBRA, 1990; Richmond et al., 2000). It was not until the Balanced Budget Act of 1997, which included the Primary Care Health Practitioner Incentive Act, that all nurse practitioners could directly bill Medicare, though at only 85% of the physician fee rate (BBA, 1997; HIPAA, 1996; HMO Acts, 1973; OBRA, 1990). Nurse practitioner and other APRN advocacy groups are still working to obtain 100% reimbursement for services that are identical to those performed by physicians.

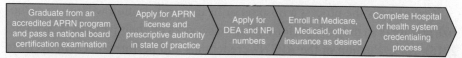

Figure 7.4. Steps in applying for an NPI number. APRN, advanced practice registered nurse; DEA, Drug Enforcement Agency; NPI, National Provider Identification.

Today, APRNs can receive reimbursement from Medicaid, Medicare, and many commercial health insurance and managed care plans. For an APRN to bill for services, a National Provider Identification (NPI) number is required. Adopted under the Health Insurance Portability and Access Act (HIPAA, 1996), the NPI number serves as a unique identifier for covered healthcare providers in financial and administrative transactions for reimbursement. The NPI application takes approximately 20 minutes to complete and is located at https://nppes. cms.hhs.gov/?userType=Provider#/(NPPES, 2018; CMS, 2015). An assigned NPI number is necessary to enroll as a Medicare provider. Medicare provider enrollment can be completed through mailing completed forms, or it can be completed through a web-based application available at https://pecos.cms.hhs. gov/pecos/login.do#headingLv1 (CMS, 2018). Medicare and Medicaid enrollment can take 2 to 6 months (see Figure 7.4).

Privileging and Credentialing

APRNs who practice in ambulatory care must gain permission or "privilege" to see their patients when hospitalized. Healthcare institutions have organizational bylaws and credentialing processes that regulate providers' privileges to deliver care in hospital or tertiary care settings. Facilities that are accredited by the Joint Commission on Accreditation of Healthcare Organizations must meet the requirement for the ongoing professional performance evaluation (OPPE) and the focused professional practice evaluation (FPPE). APRNs and other non-physician providers must meet the same evaluation standards as those set for physicians. These evaluation measures allow facilities to monitor and assess the competency of those providing care to their patients. With ongoing evaluation, hospitals can decide to whom they will grant and/or renew privilege and credentialing (Holley, 2016).

Privileging is the process a hospital or health organization will use to authorize providers so they can perform selected services on their patients (USDHHS, 2015). An evaluation of the APRN's credentials and performance will occur in order to evaluate their ability to be granted facility privileges. The credentialing process includes gathering documentation of licensure, education, training, experience, or other qualification. The healthcare organization will verify these documents by reviewing primary sources and keep this information on file. Credentialing is typically granted for a 2-year period and requires ongoing renewal.

The process can challenge an APRN's documentation of competencies since the OPPE and the FPPE include evaluation tools based on medical competencies (Wise, 2013). Each APRN role has its own professional competencies to maintain certification. Physicians have six competency domains represented in the OPPE/FPPE evaluation tools. These competencies include (1) patient care, (2) medical knowledge, (3) interpersonal and communication skills, (4) practice-based learning and improvement, (5) professionalism, and (6) systems-based practice (ACGME, 2017) (see competency-based education in Chapter 3). While the six competencies are familiar to APRN roles, many APRN programs also included American Association of Colleges of Nursing's (AACN) Essentials within their competencies, accentuating the differences in how APRN competencies are taught and evaluated. As of 2011, all APRNs and physician assistants (PAs) must use the same OPPE/FPPE process as physicians. Only those nonphysician providers who are not providing medical level of care can use an alternative pathway (The Joint Commission, 2011). APRNs should maintain records to facilitate the process of OPPE/FPPE evaluations. These evaluation processes require providers to report the specific number of times certain procedures or patient encounters were performed. APRNs need to maintain personal documentation of procedures and credentialed activities to maintain privileges (Holley, 2016).

Billing and Coding

For the provision of healthcare to receive reimbursement, it must be medically necessary and documented appropriately in the medical record, which involves the process of billing and coding. The process of billing refers to the APRN submitting a claim to a third-party payer to receive reimbursement for treatment and services. Coding refers to a standardized process of assigning alphanumeric codes that represent healthcare diagnoses, procedures, services, and equipment (Farlex, 2020). Medical diagnoses are coded using the World Health Organization (WHO) 10th revision of the *International Statistical Classification of Diseases and Related Health care Problems* (ICD-10), adopted for use in the United States in 2018 (WHO, 2020). In addition to an appropriate medical diagnoses code, the APRN must also document an E/M code along with any procedural codes to communicate to the third-party payer for what services the provider should receive reimbursement. E/M codes along with procedural codes are published and maintained by the American Medical Association (AMA) as the Current Procedural Terminology (CPT). Included in CPT is the Healthcare Common Procedure Coding System (HCPCS—often pronounced "Hick Picks") which includes three levels of codes: Level 1 consists of CPT codes which are numeric; Level II consists of supplies and nonphysician services such as ambulance services and durable medical equipment which are alphanumeric; and Level III codes are emerging technologies, services, and procedures which are also alphanumeric. For reimbursement, each patient visit must be coded for diagnoses using ICD-10 codes (Box 7.1) along with the level of visit and procedures using CPT Level I codes on an itemized form referred to as a "superbill."

BOX 7.1

▶ EXAMPLES OF COMMON ICD-10 CODES (WHO, 2019)

- I10.0—Essential (Primary) hypertension
- M48.00—Spinal stenosis, site unspecified
- E11.9—Type 2 diabetes mellitus without complications
- B20—Human immunodeficiency virus [HIV] disease
- J44.1—Chronic obstructive pulmonary disease with (acute) exacerbation
- F33.1—Major depressive disorder, recurrent, moderate
- K90.0—Celiac Disease
- J10.1—Influenza due to other identified influenza virus with other respiratory manifestations

A billable patient encounter must include the ICD-11 code of the diagnosis(es) addressed during the encounter and the E/M code that corresponds to the type and complexity of the encounter. The ICD-11 code should be documented to reflect the hierarchical condition category (HCC) as appropriate. The HCC is a risk-adjustment model designed to estimate patient healthcare costs and communicate patient complexity. E/M codes are found in the Level I CPT codes. There are E/M codes for patient encounters in an outpatient clinic, hospital setting, skilled nursing facility, home visit, urgent care, and other areas. The most common E/M codes billed are for outpatient clinics. The Centers for Medicare and Medicaid Services (CMS) released documentation guidelines for E/M coding in 1995 and 1997 (CMS, 1995; CMS 1997; CMS 2016).

The services provided at a visit must match the ICD-11 diagnoses code for reimbursement. For example, if the provider included CPT code 84443 for checking a thyroid-stimulating hormone (TSH) level but the only ICD-11 code was 1B51 streptococcal pharyngitis, then the charges would not be reimbursed because strep throat is not an indication to check a TSH. In that case, the APRN would consider using a second code, such as ICD-11 R53.83 for "other fatigue" in order to align billing with diagnoses.

Relative Value Units and Transition to Value-Based Care

Compensation for APRNs may be based on a combination of salary and relative value units (RVUs) reflecting productivity (Hicks, 2018). The Medicare reimbursement formula assigns value to physician services for specific CPT codes in the measure of RVUs. The RVU accounts for the time, complexity, practice, and professional liability expense of a specific code. For instance, a Medicare Annual Wellness visit, G0438, is 2.43 work RVUs while an episodic visit for an established patient, 99213, is 0.97 work RVUs (CMS.gov). APRN incentive compensation may be based on work RVUs over a certain threshold reflecting productivity. Compensation based on RVUs is incentivized for volume but not necessarily quality of care.

In recent years, third-party payors are shifting to value- and performance-based compensation. Quality metrics that reflect evidence-based practice, access to care, and patient satisfaction are driving incentive payments and lowering risk of financial penalties. The CMS Measure Inventory Tool and the National Quality Forum (NQF) endorse quality measures indicating evidence-based practice (https://www.cms.gov/Medicare/Quality-Initiatives-Patient-Assessment-Instruments/QualityMeasures/CMS-Measures-Inventory.html, http://www.qualityforum.org/Home.aspx). APRNs should ensure practice billing is occurring under the individual APRN's NPI number, so that the APRN's quality of care is captured.

Current and Future Challenges

As APRN roles continue to develop and expand, professional organizations must advocate for legislation to match the growing demand for access to deliver care. The future will see expanded development of APRN postgraduate residencies and fellowships as the roles continue to evolve (Al-Dossary et al., 2014; Flinter, 2005, 2011; Flinter & Hart, 2017). Statutory law in each state defines the APRN scope of practice. The purpose of regulation is to protect the public. Yet, overregulation may counterintuitively leave the public without access to the protective nature of healthcare delivery. The delivery of healthcare is continually evolving, but the demand for nurse practitioners and the capabilities of those in the role have grown faster than legislative support. Full-practice authority refers to a state licensure law that allows nurse practitioners to evaluate patients, diagnose, treat, and manage conditions to the full extent of their education and training. As of 2018, 22 states, the District of Columbia, the Veteran Affairs Administration, and the Department of Defense have authorized all nurse practitioners in their jurisdiction to practice to the full extent of their education and training. Additional states are evaluating legislation to support full-practice authority for nurse practitioners. With full-practice authority, nurse practitioners throughout the United States can serve patients, families, and populations as the role was intended, without barriers that impede access to care.

Summary

Combining advanced clinical skills with the best of nursing theory and practice, the APRN has transformed care. Through humble beginnings, APRNs have become indispensable members of the interprofessional healthcare team. With the shift from fee-for-service to value-based healthcare purchasing, APRNs are becoming a "hot commodity" in the rising team-based approach to healthcare delivery (H&HN, 2017; Jaspen, 2017). The job outlook for APRNs is excellent. The Bureau of Labor Statistics (2019) projects APRN employment to increase 36% between 2016 and 2026. The future is bright, but the responsibility is sobering. APRNs, as the pioneers before them, will shape the future of healthcare by maintaining focus on the patients, families, and populations they serve, providing the highest quality care possible.

Chapter Highlights

- The APRN Consensus Model was presented to demonstrate unique certification, licensure, and clinical practice of CNSs, nurse midwives, nurse anesthetists, and nurse practitioners.
- A brief history of the four APRN roles was provided to demonstrate the healthcare needs that each address for the nation's health.
- Core competencies of APRNs' scope of practice were reviewed with inclusion of reimbursement, privileging and credentialing, and billing and coding.
- The current and future challenges for APRNs were discussed, demonstrating continued efforts to gain consensus among all states regarding an APRN's ability to practice to their full potential.

Web Resources

- APRN Consensus Model: https://www.ncsbn.org/aprn-consensus.htm
- Centers for Disease Control (CDC): https://www.cdc.gov/
- Healthy People 2020: https://www.healthypeople.gov/
- International Classification of Diseases, Eleventh revision, Clinical Modification (ICD-11-CM): https://icd.who.int/browse11/l-m/en#/http://id.who.int/icd/entity/1642172022

Professional Organizations

- Advanced Practitioner Society for Hematology and Oncology (APSHO): https://www.apsho.org/default.aspx
- American Academy of Emergency Nurse Practitioners (AAENP): https://www.aaenp-natl.org/index.php?bypassCookie=1
- American Association of Nurse Anesthetists (AANA): https://www.aana.com/
- American Association of Nurse Practitioners (AANP): https://www.aanp.org/
- American College of Nurse Midwives: https://www.midwife.org/
- Doctors of Nursing Practice: https://www.doctorsofnursingpractice.org/
- Gerontological Advanced Practice Nurses Association (GAPNA): https://www.gapna.org/
- International Council of Nurse Practitioners (ICNP): https://international.aanp.org/
- National Association of Clinical Nurse Specialists (NACNS): https://nacns.org/
- National Association of Pediatric Nurse Practitioners (NAPNAP): https://www.napnap.org/
- National Organization of Nurse Practitioner Faculties (NONPF): https://www.nonpf.org/default.aspx
- Nurse Practitioners in Women's Health (NPWH): https://www.npwh.org/

References

AACN: American Association of Colleges of Nursing. (2011). *The essentials of master's education in nursing.* http://www.aacnnursing.org/Portals/42/Publications/MastersEssentials11.pdf

AANP: American Association of Nurse Practitioners. (2018). *Number of nurse practitioners hits a new record high.* https://www.aanp.org/press-room/press-releases/173-press-room/2018-press-releases/2190-number-of-nurse-practitioners-hits-new-record-high

AANP: American Association of Nurse Practitioners. (2019). *NP fact sheet.* https://www.aanp.org/about/all-about-nps/np-fact-sheet

ACGME: Accreditation Council for Graduate Medical Education. (2017). *Clinical competency committees: A guidebook for programs.* https://www.acgme.org/Portals/0/ACGMEClinicalCompetencyCommitteeGuidebook.pdf

ACNM: American College of Nurse-Midwives. (2019). *Essential facts about midwives.* https://www.midwife.org/acnm/files/cclibraryfiles/filename/000000007531/EssentialFactsAboutMidwives-UPDATED.pdf

Al-Dossary, R., Kitsantas, P., & Maddox, P. J. (2014). The impact of residency programs on new nurse graduates' clinical decision-making and leadership skills: A systematic review. *Nurse Education Today, 34*(6), 1024–1028.

APRN Consensus Work Group & the National Council of State Boards of Nursing APRN Advisory Committee. (2008). *Consensus model for APRN regulation: Licensure, accreditation, certification & education.* APRN Joint Dialogue Group Report. https://ncsbn.org/Consensus_Model_for_APRN_Regulation_July_2008.pdf

BBA: Balanced Budget Act. *Pub.L. 105–33, 111 Stat. 251* (1997) (enacted August 5, 1997).

BLS: Bureau of Labor Statistics, U.S. Department of Labor. (2019). *Occupational Outlook Handbook, Nurse Anesthetists, Nurse Midwives, and Nurse Practitioners*. https://www.bls.gov/ooh/health care/nurse-anesthetists-nurse-midwives-and-nurse-practitioners.htm#tab-6

Brandon, P. (1998). Barriers to Medicare reimbursement for nurse practitioners. *Oregon Nurse, 63*(3), 16.

Bullough, B. (1983). Prescribing authority for nurses. *Nursing Economics, 1*(2), 122–125.

Casey, C. (2015). *Ground-breaking NP program turns 50*. University Communications. https://cuanschutztoday.org/ground-breaking-nurse-practitioner-program-turns-50

CMS: Center for Medicare and Medicaid. (2015). *National provider identifier standard (NPI)*. https://www.cms.gov/Regulations-and-Guidance/Administrative-Simplification/National ProvIdentStand/

CMS: Centers for Medicare and Medicaid. (1995). *1995 documentation guidelines for evaluation and management services*. https://www.cms.gov/Outreach-and-Education/Medicare-Learning-Network-MLN/MLNEdWebGuide/Downloads/95Docguidelines.pdf

CMS: Centers for Medicare and Medicaid. (1997). *1997 documentation guidelines for evaluation and management services*. https://www.cms.gov/Outreach-and-Education/Medicare-Learning-Network-MLN/MLNEdWebGuide/Downloads/97Docguidelines.pdf

CMS: Centers for Medicare and Medicaid. (2016). *Evaluation and management services. (ICN 006764). Medicare learning network. Department of health and human services*. https://www.cms.gov/Outreach-and-Education/Medicare-Learning-Network-MLN/MLNProducts/Downloads/eval-mgmt-serv-guide-ICN006764.pdf

CMS: Centers for Medicare and Medicaid. (2018). *Medicare enrollment for providers and suppliers*. https://pecos.cms.hhs.gov/pecos/login.do#headingLv1

Collins, C., Ford, L. C., & Silver, H. K. (2015). *The founding of nurse practitioner education*. In *AANP celebrating 50 years of nurse practitioners* (pp. 12–15). http://assets.aanp.org/documents/2017/AANP_Celebrating_50_Years_of_NPs.pdf

DEA: Drug Enforcement Administration. (2018). *Diversion control division. U.S. Department of Justice*. https://www.deadiversion.usdoj.gov/drugreg/practioners/index.html

Dowling, R. (2019). To consult or not consult. *Medical Economics, 96*(6), 29–30. https://www.medicaleconomics.com/business/consult-or-not-consult

Farlex. (2020). *Medical coder. Segen's medical dictionary*. https://medical-dictionary.thefreedictionary.com/medical+coder

FDA: U.S. Food & Drug Administration. (2018). *Milestones in US food and drug law history. U.S. Department of Health and Human Services*. https://www.fda.gov/AboutFDA/WhatWeDo/History/FOrgsHistory/EvolvingPowers/ucm2007256.htm

Flinter, M. (2005). Residency programs for primary care nurse practitioners in federally qualified health centers: A service perspective. *The Online Journal of Issues in Nursing, 10*(3), 6.

Flinter, M. (2011). From new nurse practitioner to primary care provider: Bridging the transition through FQHC-based residency training. *The Online Journal of Issues in Nursing, 17*(1), 6.

Flinter, M. & Hart, A. M. (2017). Thematic elements of the postgraduate NP residency year and translation to the primary care provider role in a Federally Qualified Health Center. *Journal of Nursing Education and Practice, 7*(1), 95–106.

Ford, L. (1975). An interview with Loretta Ford. *Nurse Practitioner, 9*(1), 9–12.

Ford, L. (1979). A nurse for all settings: A nurse practitioner. *Nursing Outlook, 27*(8), 516–521.

Ford, L. (2015). Reflections on 50 years of change. *Journal of the American Association of Nurse Practitioners, 27*(6), 294–295. https://doi.org/10.1002/2327-6924.12271

Gandhi, T. (2017). *Improve the referral process, improve safety. Institute for Healthcare Improvement.* http://www.ihi.org/communities/blogs/improve-the-referral-process-improve-safety

Hartz, L. (2014). AK ANPs celebrate 30 years of independent practice. *Alaska Nursing Today, 2*(2), 1–2. https://www.nursingald.com/uploads/publication/pdf/1040/Alaska_6_14.pdf

Hicks, J. (2018). *Understanding relative value units.* https://www.verywellhealth.com/rvu-physician-compensation-based-on-productivity-2317026?print

HIPAA: Health Insurance Portability and Accountability Act. *HIPAA; Pub.L. 104–191, 110 Stat. 1936* (1996) (enacted August 21, 1996).

HMO: Health Maintenance Organization Act. *HMOA, Pub.L. 93–222 codified as 42 U.S.C. §300e* (1973) (enacted December 29, 1973).

Holley, S. (2016). Ongoing professional performance evaluation: Advanced practice registered nurse practice competency assessment. *The Journal of Nurse Practitioners, 12*(2), 67–74. https://www.npjournal.org/article/S1555-4155(15)00851-X/pdf

Hospitals & Health Networks. (2017). *Nurse practitioners a hot commodity; Men shying away from profession.* American Hospital Association Publication. https://www.hhnmag.com/articles/8354-nurse-practitioners-a-hot-commodity-men-shying-away-from-profession

Jaspen, B. (2017). *Nurse practitioner demand eclipses doctors as states lifts hurdles.* https://www.forbes.com/sites/brucejapsen/2017/06/04/nurse-practitioner-demand-eclipses-doctors-as-states-lift-hurdles/#1a6381aa3360

Keeling, A. (2015). Historical perspectives on an expanded role for nursing. *The Online Journal of Issues in Nursing, 20*(2), 2. https://doi.org/10.3912/OJIN.Vol20No02Man02

Kongstvedt, P. R. (2009). *Managed care: What it is and how it works* (3rd ed.). Jones and Bartlett.

Ligenza, D. (2015). Loretta Ford: The "Mother" of the nurse practitioner movement. *Healthcare News and Trends.* https://www.bartonassociates.com/blog/throwback-thursday-loretta-ford-the-mother-of-the-nurse-practitioner-movement-2

Matsusaki, T. & Sakai, T. (2011). The role of the certified registered nurse anesthetists in the United States. *Journal of Anesthesia, 25*(5), 734–740.

Montemuro, M. (1987). The evolution of the clinical nurse specialist: Response to the challenge of professional nursing practice. *Clinical Nurse Specialist, 1*(3), 106–110.

NACNS: National Association of Clinical Nurse Specialists. (2017). *Who are clinical nurse specialists? They're change leaders!* https://nacns.org/2017/09/who-are-clinical-nurse-specialists-theyre-change-leaders/

NACNS: National Association of Clinical Nurse Specialists. (2019). *What is a CNS?* https://nacns.org/about-us/what-is-a-cns/

NCSBN: National Council of State Boards of Nursing. (2020a). *APRN Campaign for consensus: Moving toward uniformity in state laws.* https://www.ncsbn.org/campaign-for-consensus.htm

NCSBN: National Council of State Boards of Nursing. (2020b). *Implementation status map.* https://www.ncsbn.org/5397.htm

NONPF: National Organization of Nurse Practitioner Faculty, Multi-organizational Work Group. (2013). *Primary care and acute care certified nurse practitioners.* http://c.ymcdn.com/sites/www.nonpf.org/resource/resmgr/consensus_model/acpcnpstatementfinal2013.pdf

NPPES: National Provider & Plan Enumeration System. (2018). *NPI registry.* https://nppes.cms.hhs.gov/?userType=Provider#/

OBRA: Omnibus Budget Reconciliation Act. *OBRA-90; Pub.L. 101–508, 104 Stat. 1388* (1990) (enacted November 5, 1990).

Perry, J. J. (2009). The rise and impact of the nurse practitioners and physician assistants on their own and cross-occupation incomes. *Contemporary Economic Policy, 27*(4), 491–511.

Phillips, S. (2018). 30th annual APRN legislative update: Improving access to health care one state at a time. *The Nurse Practitioner, 43*(1), 27–54. https://ruralprep.org/wp-content/uploads/2018/02/30th-APRN-Legislative-Update.pdf

Price, M., Martin, A., Newberry, Y., Zimmer, P., Brykczynski, K., & Warren, B. (1992). Developing national guidelines for nurse practitioner education: An overview of the product and the process. *Journal of Nursing Education, 31*(1), 10–15.

Proehl, J. (2016). What is a CNS and why do you need one? *Advanced Emergency Nursing Journal, 38*(1), 1–3. https://www.nursingcenter.com/wkhlrp/Handlers/articleContent.pdf?key=pdf_01261775-201601000-00001

Richmond, T., Thompson, H., & Sullivan-Marx, E. (2000). Reimbursement for acute care nurse practitioner services. *American Journal of Critical Care, 9*(1), 52–61.

Silver, H. & Ford, L. (1967). The pediatric nurse practitioner at Colorado. *The American Journal of Nursing, 67*(7), 1443–1444.

Silver, H., Ford, L. & Stearly, S. (1967). A program to increase health care for children: The pediatric nurse practitioner program. *Pediatrics, 39*(5), 756–760.

SSA: Social Security Administration. *Social security Amendments of 1965.* Pub.L. 89–97, 79 Stat. 286 (1965) (enacted July 30, 1965).

Stokowski, L. A. (2018). *APRN prescribing law: A state by state summary.* https://www.medscape.com/viewarticle/440315

The Joint Commission. (2011). *Standards Booster/Pak for focused professional practice evaluation/ongoing professional practice evaluation (FPPE/OPPEP).* www.jointcommissionconnect.org/NR/rdonlyres/A846669C-D456-44D5-A1AF-DC47975CEE8C/O/BP FPPEOPPE.pdf

Time, Inc. (1966). Where doctors don't reach. *Time, 88*(4), 75.

U.S. Department of Health and Human Services. (2015). *Credentialing & privileging of health center practitioners.* http://bphc.hrsa.gov/programrequirements/pdf/pin200116.pdf

Vestal, C. (2013). *Nurse practitioners slowly gain autonomy.* Stateline, July 19, 2013. The Pew Charitable Trusts. http://www.pewtrusts.org/en/research-and-analysis/blogs/stateline/2013/07/19/nurse-practitioners-slowly-gain-autonomy

Wise, R. A. (2013). *OPPE and FPPE: Tools to help make privileging decisions.* www.jointcommission.org/jc_physician_blog/oppe_fppe_tools_privileging.decisions/

World Health Organization. (2019). *ICD-10 Version: 2019.* https://icd.who.int/browse10/2019/en

World Health Organization ICD.codes. (2020). *What is ICD (international classification of diseases)?* https://icd.codes/articles/what-is-icd

8

Nurse Practitioners

Marilou Shreve · Anna Jarrett · Allison L. Scott · Kelly Vowell Johnson

LEARNING OBJECTIVES

After completing this chapter, you will be able to:

1. Understand how the role of the nurse practitioner has evolved.

2. Identify the types of nurse practitioner specialties and the population focus for each.

3. Understand the core nurse practitioner competencies.

4. Explore how population-based competencies differ for each nurse practitioner specialty.

5. Identify certification and continuing education for each type of nurse practitioner specialty.

KEY TERMS

Acute care: Short-term care provided within a hospital setting for treatment of a severe injury or episode of illness, an urgent medical condition, or during recovery from surgery.

Benevolent programs: Programs that provide care to patients or populations with the purpose of doing good.

Ethical health delivery system: A system that delivers quality healthcare to all populations to benefit the patient through collaborative decision-making and participation in care in a fair and equitable way.

Hospitalist: Providers who are specifically educated to care for the general medical needs of hospitalized patients.

Independent licensed practitioner: A licensed and credentialed professional who provides care and services within the scope of the individual's license.

Nurse practitioner: Nurses educated at the graduate level, nationally certified, and licensed in the state they practice to provide advanced care across the continuum of healthcare services to meets the needs of a specific patient population (AACN, 2018).

Primary care: Primary care includes health promotion, disease prevention, health maintenance, counseling, patient education, diagnosis, and treatment of acute and chronic illnesses in a variety of healthcare settings.

Underserved area: Areas or populations that have too few primary care providers, high infant mortality, high poverty, and/or high older adult populations. These areas or populations face economic, cultural, or linguistic barriers to healthcare.

Introduction

Nurse practitioners (NPs) are becoming more and more prevalent in the United States, with representation by multiple organizations and certification agencies specific to a variety of specialty practice population areas of focus. One organization, the American Association of Nurse Practitioners (AANP), conducts annual surveys and maintains current records of NPs. In early 2020, more than 290,000 NPs were licensed in the United States (AANP, 2020). An estimated 23,000 new NPs completed academic programs in 2015 to 2016, meaning more than 97% of NPs hold graduate degrees. In 2020, almost 90% of NPs were certified in an area of **primary care** (AANP, 2020; Fang et al., 2017). At least 80% of all practicing NPs accept Medicare and Medicaid patients (AANP, 2020). Ninety-five percent of NPs hold prescriptive authority, including controlled substances that allow NPs to prescribe medications in all 50 states and DC (AANP, 2016, 2018, 2020). In addition, over 40% of all NPs hold hospital privileges, and approximately 12% have long-term care privileges (AANP, 2016, 2018, 2020).

Economic demographics for NPs in 2019 indicated the average full-time base salary was $110,000, with 57.4% seeing three or more patients per hour. Reported demographics indicate NPs are an average age of 47 years and have been practicing for an average of 10 years (AANP, 2020). A positive reflection of professional practice was seen in low malpractice rates, with NPs being named as primary defendants in less than 2% of malpractice cases (AANP, 2018; AANP, 2020).

History and Evolution

Until the late 1930s, the NP role was influenced by the shortage of primary care physicians in rural and poor urban areas of the country, physician specialization, and consumer demand for accessible, affordable, and quality healthcare (Lusk et al., 2019). It was not until the 1960s that a distinction would be established and implemented for the role of the NP. The struggle for autonomy in practice started in the first half of the century and continues today, as the NP scope of practice varies from state to state (Lusk et al., 2019). Collaborative practice agreements are still required in some states, but more and more state boards of nursing support the removal of this requirement.

Henry Street Settlement

Lillian Wald established the Henry Street Settlement (HSS) in 1893 in the Lower East Side of Manhattan for the purpose of addressing needs of the poor (HSS, 2018). At that time, many poor individuals lived in overcrowded, unsanitary conditions. The duties of HSS nurses were to visit the ill in their homes and see patients in the nurses' dispensary in HSS. This humanitarian effort went unnoticed until the early 1900s. In 1904, the New York Medical Society, located in north Manhattan, attached a clause to the Nursing Registration Bill that prohibited nurses from practicing medicine (Lusk et al., 2019). The New York Medical Society claimed the HHS nurses were "providing ointments and giving pills" which was outside of the scope of nursing. This was the birth of nurses practicing using physician standing orders signed by physicians in these poor urban areas for emergency medications and treatments. This was but a patch for an underlying problem, but it continued until 1929 (Lusk et al.,

2019). Owing to the stock market crash, physicians were increasingly worried about competing with nurses for patients and saw these activities as an economic threat to their professional livelihood. The "uptown docs" were now interested in providing care for all. The Manchester Village Medical Group accused the HSS nurses of practicing medicine. This resulted in a meeting of the disciplines to hammer out their disagreements. Records of this meeting are not available, but HSS remained active in providing care for indigent patients and today celebrates 125 years of benevolent programs for multiple partners (Lusk et al., 2019).

Frontier Nursing Service

Frontier Nursing Service (FNS) was a group of nurses in Leslie County, Kentucky, who formed an alliance to provide midwifery service during the 1930s (Lusk et al., 2019). These midwives diagnosed, treated, and dispensed herbs and medicines (including opiates) with permission from their medical advisory committee. They worked from the now famous standing orders to dispense herbs and medications, affirming they only made tentative diagnoses for the physician. If they were incorrect, the physician corrected them and advised them how to treat the disorder. FNS purported that physicians clearly outlined what they could and could not do via standing orders. These nurses are credited with modeling the first primary care NP role.

Farm Security Administration

During the 1930s, Farm Security Administration (FSA) nurses were given latitude in their roles to provide care for migrant health clinic patients all across the United States. FSA nurses also used standing orders issued by the FSA medical offices, but had an additional requirement noting that standing orders must also be approved by local physicians. The requirement for these nurses to provide expanded practice duties included criteria that patients must be poor and marginalized and have little or no access to physician-provided care (Lusk et al., 2019).

U.S. Department of the Interior of Indian Affairs

The expansion of practice for nurses working for the U.S. Department of the Interior of Indian Affairs (formerly the Bureau of Indian Affairs [BIA]) was a result of what they called, "nursing conferences" (Lusk et al., 2019, p. 17). These included well-baby checkups, health education, and disease prevention. This practice evolved into what are known today as nurse-run clinics. Primary care problems frequently encountered were ear infections, sore throats, skin infections, and other commonly occurring illnesses.

Modern Nurse Practitioner Role

Although the NP role had previously been modeled informally, it was Loretta Ford, RN, and Henry Silver, MD, who established the first pediatric nurse practitioner (PNP) program at the University of Colorado in 1965 (Lusk et al., 2019). This 4-month pilot project funded by the Commonwealth Foundation was designed to prepare professional nurses to provide comprehensive well-child care and to manage common childhood illnesses, with an emphasis on health promotion and family-centered care. Silver and Ford (1967) measured and reported the success of the program and found these specially prepared PNPs competent in assessing and managing well and ill children in the community. Having PNPs also resulted in an increase in the number of patients served by 33%. "Documentation of the outcomes of the PNP practice established validity of NP specialties" (Lusk et al., 2019, p. 18).

Historian Susan Hagedorn, PhD, RN, FAANP, FAAN, who retired from the University of Colorado in 2006, established a foundation and repository for the history of the NP role through filmmaking. Her intent was to document and bear witness to the lives of those who went above and beyond their role as nurses for the expectations of their time. She founded *Seedworks Film Foundation* with a mission to communicate the courage, touch, human dignity, and magic of storytelling to preserve the history of the NP. The resulting film made the case that American nurses changed the face of the healthcare system by taking over access to primary care and removing the barriers that sidelined nursing as just a support system to doctors and patients. Through interviews, historical footage, and analysis from noted innovators such as Loretta Ford, Jean Steel, Julie Fairman, Jan Towers, Jamie Newland, Linda Pearson, and Michael Carter, the film examined the roots and evolution of nurse practitioners leading up to the present day (Hagedorn, 2018).

In Their Own Words

Edward E. Yackel, DNP, FNP-C, FAANP

Note: This photo was taken upon my graduation from Senior Service College a.k.a. Army War College. I received a Master's Degree in Strategic Studies.

The key points in understanding my role are… Like civilian healthcare, military healthcare is undergoing a period of rapid transformation as mandated by Congress. Knowledge of National Defense Strategy, army and healthcare policy, systems theory, evidence-based practice, healthcare transformation, and the duties of being an Army Staff Officer are foundational to everyday functioning at an expert level. Layered upon this foundation are requirements to manage healthcare quality and patient safety at the organizational level as the Chief, Quality Management for the Army Medical Command. Finally, as the family nurse practitioner (FNP) consultant to the Army Surgeon General, understanding the scope of practice for advanced practice registered nurses, the nuances of credentialing and privileging, advocating for FNP role in peacetime and during wartime, and teaching, coaching, and mentoring junior FNPs are key to influencing the direction of future FNP practice.

What keeps me coming back every day is… The "voice of nursing" needs to be represented at all levels within healthcare organizations. Advocacy for nurses, advanced practice nursing, and our patients is essential in a rapidly changing healthcare environment wherein systems and processes are built around efficiency and cost effectiveness rather than the art of healing. Helping fellow healthcare professionals "see" themselves through patient safety and quality data provides opportunities to improve how care is provided within an increasing complex system. Workflow redesign, changing policy, providing positive incentives, and involving a multidisciplinary team in designing new ways of providing care are rewarding because the patient is the ultimate recipient of improved processes.

My greatest challenge is… Work-life balance is a challenge for those who serve in the military. Not only must a service member be a medical professional, he/she must also be a military professional and a part of a family system. Being a military professional involves attending military education and training to prepare for the increased responsibility of being promoted to a senior rank as

(Continued)

well as getting ready to deploy in support of peacetime and wartime missions. As a medical professional, military nurses must also obtain advanced civilian education such as a master's degree in nursing in order to be considered for promotion to the rank of Colonel. Determination and resilience are required to balance the demands of family life with day-to-day work and the duties of being a military and medical professional.

I wish someone had told me ... Healthcare policy and measuring the quality of patient care are important in shaping the future of nursing. Understanding the important role of healthcare policy and measurement may allude novice nurses who are primarily focused on gaining competence in their craft. Experienced nurses quickly realize that working on healthcare policy and measuring the quality of nursing care directly impacts their ability to advocate for nursing as healthcare evolves. Although there are many healthcare measures, few are predictive in nature or outcome based. Achieving a deeper understanding of the complexity of these measures is requisite to developing the nursing-sensitive outcomes of the future.

I need to be a lifelong learner because ... Technological advancement and the developing field of genomics require that nurses continue to update their knowledge base. Electronic medical records and emerging monitoring technology require nursing input to develop the workflows necessary to care for patients. It is especially important for FNPs to understand the implications of genomics on the diagnoses and treatment of primary care patients. Genomics has the potential to revolutionize healthcare for underserved populations. The evolution of super bacteria and mutation of viruses will dictate the creation of new medications and nursing procedures to care for those who are infected. Education is the key to successfully adapt to the healthcare environment of the future. On the television series *Star Trek*, physicians become holograms while nurses remain human. Think about that.

Another point to understand is... It has been estimated that only one percent of U.S. citizens serve in the military. What is largely unknown by those who have not served in the military is the wide diversity that is present. Male nurses comprise approximately one-third of the Army Nurse Crops. The first male nurses were commissioned and served during the Vietnam War. Advanced Practice Registered Nursing began in the military in the 1970s, paralleling the civilian sector. The Army Nurse Corps had the first African-American female promoted to the rank of General in the United States Army. Army Nurses have served our nation proudly since 1775 and will continue to do so wherever and whenever the call comes.

Role Specifics

What began as expert nurses pushing the envelope toward independent practice with increased autonomy, responsibility, and skills has now evolved into the advanced practice nursing roles today. Central competencies of advanced practice nursing include primary criteria of graduate nursing education, certification, and practice focused on specific populations. Central competency for all advanced practice nurses is direct clinical practice. From this central competency evolved the four types of advanced practice nurses: certified nurse midwife (CNM), NP, clinical nurse specialist (CNS), and certified registered nurse anesthetist (CRNA) (Brykczynski & Mackavey, 2018).

Populations Served

The American Nurses Credentialing Center (2008) steered the advanced practice nursing profession toward uniformity and simplification by publishing the advance practice registered nurse (APRN) Consensus Model. This model addressed the lack of common definitions for APRN roles and population foci by identifying four APRN roles and requiring national certification in one or more of six patient population foci: (1) family/individual across the lifespan, (2) adult-gerontology, (3) neonatal, (4) pediatrics, (5) women's health/gender-related, and (6) psychiatric/mental health.

The role of the NP has become more specialized with higher levels of skills acquisition and competency requirements. Population- and specialty-based NP roles have led to the development of advanced practice certifications in acute care, adult health, family health, gerontology health, neonatal health, oncology, pediatric/child health, psychiatric/mental health, and women's health (Tracy & O'Grady, 2018). Table 8.1 illustrates the distribution of clinical settings by NP certification.

Services Provided

NPs diagnose, treat, and address disease prevention and health management. Depending on each state, NPs collaborate with physicians and other healthcare providers to provide a full range of primary, acute, and specialty healthcare services. Generally, NPs provide billable services that include ordering, performing,

Table 8.1. Distribution, Top Practice Setting, and Clinical Focus Area by Area of NP Certification

Population	Percent NPs	Top Practice Setting	Top Clinical Foci
AGACNP	2.0	Hospital Inpatient Clinic (43.3%)	Surgical (13.3%)
AGPCNP	4.4	Hospital Outpatient Clinic (18.7%)	Primary Care (46.6%)
FNP	60.6	Private Group Practice (12.7%)	Primary Care (46.2%)
NNP	1.3	Hospital Inpatient (69.1%)	Neonatal (57.8%)
PNP-AC	0.6	Hospital Inpatient (38.2%)	Other (19.7%)
PNP-PC	4.6	Hospital Outpatient Clinic (18.7%)	Primary Care (55.6%)
PMHNP	1.7	Psych/Mental Health Facility (23.0%)	Psychiatric (93.6%)
WHNP	3.4	Hospital Outpatient Clinic (15.7%)	OB/GYN (64.1%)

Reprinted with permission American Association of Nurse Practitioners (2018). *NP Fact Sheet*. https://www.aanp.org/all-about-nps/np-fact-sheet.
AGACNP, adult-gerontology acute care nurse practitioner; AGPCNP, adult-gerontology primary care nurse practitioner; FNP, family nurse practitioner; NNP, neonatal nurse practitioner; NP, nurse practitioner; OB/GYN, obstetrics and gynecology; PMHNP, psychiatric/mental health nurse practitioner; PNP, pediatric nurse practitioner; PNP-AC, acute care PNP; PNP-PC, primary care PNP; WHNP, women's health nurse practitioner.

and interpreting diagnostic tests such as laboratory work and x-rays; diagnosing and treating acute and chronic conditions such as diabetes, high blood pressure, infections, and injuries; prescribing medications and other treatments; managing patients' overall care; and counseling and educating patients on disease prevention, health promotion, and lifestyle choices.

Family Nurse Practitioner

The family nurse practitioner (FNP) is often called a primary care NP, but this is a misnomer. Primary care is not consistent with the Consensus Model's (ANCC,

2008) population-focused nomenclature. FNPs perform and document health history and comprehensive physical examination on all individuals and families across the lifespan. They identify health and psychosocial risk factors and plan interventions to promote health in individuals and families. They distinguish and assess the impact of normal changes and acute and chronic illnesses or conditions throughout the lifespan and are the collectors of tests, referrals, and diagnostic results for each patient. They manage chronic conditions and oversee health and wellness of women, including preconception and prenatal care. On any given day, an FNP may treat minor acute injuries, provide health and wellness care to infants and children, and provide episodic care for acute illnesses of all ages.

Adult-Gerontology Nurse Practitioner

Adult-gerontology NPs evolved from what were formerly known as adult NPs and geriatric NPs. Two types of adult-gerontology NPs exist. Adult-gerontology primary care nurse practitioners (AGPCNPs) typically provide care in settings consistent with adult-gerontology populations. Adult-gerontology acute care nurse practitioners (AGACNPs) focus on acute and critical care for adult-gerontology populations.

Adult-Gerontology Primary Care Nurse Practitioner

The AGPCNP role evolved due to patient needs and a rapidly growing senior population in the United States. The AGPCNP manages common acute and chronic health problems for patients from the age of 13 years throughout the senior years. The focus is a long-term relationship in order to deliver high-quality, cost-effective care, emphasizing disease prevention and health promotion. AGPCNPs understand the complex developmental stages and transitions of life from adolescents to autonomous adults to older adults benefiting from more assistance (National Organization of Nurse Practitioner Faculty [NONPF], 2016). The practice of the AGPCNP is based on patient need and is not setting specific (NONPF, 2012).

Adult-Gerontology Acute Care Nurse Practitioner

The role of the AGACNP emerged as a certification and specialty practice in 1995 as a result of increased pressure on acute care facilities to utilize resources effectively. This became increasingly important when medical residency programs restricted the total hours medical students and residents were allowed to work. This left a large gap in provider coverage in acute care facilities. The AGACNP's focus is patients who are "physiologically unstable, technologically dependent, and/or are highly vulnerable to complications" (NONPF, 2016, p. 5). AGACNPs must quickly assess complex problems in acutely ill patients. Over time, the most likely home for the AGACNP will be acute care facilities in roles such as hospitalist APRN, intensivist APRN, and urgent care APRN. The population focus for this role is young adults through older adults. The exact age of young adulthood has not been clearly established, although typically the AGACNP population includes acute and critically ill individuals aged 18 years and older. They are frequently part of critical care teams, rapid response teams, and specialty services.

Neonatal Nurse Practitioner

The neonatal nurse practitioner (NNP) certification was developed in 1983 in response to the demand for nurses with advanced skills in caring for the growing numbers of infants admitted to neonatal special care units (National Association of Neonatal Nurses, 2012). Today, they are certified by the National Certification Corporation (NCC, 2020). The role of the NNP has increased to include care post-discharge and primary care of infants previously in neonatal special care units. NNPs commonly practice in hospital settings, but also in specialty clinics and primary care pediatric clinics.

Pediatric Nurse Practitioner

Advanced education in assessment, diagnoses, and treatment of illnesses was provided to pediatric nurses as a way to increase healthcare to rural and underserved children in Colorado in the 1960s (Aruda, Griffin, Schartz, & Geist, 2015). The evolution of the pediatric nurse practitioner (PNP) has included expanding the patient population beyond rural and underserved areas. PNPs provide healthcare to children from birth to young adulthood (Pediatric Nursing Certification Board [PNCB], 2018). The scope of practice for PNPs includes assessment, diagnosis, and management of both patients and their families (Scope and Standards of Practice, 2015), as well as meeting the physiologic and psychological needs of the pediatric patient through health promotion and maintenance and management of diseases processes. These needs are met through a comprehensive therapeutic plan including the use of pharmacological and nonpharmacological treatments. Treatment plans need to include educating family and patient (when developmentally appropriate), monitoring disease process, monitoring growth and development, and advocating for patient rights. The role of the PNP has evolved into two areas of focus: the primary care PNP and the acute care PNP. Both primary care and acute care PNPs must hold a minimum of a master's degree, have passed the certification examination for each respective area of practice, and have the appropriate credentials as determined by the state boards of nursing (Scope and Standards of Practice, 2015).

Acute Care Pediatric Nurse Practitioner

The acute care PNP (PNP-AC) provides comprehensive healthcare to those infants and children who are considered acutely, critically, or chronically ill (Scope and Standards of Practice, 2015). The PNP-AC is not limited to inpatient care and provides healthcare in a number of settings that includes but is not limited to inpatient settings including critical care units and emergency rooms, and subspecialty practice clinics (Scope and Standards of Practice, 2015). Currently the only certifying body to certify PNP-ACs is the PNCB.

Primary Care Pediatric Nurse Practitioner

The primary care PNP (PNP-PC) focuses on providing comprehensive healthcare to infants and children through the prevention and management of common pediatric acute illness and chronic conditions (PNCB, 2018). PNP-PCs serve in a number of settings that include but are not limited to community health centers, school settings, ambulatory clinics, and camp settings. PNP-PCs may extend their practice into the inpatient setting based on patient need. Currently, like the PNP-AC, PNP-PCs can only be certified by the PNCB, publicly supported by the National Association of Pediatric Nurse Practitioners (NAPNAP). The American Nurses Credentialing Center (ANCC) no longer offers the PNP certification examination as of December 31, 2018 (NONPF, 2013; Scope and Standards of Practice, 2015).

Women's Health Nurse Practitioner

In 1969, the Nurses Association of American College of Obstetricians and Gynecologists (NAACOG) was formed within the American College of Obstetricians and Gynecologists. The purpose of the organization was to provide education and establish standards of practice for nurses specializing in women's health, obstetrics, and neonatal care. In 1972, the role was formally defined

(Kass-Wolff & Lowe, 2009). In 1980, the first certification examination for women's health nurse practitioners (WHNPs) was written. In that era, the name of the National Association of Nurse Practitioners in Reproductive Health was changed to the National Association of Nurse Practitioners in Women's Health (NPWH) to more accurately reflect the scope of this specialty. In the 1990s, the role of this specialty became standardized (Kass-Wolff & Lowe, 2009). Box 8.1 depicts specific services WHNPs provide as specified by Women's Health Nurse Practitioner (NPWH, 2018).

BOX 8.1

▶ SPECIFIC WOMEN'S HEALTH SERVICES PROVIDED BY WHNPS

Adolescent healthcare

Well-woman examinations

Breast cancer screening and problem evaluation

Pap smears, human papillomavirus (HPV) screening

Health and wellness counseling

Contraceptive care, sexually transmitted disease (STD) screening, treatment, and follow-up

Pregnancy testing

Health management during the childbearing year including optimizing preconception health, prenatal visits, and after pregnancy care

Problems with menstruation—too much, too little, too many, too few

Fertility evaluation

Evaluation and treatment of common infections

Urinary tract problems like incontinence or infections

Menopause health promotion and problem management

Screening for general health problems

Psychiatric/Mental Health Across the Lifespan Nurse Practitioner

The psychiatric/mental health nurse practitioner (PMHNP) offers primary care that is focused on psychiatric/mental health issues for patients across the lifespan (American Psychiatric Nursing Association, 2017). Care may include a range from mild mental health concerns to complex psychiatric conditions such as schizophrenia. Consistent with other nurse practitioners, PMHNPs assess, diagnose, and treat individuals who have or are at risk for mental health disorders. Treatments of psychiatric/behavioral health problems consist of psychopharmacological or psychotherapy with prescriptive authority. PMHNPs function in a variety of settings including but not limited to community health centers, hospitals, residential settings, home health, and primary care settings.

Professionalism

The National Organization of Nurse Practitioner Faculties (NONPF) developed nine core competencies for all nurse practitioners regardless of population focus. The nine areas require competency in scientific foundation, leadership, quality, practice inquiry, technology and information literacy, policy, health delivery system, ethics, and independent practice (NONPH, 2017).

Competencies

Scientific foundation is the first of the nine core competencies (see Table 8.2). It is the process of integrating the humanities and sciences knowledge to nursing science. This process uses critical data analysis and translates research to improve practice processes, develop new practice approaches, and improve outcomes based on practice knowledge, research, and theory.

According to the National Organization of Nurse Practitioner Faculty (NONPF) (2017), *leadership* is demonstrated at the advanced level by using reflective and critical thinking to promote change at all levels. Leaders promote collaboration with multiple stakeholders to improve healthcare by advocating for quality, cost-effective, and accessible healthcare. Participating in professional organizations and activities and showing effective communication both orally and in writing advance the practice by developing and implementing innovations that incorporate principles of change that improve healthcare.

Table 8.2. Nurse Practitioner Competencies

Competency Area	NP Core Competencies
Scientific Foundation Competencies	Critically analyzes data and evidence to improve advanced nursing practice. Integrates knowledge from humanities and sciences within the context of nursing science. Translates research and other forms of knowledge to improve practice processes and outcomes. Develops new practice approaches based on the integration of research, theory, and practice knowledge.
Leadership Competencies	Assumes complex and advanced leadership roles to initiate and guide change. Provides leadership to foster collaboration with multiple stakeholders. Demonstrates leadership that uses critical and reflective thinking. Advocates for improved access, quality, and cost-effective healthcare. Advances practice through development and implementations of innovations incorporating principles of change. Communicates practice knowledge effectively, both orally and in writing. Participates in professional organizations and activities that influence advanced practice nursing and/or health outcomes for populations.
Quality Competencies	Uses best available evidence to continuously improve quality of clinical practice. Evaluates the relationships among access, cost, quality, and safety and their influence on healthcare. Evaluates how organizational structure, care processes, finances, marketing, and policy decisions impact the quality of healthcare. Applies skills in peer review to promote a culture of excellence. Anticipates variations in practice and is proactive in implementing interventions to ensure quality.

(Continued)

Table 8.2. Nurse Practitioner Competencies   (continued)

Competency Area	NP Core Competencies
Practice Inquiry Competencies	Provides leadership in the translation of new knowledge into practice. Generates knowledge from clinical practice to improve practice and patient outcomes. Applies clinical investigative skills to improve health outcomes. Leads practice inquiry, individually or in partnership with others. Disseminates evidence from inquiry to diverse audiences using multiple modalities. Analyzes clinical guidelines for individualized application into practice.
Technology and Information Literacy Competencies	Integrates appropriate technologies for knowledge management to improve healthcare. Translates technical and scientific health information appropriate for various users' needs. Assesses the patient's and caregiver's educational needs and coaches them to provide effective, personalized healthcare. Demonstrates information literacy skills in complex decision-making. Contributes to the design of clinical information systems that promote safe, quality, and cost-effective care. Uses technology systems that capture data on variables for the evaluation of nursing care.
Policy Competencies	Demonstrates an understanding of the interdependence of policy and practice. Advocates for ethical policies that promote access, equity, quality, and cost. Analyzes ethical, legal, and social factors influencing policy development. Evaluates the impact of globalization on healthcare policy development. Advocates for policies for safe and healthy practice environments.

Table 8.2. Nurse Practitioner Competencies   (continued)

Competency Area	NP Core Competencies
Health Delivery Systems Competencies	Applies knowledge of organizational practices and complex systems to improve healthcare delivery. Effects healthcare change using broad-based skills including negotiation, consensus-building, and partnering. Minimizes risk to patients and providers at the individual and systems level. Facilitates the development of healthcare systems that address the needs of culturally diverse populations, providers, and other stakeholders. Evaluates the impact of healthcare delivery on patients, providers, other stakeholders, and the environment. Analyzes organizational structure, functions, and resources to improve delivery of care.
Ethics	Integrates ethical principles in decision-making. Evaluates the ethical consequences of decisions. Applies ethically sound solutions to complex issues related to individuals, populations, and systems of care.
Independent Practice	Functions as a licensed independent practitioner. Demonstrates the highest level of accountability for professional practice. Practices independently managing previously diagnosed and undiagnosed patients. Provides patient-centered care recognizing cultural diversity and the patient or designee as a full partner in decision-making. Educates professional and lay caregivers to provide culturally and spiritually sensitive, appropriate care. Collaborates with both professional and other caregivers to achieve optimal care outcomes. Coordinates transitional care services in and across care settings. Participates in the development, use, and evaluation of professional standards and evidence-based care.

From National Organization of Nurse Practitioner Faculties (2017). *Nurse practitioner core competencies content.* https://c.ymcdn.com/sites/nonpf.site-ym.com/resource/resmgr/competencies/20170516_ NPCoreCompsContentF.pdf: Nurse Practitioner Core Competencies Content.

The *quality of care* competency uses skills acquired in peer review to evaluate access, cost, and safety to promote a culture of excellence (NONPF, 2017). This is accomplished by being proactive in anticipating variations of practice and implementing interventions that promote quality. Recognizing that organizational structure, financing, marketing, policy, and care processes need to be evaluated is part of the quality of care competency.

NONPF (2017) identifies *practice inquiry* as the process of translating newly generated knowledge to improve practice and ultimately patient outcomes. NPs must apply inquiry and investigative skills at the clinical level to analyze how the application clinical guidelines are best put into practice at the individual level. Using multiple modalities, NPs disseminate evidence of practice inquiry to diverse audiences.

NPs must be able to *integrate technology* and translate scientific health information to assess the needs of education and the effectiveness of personalized healthcare of the patient (NONPF, 2017). Technology assists the provider to coach the patient to promote positive behavioral change.

Health *policy* and practice are interdependent, and NPs should analyze the implications of policy across disciplines and globally. NPs need to be involved in policy development and analysis. NPs are well equipped to use critical thinking skills to address social and legal factors that influence policy development to create safe practice environments. Promoting access to quality healthcare through a focus on the development and critical assessment of current policies and procedures is a key component of the NP's role.

The evaluation and analysis of the delivery of care is based on the organizational structure, function, and resource allocations. Collaboration at the systems level includes partnering, consensus-building, and negotiating to develop a *healthy delivery system* with a focus on *ethics*.

In order to have an *independent practice* as an independent licensed practitioner, nurse practitioners need to "demonstrate the highest level of accountability for professional practice" (NONPF, 2017, p. 13). Appropriate care that spans services as well as settings should be patient centered, culturally and spiritually sensitive, and in collaboration with caregivers and other professionals. Professional standards and evidence-based care should be used and evaluated when managing previously diagnosed and undiagnosed patients. NPs should participate in the development and education of professional standards and evidence-based care. Core competencies are shared across specialties, but differences are present depending on the specific focus of populations.

Competencies across specialty practice NP organizations were compared for similarities and differences. Literature abounds about core competencies, but differences between specialties have not been clearly delineated. Table 8.3 contains data compiled from different sources to show the differences between NPs according to certification bodies specific to each specialty.

Table 8.3. Competency Differences	
Competency	**Examples of Competency Standards by NP Specialty**
Scientific Knowledge	**PNP-PC:** Knowledge development, quality improvement, program evaluation, translation and dissemination of evidence to improve child- and family-centered care. **PNP-AC:** Knowledge development, quality improvement, program evaluation, translation and dissemination of evidence to improve child- and family-centered care. **AGACNP:** Knowledge development, quality improvement, program evaluation, translation and dissemination of evidence to improve adult-gerontology care. **WHNP:** Integrates research, theory, and evidence-based practice knowledge to develop clinical approaches and improve practice to address women's responses to physical and mental health and illness across the lifespan.
Leadership Scientific Foundation	**FNP:** Works with individuals of other professions to maintain a climate of mutual respect and shared values. **PNP-PC:** Advocates for unrestricted access to quality cost-effective care within healthcare agencies for children and families. **AGACNP:** Provides leadership to facilitate the highly complex coordination and planning required for the delivery of care to young adults (including late adolescents), adults, and older adults. **NNP:** Interprets the role of the neonatal nurse practitioner (NNP) to the infant's family, other healthcare professionals, and the community. **PMHNP:** Advocates for complex patient and family medicolegal rights and issues.

(Continued)

Table 8.3. Competency Differences   (continued)

Competency	Examples of Competency Standards by NP Specialty
Quality Competencies	**PNP-PC:** Recognizes the importance of collaborating with local, state, and national child organizations to foster best practices and child safety. **PNP-AC:** Articulates the importance of collaborating with local, state, and national child organizations to foster best practices and child safety. **AGACNP:** Implements evidence-based practice interventions to promote safety and risk reduction for young adults, adults, and older adults with acute, critical, and complex chronic illness needs. **PMHNP:** Evaluates the appropriate uses of seclusion and restraints in care processes.
Practice Inquiry Competencies	**PNP-PC:** Promotes research that is child-centered and contributes to positive change in the health of or the healthcare delivered to children. **PNP-AC:** Ensures pediatric assent and consent, and/or parental permission when conducting clinical inquiry. **WHNP:** Evaluates gender-specific interventions and outcomes.
Technology and Information Literacy Competencies	**PNP-PC:** Promotes development of information systems to assure inclusion of data appropriate to pediatric patients, including developmental and physiologic norms. **PNP-AC:** Evaluates information systems to assure the inclusion of data appropriate for pediatric patients. **AGACNP:** Synthesizes data from a variety of sources, including clinical decision support technology, to make clinical decisions regarding appropriate management, consultation, or referral for acutely and critically ill patients. **WHNP:** Uses health information and technology tools in providing care for women across the lifespan to communicate, manage knowledge, improve access, mitigate error, and support clinical decision-making locally and globally.

Table 8.3. Competency Differences (continued)	
Competency	Examples of Competency Standards by NP Specialty
Policy Competencies	**PNP-PC:** Applies knowledge of family, child development, healthy work environment standards and organizational theories, and systems to support safe, high-quality, and cost-effective care within healthcare delivery systems. **PNP-AC:** Advocates for unrestricted financial and legislative access for children and families to quality, cost-effective healthcare. **AGACNP:** Participates in the design and/or implementation, and evaluation of evidence-based, age-appropriate professional standards and guidelines for care impacting acute, critical, and complex chronically ill patients. **WHNP:** Advocates for healthcare policies and research that support accessible, equitable, affordable, safe, and effective healthcare for women both locally and globally. **PMHNP:** Employs opportunities to influence health policy to reduce the impact of stigma on services for prevention and treatment of mental health problems and psychiatric disorders.

AGACNP, adult-gerontology acute care nurse practitioner; FNP, family nurse practitioner; NNP, neonatal nurse practitioner; NP, nurse practitioner; PMHNP, psychiatric/mental health nurse practitioner; PNP-AC, acute care pediatric nurse practitioner; PNP-PC, primary care pediatric nurse practitioner; WHNP, women's health nurse practitioner.

Scope of Practice

The APRN profession encompasses a wide variety of advanced nursing specialties and scope of practice (The National Council of State Boards of Nursing[NCSBN], 2018). The main scope of practice issue across all APRN specialties is independent practice. As of 2018, 23 states allow NPs to diagnose and treat without physician involvement (AANP, 2018). APRNs collaborate, consult with, or refer to physicians. The scope of practice for APRNs varies widely by state and specialty and varies from state to state based on each State Board of Nursing's Nurse Practice Act (NCSBN, 2018).

Certification Prerequisites and Licensure

All APRNs must hold a registered nurse (RN) license and be nationally certified and state licensed to practice as an NP. ANCC (2017) initial certification requires the equivalent of 2 years full time as a nurse and a minimum of 2000 hours of specialty practice in nursing within the last 3 years for all NP certification candidates. Prior to being qualified for licensure, NPs must apply and sit for a national certification as an NP in their specialty. The ANCC and AANP are the credentialing agencies. Requisites for NP certification require at least a Master's of Science in Nursing (MSN or MNSc) in their role specialty which is accredited by the Accreditation Council for Nursing Education (ACEN) or the Commission on Collegiate Nursing Education (CCNE) (AANP, 2018; ANCC, 2018; NCC, 2020; PNCB, 2018).

In addition, the clinical hour requirement is certification specialty specific. The minimum hours required for NPs are 500 hr, but some specialties and academic programs may require additional hours. APRN core courses, commonly known as the three P's, include advanced physiology/pathophysiology across the lifespan; physical assessment inclusive of all body systems using advanced assessment concepts, approaches, and techniques; and pharmacology, which must include pharmacokinetics, pharmacotherapeutics, and pharmacodynamics (ANCC, 2018). After a successful attempt to pass the certification examination, one may apply for state licensure with/without prescriptive authority.

An important decision for the graduate nurse wishing to sit for certification is to ask prospective employers which certification is required for the institution. In one small city, two community hospitals may require different certification organizations for NPs. In a similar situation, it may be advantageous to sit for both examinations until a professional working alliance has been developed in a specific healthcare system (AANP, 2018). Table 8.4 compares certification requirements across specialties by certifying organization.

Table 8.4. NP Certification Requirements for Graduate Nursing Students

Role	ANCC				AANP	PNCB		NCC	
	FNP	AGPCNP	AGACNP	PMHNP	FNP	PNP-PC	PNP-AC	NNP	HNP
Education Requirements: MSN, MNSc, PostGraduate Certificate, DNP (in Role Specialty)	✓	✓	✓	✓	✓	✓	✓	✓	✓
Graduate Curricula Advanced Course Requirements: • Pathophysiology • Pharmacology • Physical Assessment	✓	✓	✓	✓	✓	✓	✓	✓	✓
Specific Graduate Curricula Requirements: • Health Promotion/Maintenance • Differential Diagnosis and Disease Management With Pharmacologics/Nonpharmacologics	✓	✓	✓	✓	--	--	--	--	--
Clinical Hour Requirement: 500 Faculty-Supervised Direct Patient Care Clinical Hours	✓	✓	✓	✓	✓	✓	✓	✓	✓

AANP, American Association of Nurse Practitioners; AGPCNP, adult-gerontology primary care nurse practitioner; ANCC, American Nursing Credentialing Corporation; FNP, family nurse practitioner; HNP, health nurse practitioner; NCC, National Certification Corporation; NNP, neonatal nurse practitioner; NP, nurse practitioner; PMHNP, psychiatric/mental health nurse practitioner; PNCB, Pediatric Nursing Certification Board; PNP, pediatric nurse practitioner; PNP-AC, acute care PNP; PNP-PC, primary care PNP.

Continuing Education and Recertification

Continuing education is essential to maintain competent practice through ongoing knowledge development. Practice guidelines change frequently. It is important to know the current guidelines, as well as why the guidelines have changed. This can be accomplished through professional conferences, online learning modules, or formal classroom experiences.

To maintain national recertification, ongoing continuing education requirements have been established (AANPCB, 2018). To be eligible for all renewal certifications, nurse practitioners must hold an active current RN license.

ANCC requires 75 contact hours of advanced practice continuing education specific to the population certification. Additionally, a minimum of 25 of the 75 contact hours must be in pharmacotherapeutics. A renewal application must also include one of the eight categories: (1) contact hours; (2) academic credits; (3) presentations; (4) evidence-based quality improvement projects, publications, research, or thesis or other doctoral project; (5) preceptor hours; (6) professional service; (7) 1,000 practice hours in clinical role specialty immediately preceding renewal date; and (8) re-sit for the certification examination (ANCC, 2017). New in 2017, 1,000 practice hours in clinical specialty is now an alternative instead of a required category.

AANP (2018) requirements include Option 1 and Option 2. One hundred contact hours plus 25 pharmacology hours are required, but 25 of the 100 non-pharmacology hours may include precepting NP students. Renewal requirements may differ according to role specialty and certifying organization. Table 8.5 compares recertification requirements across specialties by certifying organization.

Subspecialties

In addition to specialty NP roles, scope of practice, and population focus certification, subspecialty areas may include allergy and immunology, cardiovascular, dermatology, emergency, endocrinology, gastroenterology, hematology, neurology, occupational health, orthopedics, pulmonology, sports medicine, or urology (AANP, 2018). Concerns have been voiced that subspecialty practice by NPs may in fact mirror the traditional evolution of physicians away from primary care practice (Petterson, Phillip, Bazemore, & Koinis, 2013).

Table 8.5. NP Recertification Requirements

Role	Renewal Certification Time Period	Contact Hours in Certification Specialty Including Pharmacology Hours	One Requirement in Categories 2–8	1,000 Practice Hours in Role Specialty	Reexamination
ANCC					
FNP	5 years	75	✓	Category 7	Category 8
AGPCNP	5 years	75	✓	Category 7	Category 8
AGACNP	5 years	75	✓	Category 7	Category 8
PMHNP	5 years	75	✓	Category 7	Category 8
AANP					
FNP	5 years	Option 1:100	N/A	Option 1	**OR** Option 2

(Continued)

Table 8.5. NP Recertification Requirements   (continued)

Role	Renewal Certification Time Period	Contact Hours in Certification Specialty Including Pharmacology Hours	One Requirement in Categories 2–8	1,000 Practice Hours in Role Specialty	Reexamination
PNCB					
PNP-PC	1 year	15 per year, 15 pharmacology every 7 years	4 PNCB modules: 2—primary care 2—choice	N/A	N/A
PNP-AC	1 year	15 per year, 15 pharmacology every 7 years	4 PNCB modules: 2—acute care 2—choice	N/A	N/A
NCC					
NNP	3 years	Based on examination results	N/A	N/A	Required to evaluate competency
WHNP	3 years	Based on examination results	N/A	N/A	Required to evaluate competency

AANP, American Association of Nurse Practitioners; AGPCNP, adult-gerontology primary care nurse practitioner; ANCC, American Nursing Credentialing Corporation; FNP, family nurse practitioner; NCC, National Certification Corporation; NNP, neonatal nurse practitioner; NP, nurse practitioner; PMHNP, psychiatric/mental health nurse practitioner; PNCB, Pediatric Nursing Certification Board; PNP, pediatric nurse practitioner; PNP-AC, acute care PNP; PNP-PC, primary care PNP; WHNP, women's health nurse practitioner.

Professional Organizations

The AANP formed in 2013 with the merging of the American Academy of Nurse Practitioners (founded in 1985) and the American College of Nurse Practitioners (ACNP, founded in 1995). This organization is considered the organization for all NPs (NP Schools, 2014). International, national, and state NP organizations have also been established. In addition to AANP, several well-known national NP organizations include Doctors of Nursing Practice (DNP), Gerontological Advanced Practice Nurses Association (GAPNA), NONPF, NPWH, NAPNAP, Advanced Practitioner Society for Hematology and Oncology (APSHO), National Academy of Dermatology Nurse Practitioners (NADNP), and the American Academy of Emergency Nurse Practitioners (AAENP). International organizations consist of the International Council of Nurse Practitioners, the Australian College of Nurse Practitioners, the Canadian Association of Advanced Practice Nurses, and the Association of Occupational Health Nurse Practitioners (United Kingdom) (NP Schools, 2014).

The role of the NP has evolved and become more specialized. The political influence of NPs has grown exponentially since 1965, with strong professional organizations supporting the autonomy, authority, and obligation to patients to practice to the full extent of education, certification, and licensure in the United States.

In Their Own Words

Michele Kilmer, DNP, APRN, CPNP-PC

The key points in understanding my role are... Pediatric nurse practitioners are not just excellent care providers; they are advocates for change and the voice of a vulnerable population. PNPs specialize in understanding the complexities inherent in childhood health promotion and disease promotion,

(Continued)

enabling them to lead initiatives that improve the care management of pediatric patients by incorporating evidence into practice, create a culture of accountability and encouragement, involve parents or guardians into the plan of care, and understand that pediatric patients deserve to be partners in their care management.

What keeps me coming back every day is . . . I love kids! It is not uncommon for healthcare providers to feel overworked and underappreciated in their jobs. I feel recharged when one of my patients gives me a big grin, hugs me when I walk into the room, or colors a picture for me to hang in my office. I love to hear their success stories, whether they are about sports, grades, other hobbies, or relationships. I feel that a part of my job is to instill them with hope for the future and a belief that they are valuable and appreciated.

My greatest challenge is... It is difficult to work in a place that does not agree with your vision for pediatric care. So many challenges arise related to variation of practice between colleagues and expectations of administration for the site's provider. The working environment plays a vital role in your mental health so choose wisely. I have excelled as a provider when I work at a site that shares similar healthcare values as I do.

I wish someone had told me... I wish someone had told me to investigate noncompliance concerns with an open mind and gentle spirit. There are many reasons why a parent or caregiver may not be following the plan of care as directed. Noncompliance is a complex issue; very few times is straightforward neglect the cause for concern. I have found that spending time assessing the socioeconomic anxieties is just as important as time spent evaluating the chief complaint of the visit.

I need to be a lifelong learner because... I need to be a lifelong learner because things are constantly changing in the field of pediatric care. When I first started out in nursing, there were several pediatric conditions that severely limited the quality of life and lifespan of the patients. Advances in medicine have improved both of those factors, and new innovations are always around the corner. My job is to provide the best evidence-based care to my patients that I possibly can provide. Their lives are important enough for me to spend extra time in keeping up with changes in healthcare.

(Continued)

> **Another point to understand is…** The responsibility of being an advocate for pediatric patients should not be undervalued. There are so few who are willing to step into this position. Families and patients need PNPs to be involved in legislative agendas that promote pediatric care at local, state, and national levels. Also, many times patients need the PNP to advocate for special services to be offered during the school year. It is vital that PNPs collaborate with community resources to ensure the patient is receiving consistent, evidence-based care that will benefit that patient now and in years to come.

Summary

Although the NP role had been modeled informally in the 1930s, it was Loretta Ford, RN, and Henry Silver, MD, who established the first PNP program at the University of Colorado in 1965 (Lusk et al., 2019). From there, the NP role has gained momentum in gaining a strong presence in the provision of healthcare within the United States. Multiple roles and specializations exist for nurse practitioners as identified in this chapter.

The Consensus Model defined APRN roles and population foci by identifying four APRN roles and requiring national certification in one or more of six patient population foci: (1) family/individual across the lifespan; (2) adult-gerontology; (3) neonatal; (4) pediatrics; (5) women's health/gender-related; and (6) psychiatric/mental health. The consensus model sets national expectations for practice.

Major competency areas for all NPs include competencies specific to scientific inquiry, leadership, quality, practice inquiry, technology and information literacy, policy, ethics, and independent practice. NP core competencies are shared across specialties, but differences are present depending on the specific focus of populations.

The scope of practice for APRNs varies widely by state and specialty and varies from state to state based on each State Board of Nursing's Nurse Practice Act (NCSBN, 2018). NPs and professional organizations continue to remain involved in political activism to allow NPs to work to the full scope of practice.

Chapter Highlights

- What began as expert nurses pushing the envelope toward independent practice with increased autonomy, responsibility, and skills has now evolved into the advanced practice nursing roles today.
- Although the NP role was modeled informally in the 1930s, it was Loretta Ford, RN, and Henry Silver, MD, who established the first PNP program at the University of Colorado in 1965 (Lusk et al., 2019).
- The role of the NP has become more specialized with higher levels of skills acquisition and competency requirements.
- Population-and specialty-based NP roles have led to the development of advanced practice certifications in acute care, adult health, family health, gerontology health, neonatal health, oncology, pediatric/child health, psychiatric/mental health, and women's health.
- NPs diagnose, treat, and address disease prevention and health management. Depending on each state, NPs collaborate with physicians and other healthcare providers to provide a full range of primary, acute, and specialty healthcare services.
- The National Organization of Nurse Practitioner Faculties (NONPF) developed nine core competencies for all nurse practitioners regardless of population focus. The nine areas require competency in scientific foundation, leadership, quality, practice inquiry, technology and information literacy, policy, health delivery system, ethics, and independent practice.
- The Consensus Model defined APRN roles and population foci by identifying four APRN roles and requiring national certification in one or more of six patient population foci: (1) family/individual across the lifespan; (2) adult-gerontology; (3) neonatal; (4) pediatrics; (5) women's health/gender-related; and (6) psychiatric/mental health.
- The main scope of practice issue across all APRN specialties is independent practice. As of 2019, 23 states allow NPs to diagnose and treat without physician involvement.
- Central competency for all advanced practice nurses is direct clinical practice. From this central competency evolved the four types of advanced practice nurses: CNM, NP, CNS, and CRNA (Brykczynski & Mackavey, 2018).

Questions to Ask Yourself

1. Why do I want to be a nurse practitioner?
2. Which APRN role fits my experience, personality, and lifestyle?
3. What population would I feel most competent to serve?
4. Am I willing to adhere to my state board of nursing regulations regarding advanced nursing practice?
5. In which professional organization will I be an active participant that promotes my practice?
6. Which professional organization can support my career growth and expertise?

Certification and Professional Organizations

NP Certification Organizations

- American Academy of Nurse Practitioners Certification Board: https://www.aanpcert.org/
- American Association of Critical Care Nurses: https://www.aacn.org/
- American Nurses Credentialing Center: https://www.nursingworld.org/ancc/
- Pediatric Nursing Certification Board: https://www.pncb.org/
- National Certification Corporation for the Obstetric, Gynecologic and Neonatal Nursing Specialties: https://www.nccwebsite.org/

National Organizations

- Association of Advanced Practice Psychiatric Nurses: https://www.aappn.org/
- American Association of Nurse Practitioners: https://www.aanp.org/
- Gerontological Advanced Practice Nurses Association: https://www.gapna.org/
- National Organization of Nurse Practitioner Faculties: https://www.nonpf.org/
- Nurse Practitioners in Women's Health: https://www.npwh.org/
- National Association of Pediatric Nurse Practitioners: https://www.napnap.org/
- Advanced Practitioner Society for Hematology and Oncology: https://www.apsho.org/
- National Academy of Dermatology Nurse Practitioners: http://www.nadnp.net/
- American Academy of Emergency Nurse Practitioners: https://aaenp-natl.org/

(Continued)

Web Resources

State Organizations

- Central Alabama Nurse Practitioner Association: https://canpa.enpnetwork.com/
- North Alabama Nurse Practitioner Association: https://northalabamanpa.enpnetwork.com/
- Alaska Nurse Practitioner Association: https://anpa.enpnetwork.com/
- Arizona Nurse Practitioner Council: https://arizonanp.enpnetwork.com/
- Arkansas Advanced Practice Nurse Council: https://anpassociation.enpnetwork.com/
- California Association for Nurse Practitioners: https://canpweb.org/
- Colorado Society of Advanced Practice Nurses: https://csapn.enpnetwork.com/
- Connecticut Advanced Practice Registered Nurse Society: https://ctaprns.enpnetwork.com/
- The Advanced Practice Nurse Council of Delaware: http://www.delapn.org/
- Nurse Practitioner Association of the District of Columbia: https://npadc.enpnetwork.com/
- United Advanced Practice Registered Nurses of Georgia: https://uaprn.enpnetwork.com/
- Hawaii Association of Professional Nurses: https://www.hapnhawaii.org/
- Nurse Practitioners of Idaho: https://npidaho.enpnetwork.com/
- Illinois Society for Advanced Practice Nurses: https://www.isapn.org/
- Coalition of Advanced Practice Nurses of Indiana: https://capni.enpnetwork.com/
- Iowa Nurse Practitioner Society: https://www.iowanpsociety.org/
- Kansas State Nurses Association, APRN Task Force: http://www.ksnurses.com/ks-aprn/
- Kentucky Coalition of Nurse Practitioners and Nurse Midwives: https://www.kcnpnm.org/
- Louisiana Association of Nurse Practitioners: https://lanp.enpnetwork.com/
- Maine Nurse Practitioner Association: https://www.mnpa.us/
- Nurse Practitioner Association of Maryland: https://www.npamonline.org/
- Michigan Council of Nurse Practitioners: https://www.micnp.org/
- Minnesota Nurse Practitioners: https://www.mnnp.org/
- Mississippi Nurses Association: https://www.msnurses.org/
- Missouri Nurses Association: http://www.missourinurses.org/
- Montana Nurses Association: https://mtnurses.nursingnetwork.com/
- Nebraska Nurse Practitioners: https://nebraskanp.com/
- Nevada Nurses Association: https://www.nvnurses.org/
- Forum of Nurses in Advanced Practice (New Jersey Nurses State Nurses Association): https://njsna.org/forums/fnap/
- The Nurse Practitioner Association New York State: https://www.thenpa.org/
- Council of Nurse Practitioners (North Carolina Nurses Association): https://ncnurses.org/networking/councils-and-commissions/nurse-practitioner-council/

- North Dakota Nurses Association: https://ndna.nursingnetwork.com/
- Ohio Association of Advanced Practice Nurses: https://oaapn.org/
- Association of Oklahoma Nurse Practitioners: https://npofoklahoma.com/events/EventDetails.aspx?id=1051420
- Nurse Practitioners of Oregon: https://www.nursepractitionersoforegon.org/
- Pennsylvania Coalition of Nurse Practitioners: https://www.pacnp.org/
- Nurse Practitioner Alliance of Rhode Island: https://npari.enpnetwork.com/
- South Carolina Nurses Association APRN Chapter: https://www.scnurses.org/page/APRN
- Nurse Practitioner Association of South Dakota: https://npasd.enpnetwork.com/
- Tennessee Nurses Association Advanced Practice Council: https://www.tnaonline.org/aprn-issues-and-updates-2/
- Texas Nurse Practitioners: https://www.texasnp.org/
- Utah Nurse Practitioners: https://utahnp.enpnetwork.com/
- Vermont Nurse Practitioners Association: https://vtnpa.enpnetwork.com/
- Virginia Council of Nurse Practitioners: https://www.vcnp.net/
- ARNPs United of Washington State: https://auws.enpnetwork.com/
- Puget Sound Nurse Practitioner Association: https://psnpa.enpnetwork.com/
- West Virginia Nurses Association: https://wvnurses.nursingnetwork.com/
- Wisconsin Nurses Association: https://www.wisconsinnurses.org/
- Wyoming Nurses Association: https://wyonurse.nursingnetwork.com/

References

2018 American Association of Nurse Practitioners. (2018). *NP fact sheet*. https://www.aanp.org/all-about-nps/np-fact-sheet

American Association of Collegs of Nursing (AACN). (2008). *Consensus model for APRN regulation: Licensure, accreditation, certification & education*. https://www.aacn.org/~/media/aacn-website/nursing-excellence/standards/aprnregulation.pdf?la=en

American Association of Critical Care Nurses. (2018). *Advanced practice*. https://www.aacn.org/certification/advanced-practice

American Association of Nurse Practitioner Certification Board (AANPCB). (2018). *NP recertification certificant handbook ANP-C, AGNP-C, FNP-C, GNP-C*. American Academy of nurse practitioners certification board. https://www.aanpcert.org/resource/documents/Recertification%20Handbook.pdf

American Association of Nurse Practitioners. (2016). *2016 AANP national nurse practitioner sample survey*. https://www.aanp.org/images/documents/research/2016%20np%20sample%20survey%20report_final.pdf

American Association of Nurse Practitioners. (2020). *NP fact sheet*. https://www.aanp.org/about/all-about-nps/np-fact-sheet

American Nurses Association. (2015). *Pediatric nursing: Scope and standards of practice* (2nd ed.) National Association of Pediatric Nurse Practitioners (NAPNAP) and the Society of Pediatric Nurses (SPN).

American Nurses Credentialing Center. (2018). *Consensus model for APRN regulation: Licensure, accreditation, certification and education.* http://www.nursecredentialing.org/APRN-ConsensusModelReport.aspx

American Nurses' Credentialing Center. (2017). *2017 Certification renewal requirements.* https://www.nursingworld.org/~4abfd7/globalassets/certification/renewals/RenewalRequirements

American Psychiatric Nursing Association. (2017). *FAQS about advanced practice psychiatric nurses.* https://www.apna.org/i4a/pages/index.cfm?pageID=3866#5

Aruda, M. M., Griffin, V. J., Schartz, K., & Geist, M. (2015). Evolving role of pediatric nurse practitioners. *Journal of the American Association of Nurse Practitioners, 28*(2), 68–74.

Brykczynski, K. A., & Mackavey, C. L. (2018). Role development of the advanced practice nurse. In M. F. Tracy & E. T. O'Grady (Eds.), *Hamric and Hanson's advanced practice nursing: An integrative approach* (6th ed., pp. 80–107). Elsevier.

Fang, D., Li, Y., Kennedy, K. A., & Trautman, D. E. (2017). *2016–2017 Enrollment and graduations in baccalaureate and graduate programs in nursing.* AACN.

Hagedorn, S. (2018). *Inventing the nurse practitioner in America.* Keynote address presented at national conference for nurse practitioners. Lippincott Williams & Wilkins.

Henry Street Settlement, Inc. (2018). *History of Henry Street settlement.* https://www.henrystreet.org/about/our-history/

Kass-Wolff, J. H. & Lowe, N. K. (2009). A historical perspective of the women's health nurse practitioner. *Nursing Clinics of North America, 44*(3), 271–280. https://doi.org/10.1016/j.cnur.2009.06.006

Lusk, B., Cockerham, A. Z., & Keeling, A. W. (2019). Highlights from the history of advanced practice nursing in the United States. In M. Tracy & E. O'Grady (Eds.), *Hamric and Hanson's advanced practice nursing: An integrative approach* (pp. 1–24). Elsevier.

National Association of Neonatal Nurses. (2012). *Neonatal nurse practitioner workforce position statement #3058.* http://nann.org/uploads/About/PositionPDFS/NNP_Workforce_Position_Statement_01.22.13_FINAL.pdf

National Association of Women's Health. (2018). *What specific women's health services do nurse practitioners provide?* https://www.npwh.org/pages/about/NPfacts

National Certification Corporation. (2020). *Core NP-BC nurse practitioner board certified.* 2018 certification examination (p. 29). https://www.nccwebsite.org/content/documents/cms/exam-np-bc.pdf

National Council of State Boards of Nursing. (2018). *Scope of practice FAQs for consumers.* https://ncsbn.org/APRNS_Scope_of_Practice_FAQs_for_Consumers.pdf

National Organization of Nurse Practitioner Faculties. (2012). *Nurse practitioner core competencies.* The National Organization of Nurse Practitioner Faculties.

National Organization of Nurse Practitioner Faculties. (2013). *Population focused nurse practitioner competencies: Pediatric acute care and pediatric primary care competencies.* https://cdn.ymaws.com/www.nonpf.org/resource/resmgr/competencies/populationfocusnpcomps2013.pdf

National Organization of Nurse Practitioner Faculties. (2017). *Nurse practitioner core competencies content.* https://c.ymcdn.com/sites/nonpf.site-ym.com/resource/resmgr/competencies/20170516_NPCoreCompsContentF.pdf

National Organization of Nurse Practitioner Faculty. (2016). *Adult-Gerontology acute care and primary care NP competencies.* https://cdn.ymaws.com/www.nonpf.org/resource/resmgr/competencies/NP_Adult_Geri_competencies_4.pdf

National Organization of Nurse Practitioner Faculty. (2018). *NP certifying bodies.* https://www.nonpf.org/general/custom.asp?page=18

NP Schools. (2014). *List of national, international and state NP associations.* https://www.nurse-practitionerschools.com/blog/np-associations-list

Pediatric Nursing Certification Board. (2018). *The primary care CNPN (CPNP-PC).* https://www.pncb.org/cpnp-pc-role

Petterson, S. M., Phillips, R. L., Bazemore, A. W., Burke, B. T., & Koinis, G. T. (2013). Relying on NPs and PAs does not avoid the need for policy solutions for primary care. *American Family Physician, 88*(4), 230. https://www.aafp.org/afp/2013/0815/p230.html

Silver, H., & Ford, L. (1967). The pediatric nurse practitioner at Colorado. *American Journal of Nursing. 67*(7):1365–1366.

The Regents of the University of Colorado. (2013). *Sue Hagedorn: Recipient of the distinguished alumni award.* http://www.ucdenver.edu/academics/colleges/nursing/about-us/news/Pages/2014/Sue-Hagedorn.aspx

Tracy, M. F., & O'Grady, E. T. (2018). *Hamric and Hanson's advanced practice nursing: An integrative approach* (6th ed.). Elsevier.

9

Certified Nurse Midwives

Kim Amsley-Camp

LEARNING OBJECTIVES

After completing this chapter, you will be able to:

1. Describe the history of nurse midwifery in the United States.

2. Explain the difference between the midwife and the obstetrician.

3. Discuss the barriers to midwifery care in our current healthcare system.

4. Describe practice authority for midwives in the United States.

5. Classify the core competencies of nurse midwifery.

KEY TERMS

American College of Nurse-Midwives (ACNM): The professional association that represents certified nurse midwives (CNMs) and certified midwives (CMs) in the United States.

American College of Obstetricians and Gynecologists (ACOG): Professional association of physicians specializing in obstetrics and gynecology in the United States.

Direct-entry midwives: Term used to describe a person who enters a midwifery program without first being educated as a registered nurse.

Freestanding birth center: An independent facility offering a more natural, family-centered childbirth experience without routine interventions.

Granny midwives: Predominantly African-American women who, in the earliest history of the United States, provided birthing care to women in communities throughout the southeastern United States until the middle of the 20th century.

Indian Health Service (IHS): The federal health program for American Indians and Alaska Natives.

Infant mortality rate: The number of infants who die before reaching 1 year of age per 1,000 live births.

Lay midwifery: Connotes domiciliary such as home birth practice and informal training that is founded in experience (Rooks, p. 8).

Introduction

The American College of Nurse Midwives (2019) reports more than 12,000 certified nurse midwives (CNMs) are practicing in the United States. In 2017, these midwives attended 351,968 births. CNMs are registered nurses who have earned graduate degrees, completed nurse midwifery education programs accredited by the Accreditation Commission for Midwifery Education (ACME), passed a national certification examination administered by the American Midwifery Certification Board (AMCB), and met criteria for certification by the American College of Nurse-Midwives (ACNM) to receive the professional designation of CNM (Table 9.1). CNMs are responsible not only for perinatal care but are also educated to provide primary care services to women. A CNM is an exciting role that is characterized by autonomy and a high level of career satisfaction.

As the key terms suggest, not all midwives in the United States are CNMs. Some midwives have entered the educational pathway without obtaining an RN license, while others may have high school or undergraduate educational preparation. Table 9.1 presents major differences between the multiple midwifery titles.

Table 9.1. Differences Between Certified Nurse Midwives (CNMs), Certified Midwives (CMs), and Certified Professional Midwives (CPMs)

	Certified Nurse Midwife (CNM)	Certified Midwife (CM)	Certified Professional Midwife (CPM)
Minimum degree for certification	Master's degree	Master's degree	Academic degree not required but ranges from associate degree to master's degree
Minimum degree for admission to midwifery education program	Bachelor's degree in nursing or higher from an accredited college/university	Bachelor's degree or higher from an accredited college/university	High school diploma or equivalent
Licensure	Earn RN license prior to or within midwifery education program	May or may not earn RN license prior to or within midwifery education program; licensure limited to DE, ME, NJ, NY, and RI	Licensed and trained in midwifery only; licensure requires PEP (portfolio evaluation process)
Scope of practice	Can practice in all 50 states + DC; scope varies from state to state; can deliver in all settings depending on state regulations; can provide care from "menarche through menopause"; needs physician oversight in most states; can write prescriptions; eligible for third-party reimbursement	Practice limited to a few states; can practice in all settings; provides full range of primary healthcare services from women from adolescence beyond menopause; has prescriptive authority in NY, RI, and ME; eligible for third-party reimbursement	Can practice in most states but some states will not license CPMs; does not require physician oversight; cannot write prescriptions; care is limited to pregnant or postpartum women in some states; other states allow well-woman care

Table 9.1. Differences Between Certified Nurse Midwives (CNMs), Certified Midwives (CMs), and Certified Professional Midwives (CPMs) (continued)

Certification	Graduate of midwifery program accredited by ACME	Graduate of midwifery program accredited by ACME	Completion of NARM's PEP, graduate of midwifery program accredited by the Midwifery Education Accreditation Council (MEAC) or AMCB-certified CNM/CM with at least 10 community-based birth experiences or completion of an equivalent state licensure program (all applicants must also submit evidence of current adult CPR and neonatal resuscitation or course completion)
Recertification	Every 5 y	Every 5 y	Every 3 y
Professional association	American College of Nurse-Midwives (ACNM)	American College of Nurse-Midwives (ACNM)	National Association of Certified Professional Midwives (NACPM)

ACME, Accreditation Commission for Midwifery Education; AMCB, American Midwifery Certification Board; CPR, Cardiopulmonary resuscitation; NARM, North American Registry of Midwives.
Adapted from American College of Nurse-Midwives. (2017). *Comparison of certified nurse-midwives, certified midwives, certified professional midwives clarifying the distinction among professional midwifery credential in the U.S.* http://www.midwife.org/acnm/files/ccLibraryFiles/FILENAME/000000006807/FINAL-ComparisonChart-Oct2017.pdf and Veteto, K. J. (2015). *Certified professional midwife vs. certified nurse midwife.* http://www.kristaveteto.com/certified-professional-midwife-vs-certified-nurse-midwife-cpm-vs-cnm/. Comparison of Certified Nurse-Midwives, Certified Midwives, Certified Professional Midwives clarifying the distinction among professional midwifery credential in the U.S.

Overview to the Role

The English word *midwife* means "with" (*mid*) "wife" or "woman" (*wif*). The term was used beginning in 1303 to refer to the care provided to women during childbirth (Rooks, 1997). The midwife is even referenced in the Holy Bible in the Book of Genesis: "And it came to pass, when she was in hard labour, that the midwife said unto her, Fear not"…*Genesis 35:17*. At that time, most midwives were women, so the term referred to a *female birth attendant*.

CNMs must demonstrate completion of the *Core Competencies for Basic Midwifery Practice* of the American College of Nurse-Midwives (ACNM, 2012) upon completion of their midwifery education programs. These competencies meet or exceed the global competencies and standards of the practice of midwifery defined by the International Confederation of Midwives (2017). CNMs must be recertified every 5 years through AMCB and must meet continuing education requirements as designated by each state in nursing and in midwifery (American Midwifery Certification Board, 2018).

The name nurse midwife specifies who they are and what they are. The word *nurse* recognizes the requisite nursing education, which distinguishes them from the lay midwife. The term *midwife* recognizes the additional, highly specialized training and preparation in the field of the medical aspect of normal obstetrics. While nurse midwives were criticized for trying to be physicians, they believe strongly in how who they are and what they have to offer distinguishes them from physicians. These challenges to acceptance have contributed to making nurse midwifery a field that attracts professionals who are deeply committed to the improvement and delivery of exemplary care to women and infants.

At their core, nurse midwives believe in physiologic birth and the power of women to make sound decisions on where and how to birth their babies. The relationship between the nurse midwife and the woman is paramount to the strength of the profession. Women who are allowed to make choices regarding their birth are stronger as people and pass that strength and confidence to mothering their children. This passion changes our culture for the better and bonds women to their nurse midwives.

Early in the 20th century, American obstetric care became highly medicalized for the pregnant woman, in particular during childbirth. This expensive approach to childbirth resulted in increased cesarean sections and other interventions that were harmful to women and their newborns (Rooks, 1997). This philosophy of care focuses on the potential pathology of birth. Midwifery is considered an alternative model of birth in the United States that focuses instead on a more holistic approach to care. The greatest distinction between the midwife and the physician or obstetrician gynecologist (OB/GYN) is that the midwife is expert in the physiology of birth and the physician, in the pathology of birth. Because midwives are positioned to provide optimal maternity care globally, they should be the provider of choice for childbearing women (Edmonds et al., 2020). Vedam and associates (2018) report other high-resource nations have anywhere from 50% to 75% of births attended my midwives compared with approximately 10%

within the United States where midwives additionally face barriers to practice, including inability to obtain third-party reimbursement and other regulatory and legal restrictions (Vedam et al., 2018).

Unlike in many developed countries, in most parts of the United States, midwifery is part of nursing programs and not its own specialty. Midwives without a nursing degree, including **lay midwives** and direct-entry midwives, are often known as certified midwives (CMs). CMs are only legal in a few states in the United States. Efforts to unify the profession have proved difficult as many of the lay midwives or "granny midwives" provided the entry point for CNMs in the United States. ACNM has been working with midwives who serve as unlicensed birth attendants to unify the profession and find pathways to certification (Box 9.1). Many communities still value the apprenticeship model of midwifery and hold firm to their traditions of training, which often exclude formalized, standard curricula. In rural areas, these birth attendants provide much needed care for women who would otherwise be unserved during pregnancy.

The argument for the medical model of birth attended by physicians in hospitals has been supported by the high maternal mortality rate in the early 20th century. However, with the development of antibiotics, blood transfusions, and medications to treat pregnancy-induced hypertension, the risks related to pregnancy and childbirth that women once faced have changed. Mayer and associates (2019) assert that in contrast to other developed nations, the maternal mortality rate in the United States has been increasing over the past decade, as presented in Figure 9.1. The authors cite multiple factors as contributing to this increase, including chronic diseases, disparities in access to care, racial and ethnic disparities, income, housing, and education.

Questions to Ask Yourself

1. Would I enjoy providing primary care to women and their newborns?
2. Am I comfortable assuming the responsibility for providing prenatal care and attending the birth process?
3. Do I have good listening, observational, and communication skills?
4. Would I enjoy an autonomous practice that also needs to function within a team?
5. Do I have patience as well as the ability to act quickly?

BOX 9.1

▶ ACNM CORE COMPETENCIES

I. **Hallmarks of Midwifery.** The art and science of midwifery are characterized by the following hallmarks: recognition of menarche, pregnancy, birth, and menopause as normal physiologic and developmental processes.

II. **Components of Midwifery Care: Professional Responsibilities of CNMs.** The professional responsibilities include but are not limited to the following: promotion of the hallmarks of midwifery and knowledge of the history of midwifery and to collaborate in research.

III. **Components of Midwifery Care: Midwifery Management Process.** The midwifery management process is used for all areas of clinical care and consists of the following steps: investigate by obtaining all necessary data and healthcare needs based on correct interpretation of the subjective and objective data, anticipate potential problems, evaluate the effectiveness of the care given, and recycling through the management process for any aspect of care that has been ineffective.

IV. **Components of Midwifery Care: Fundamentals.** Anatomy and physiology, including pathophysiology, normal growth and development, psychosocial, sexual and behavioral development, pharmacokinetics, and pharmacotherapeutics.

V. **Components of Midwifery Care of Women.** Independently manages primary health screening, health promotion, and care of women from the perimenarcheal period through the lifespan using the midwifery management process. While the woman's life is a continuum, midwifery care can be divided into primary, preconception, gynecologic, antepartum, and postpregnancy care.

U.S. Women Are More Likely to Die in Pregnancy and Childbirth Than Those in Other Wealthy Nations

Maternal mortality ration (maternal deaths/100,000 live births) among women ages 15–49

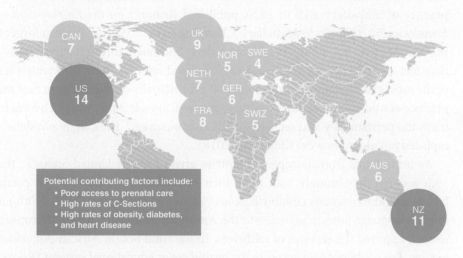

CAN 7
UK 9
NOR 5
SWE 4
NETH 7
GER 6
US 14
FRA 8
SWIZ 5
AUS 6
NZ 11

Potential contributing factors include:
• Poor access to prenatal care
• High rates of C-Sections
• High rates of obesity, diabetes, and heart disease

Data: The data reflect UNICEF estimates because of missing internationally comparable data for the U.S. National statistics are available for most countries from the OECD.

Source: Murina Z. Gunja et al., *What Is the Status of Women's Health and Health Care in the U.S. Compared to Ten Other Countries?* (Commonwealth Fund, Dec. 2018). https://doi.org/10.26099/wy8a-7w13

Figure 9.1. Comparison of pregnancy and childbirth mortality rates.

Early History

Varney and associates (2003) report the history of midwifery in the United States began in the colonial times. Most likely there were midwives among the Native Americans, but their history is generally unknown and unresearched. Colonial midwives were vital to their communities, treated with respect and dignity, and extended special privileges such as housing, land, food, and salary. Town records and charters from the mid-17th century document midwifery services. In addition to attending births, midwives cared for the sick and dying and prepared the body for death.

Midwifery Through the 1800s

In the early 18th century, salary for midwives was substandard, decreasing the economical feasibility for midwives to practice, especially in cities. In Europe, by the late-18th century, obstetrical care by physicians became popular. Soon this practice arrived in the United States, where medicine became highly competitive and male dominated. Harvard physician Dr. Walter Channing denounced the practice of midwifery and, in 1820, published *Remarks on the Employment of Females as Practitioners in Midwifery*. Channing wrote, "Women seldom forget a practitioner who has conducted them tenderly and safely through parturition—they feel a familiarity with him, a confidence and reliance upon him which are of the most essential mutual advantage...It is principally on this account that the practice of midwifery becomes desirable to physicians. It is this which ensures to them the permanency and security of all other business." Thus, male physicians replaced female midwives (King et al., 2018).

As immigrants from European countries arrived in the United States in the 19th century, they brought with them their own midwives from the "old country" to attend to women's childbirth needs (Varney & Thompson, 2016). Without English language fluency or access to the American healthcare system, European women required the services of midwives. In the rural South, African-American women also could not gain access to the healthcare or educational systems (Rooks, 1997). "Granny midwives" who passed the practice of midwifery through the generations of female family members relied on experience, patience, home remedies, and prayer. Lack of licensure, organization, and formal education prevented urban immigrant midwives and black midwives in the rural South from becoming part of the U.S. healthcare system (Varney & Thompson, 2016). Meanwhile, pioneer women crossing the country with their families provided birth assistance to other women in the wagon trains (King et al., 2018).

During the 19th century, the status of American women was at an all-time low. Midwifery was reduced from an honorable profession to one of disrespect. Religious attitudes, economics, replacement of midwives by physicians, lack of education and organization, an increase in immigrants in the United States, and the disenfranchisement of all women contributed to this shift (King et al., 2018) (Box 9.2).

Midwifery in the Early 20th Century

In the early 1900s, healthcare for women began to change with the establishment of the Children's Bureau in Washington, DC, and the Maternity Center Association (MCA) in New York City (King et al., 2018). These organizations made women's health and newborn care a priority by focusing on maternal and infant mortality, regardless of who was providing the care. The first order of

BOX 9.2

▶ KEY DATES IN U.S. NURSE MIDWIFERY HISTORY

	Event
1915	Maternity Center Association (MCA) in New York City identified the connection between mortality and lack of prenatal care. As a result, 30 maternity centers were established in NYC to care for women. MCA collaborated with Henry Street Visiting Nurse Association to study maternity care.
1925	Mary Breckinridge, British-trained nurse midwife, established the Frontier Nursing Service (FNS) in Kentucky.
1932	Manhattan Midwifery School in NYC becomes the first school for education of graduate nurses to become midwives.
1960s	Only New Mexico, Kentucky, and NYC legally recognized nurse midwifery practice.
1968	Nurse midwives were hired by the Maternal-Infant Care (MIC) nurse midwifery program in NYC to practice in community clinics.
1969	The Indian Health Service allowed nurse midwives to practice.
1971	A joint statement from the American College of Obstetricians and Gynecologists, the Nurses Association of the American College of Obstetricians and Gynecologists, and the American College of Nurse-Midwives supported the expansion of midwifery services.
1984	Nurse midwives were practicing in all 50 states plus the District of Columbia, Guam, Puerto Rico, and the Virgin Islands.
2010	Congress passed the Patient Protection and Affordable Care Act (ACA), recognizing nurse midwives as critical members of the healthcare workforce.
2012	Institute of Medicine finds expenditures to educate OB/GYN residents were $500 million, while only $2 million was spent educating nurse midwives.
2017	The American College of Nurse-Midwives released a position statement recognizing the role of nurse midwives as primary care providers as well as leaders of Maternity Care Homes.

business was to conduct a study of infant death. In 1912, the infant mortality rate was 124 per 1,000 live births (compared with 5.9/1,000 in 2016). The Centers for Disease Control and Prevention (CDC) defines infant mortality as the number of infant deaths prior to their first birthday. The Children's Bureau identified the link between infant health and maternal health during the maternity period. This outlined the relationship between early and continuous prenatal care and the ability to save women and children from sickness and death.

In 1915, the MCA identified the connection between mortality and lack of prenatal care. The New York health commissioner established 30 maternity centers in New York City to care for women. Teaching materials were developed, and educational exhibits presented throughout the city to demonstrate maternity and prenatal care. MCA and the Henry Street Visiting Nurse Association collaborated to study maternity care from a public health perspective and compared it with how other countries provided obstetrical care. This led to the understanding of the need to prepare nurses who provide routine obstetric care, and the idea of a school of nurse midwifery was born (King et al., 2018).

A debate ensued over the value of midwifery to provide for women's healthcare needs. Nurse midwifery educational programs opened, and European nurse midwives who were an integral part of the European healthcare system with a proven track record of excellence were introduced in the United States. The first nurse midwives to practice in the United States were British trained and brought in by Mary Breckinridge in 1925 to care for the women of the Kentucky mountains. The Frontier Nursing Service (FNS) involved outpost nursing centers staffed by nurse midwives and backed by a medical doctor located in a rural hospital. Prior to the opening of the FNS, a study of births and deaths in the region was conducted to provide baseline data (King et al., 2018). This work was monumental in changing obstetrical care in the United States. In 1951, the FNS statistics indicated that among the 8,596 registered nurse-midwifery patients delivered in primitive homes, the maternal death rate was 1.2 per 1,000 compared with the national maternal death rate of 6.73 per 1,000. These improved outcomes were not a result of a nurse midwifery education program but rather from the implementation of a midwifery model of care during delivery (King et al., 2018).

The first school for educating graduate nurses to be midwives was the Manhattan Midwifery School in New York City. The Manhattan Midwifery School only existed briefly and was replaced by the Lobenstine Midwifery

School, named after the charter member Dr. Ralph Waldo Lobenstine. The curriculum was based on the British curriculum and modified to meet the needs of American cultural patterns and the healthcare system in the United States. Hattie Hemschemeyer, a public health nurse educator, was named the first director of the Lobenstine Midwifery Clinic and School. From 1932 to 1958, the school and clinic attended 7,099 deliveries, 6,116 in the patient's homes, with a maternal mortality rate of 0.9 per 1,000 live births, in contrast to a maternal death rate of 10.4 per 1,000 live births in the same geographic district for leading hospitals in New York City (Varney & Thompson, 2016).

In Their Own Words

Victoria L. Asturrizaga, MSN, CNM

The key points in understanding my role are… One of the key points to understanding my role is being aware that midwifery is not obstetrics or gynecology. Similar to an OB/GYN, midwives are able to care for patients from menarche through menopause and beyond. We also care for those who become pregnant and their families from their first prenatal appointment through their postpartum period. CNMs specialize in care of the low-risk pregnancy and well woman, while the physician is the expert in high-risk pregnancies, gynecologic complications, and surgery. We tend to practice more holistically and not only incorporate the whole person into our care plan but the family as well. We, as midwives, tend to spend more quality time with our patients to get better acquainted with them in order to provide a more personalized care plan. Physicians and midwives are both experts in our fields and while they overlap in many instances, they are very different. We work together to provide a cohesive environment and seamless care that includes the best of both worlds. Many, if not all, CNMs have collaborative practice agreements with physicians to ensure continuity of care when complications arise. We can consult, collaborate, and refer to an OB/GYN if need be and still remain part of the care team to provide continuity of care and support for the patient and family.

Another point to understand is that there are different types of midwives and the rules and regulations that govern our practices vary from state to state. It is important for each midwife to know their state's practice acts and scope of

(Continued)

practice. Some states have independent practice and others require a written agreement with a physician in order to practice. Practicing within our license and scope enables us to provide the highest quality of care possible.

What keeps me coming back every day are… What keeps me coming back every day are the patients and families I care for. Midwifery care tends to be a more personal experience. We develop relationships with those we care for. We are there at some of the best and/or worst times of their lives while supporting them through it and walking alongside them. They may not remember myself or the nurses and maybe not even the room or hospital they were in; but they will remember how safe, supported, and empowered they felt during their visit or stay. It is very rewarding to enable families to have the experiences they are looking for.

My greatest challenge is… My greatest challenge is to dispel the myths of midwifery. Most of society views midwives as Birkenstock-wearing, crunchy-granola women who attend home births and dabble with herbs. Many believe that we only care for women during pregnancy and labor. While we can be and do all of these, we also attend hospital births and call for epidurals, we support during cesarean sections and educate on formula feeding, and we see patients for annual exams and provide education on contraception and abortion. We are whatever the families we serve need us to be. Historically, we were made out to be dirty, disease-spreading, ignorant witches placing mothers' and babies' lives at risk. The reality is far from the truth. We have always brought the best, most comprehensive care to wherever the need is; whether the setting is a home in the hills of Kentucky, a private practice office, or a busy intercity hospital obstetric unit. The statistics show that compared with care provided by other providers, midwifery care excels in many areas. The patients we care for experience higher rates of normal vaginal birth, breastfeeding, satisfaction with their birth experience and lower rates of labor interventions, cesarean sections, episiotomies, and significant vaginal tearing. These are the facts of midwifery.

I wish someone had told me… I wish someone had told me how much I would fall in love with my career choice. Prior to becoming a CNM, I was a labor and delivery registered nurse for over 13 years. I thoroughly enjoyed caring for these patients during what would be one of the most memorable times in their lives. It was amazing to see the strength and courage these women displayed. I worked with many talented and compassionate providers and learned what true "being with woman" is. I learned what midwifery care was and the benefits

(Continued)

these patients received from such care and I wanted to be able to provide that kind of care. When patients put their trust in me and are happy with the care they receive that means more to me than anything. There are so many opportunities to educate and empower our patients through the different stages of their lives and get to know them, as well as their families, over the years. This relationship between patient and midwife is like no other.

I need to be a lifelong learner because… Midwives practice evidence-based care which means that we never stop learning. We need to keep our knowledge base up-to-date with the most clinically relevant information and recommendations that are made based on that information. Following studies, looking at the evidence to develop recommendations and plans of care is how we deliver the best possible care to those we serve. As newer evidence emerges, our care must adapt to these new standards. Midwives are constantly reading journals, attending conferences and workshops, and networking with peers to seek out learning experiences to continue to provide the best care for those that we care for.

Another point to understand is… Midwifery is both an art and a science. It is the science of researching and relaying the pertinent clinical information along with the art of compassion and support. Our job is not to dictate care or direct the patients in what course of action, or inaction to take. Our job is to provide them with the information and tools they need to make the decisions regarding their healthcare plan for themselves while providing emotional and physical support needed during the decision-making process. Only the patient knows what works best for them and their family, we provide safe options in every scenario and discuss their values, fears, and desires as they relate to those options. This is patient-centered shared decision-making and is one of the hallmarks of midwifery care.

Midwifery in the Late 20th Century

Practice opportunities were limited for early-1960s midwifery graduates. Only two states and one city legally recognized nurse midwifery practice: New Mexico, Kentucky, and New York City. Maryland allowed nurse midwives to practice under a "granny midwife" law. Nurse midwives could join the faculties of existing midwife education programs or practice overseas doing mission work. Early graduates went into teaching or supervisory or administrative roles in healthcare.

In the late 1950s and early 1960s, nurse midwives made a deliberate effort to gain access to hospitals where the majority of births were performed. They moved toward family-centered maternity care and became consumer advocates to childbearing women. At this time, nurse midwives were successful in working in and out of the hospital. Nurse midwives in 1968 were hired by the Maternal-Infant Care (MIC) nurse midwifery program in New York City to practice in community clinics. In addition to attending births, midwives provided well-woman care, including birth control counseling and placement. In 1969, the Indian Health Service allowed nurse midwives to practice (King et al., 2018). Despite their low maternal and infant mortality and high patient satisfaction, nurse midwife practices were not growing.

Many barriers existed to the acceptance of nurse midwives including misconceptions and stereotypes, very often among physicians and nurses. Varney and associates (2003) summarize this challenge:

> When only the word midwife is used, the word conjures up a negative image…of the good-hearted, loving but untrained midwife either of past history or in rural areas of the South…leading to the irrational conclusion that nurse-midwives are an uneducated menace representing a backward step into illiteracy in the provision of maternal-infant healthcare.
>
> (p. 14)

In the 1970s, more women were demanding nurse midwifery services. The U.S. healthcare system was struggling to meet the workforce demands, and it became clear that nurse midwives were not only safe but valued (Varney & Thompson, 2016). During this time of rapid growth, 22 nurse midwifery educational programs were developed.

A number of factors contributed to the growing acceptance of midwives. In a 1971 joint statement, the American College of Obstetricians and Gynecologists, the Nurses Association of the American College of Obstetricians and Gynecologists, and the American College of Nurse-Midwives (ACNM) supported the expansion of midwifery services. The women's movement and the rise of feminism increased women's feelings of self-worth and confidence. They gravitated to nurse midwives who embraced natural and normal birth processes, family-centered care, and the right to self-determination. Public awareness of the nurse midwife role increased with articles in *Life, Redbook, Newsweek, McCall's,* the *New York Times,* and *The Wall Street Journal.* Consumer awareness and satisfaction from women who were served by nurse midwives increased the demand in ways never expected. Nurse midwives were now present in federally funded projects such as MIC, Family Planning (314E), and other projects geared toward improving maternal-infant health and family planning services.

The post–World War II baby boom resulted in an insufficient number of obstetricians to care for all of the childbearing women in the United States (Varney & Thompson, 2016). After years of struggling for recognition, nurse midwives were now the preferred providers of care by many women. The resulting shortage and increased demand for services by women who did not want to deliver in a hospital setting led to the development of lay midwifery. Lay midwifery is a term that still exists and refers to midwives who enter the profession through apprenticeship to a practicing midwife as opposed to through a formal educational program (Davis-Floyd & Johnson, 2006).

In Their Own Words

Cathy Collins-Fulea, DNP, CNM, FACNM
President, American College of Nurse-Midwives
Assistant Professor, Frontier Nursing University

The key points in understanding my role are… As president of the American College of Nurse-Midwives, it is my role to represent the interests of certified nurse-midwives and certified midwives as well as advance the practice of midwifery, achieving optimal health for the people we serve throughout their lifespan. I do this by promoting education, research, and advocacy that advances clinical excellence; advocating for the expansion of a diverse midwifery workforce; and lobbying for equitable legislation, regulation, and institutional policies that establish midwifery as the standard of care for women. I lead a board of dedicated midwives who set the agenda for how we will accomplish this and together with a national office staff and a robust volunteer structure, we work to accomplish our vision of a midwife for every woman.

What keeps me coming back every day is… knowing that I can make a difference. That one dedicated person can inspire others to greatness.

My greatest challenge is… creating a sense of belong among all midwives that there is value in belonging to a community of midwives who are working

(Continued)

collectively to advance the profession. Everyone is so busy with their own lives that they forget that we need to put effort into maintaining the gains we have and to pushing forward to ensure full autonomy in practice. We can do this by belonging to the community of midwives.

I wish someone had told me… how hard it is to maintain a work-life balance when you volunteer to lead. There is always something that needs done, a new crisis that needs attention. I could spend 25 hours a day and still there would be more to do. To be able to accomplish what needs done you must keep a laser focus on the goal. To be able to do this you must be healthy yourself which means taking time for yourself and your family. You will have more energy and more focus if you are centered and grounded.

I need to be a lifelong learner because… there is always more to learn. New information that needs assimilated. New ways of looking at old knowledge. Times change, people change, the environment changes. To understand how to adapt, you need to be open to new ideas, which means continuous learning. It is not just the science that is changing as we conduct more research to identify best practices. It is how we interact with others, how we motivate others, how we honor others. Life is a journey. Every person we come in contact with along the way can teach us from their life experiences and we can learn through them. So the learning never stops. It helps us to grow as an individual and as a leader.

Another point to understand is… leading is not easy. You need to be open to listening to others and learning from others. Leaders need to be able to see into the future and communicate that in a way that inspires others to want to join the journey. It is only when we work together that we can see the true transformative change that is possible. None of us is as strong as all of us.

Nurse midwives were now practicing in clinics, federally funded programs, health maintenance organizations (HMOs), and hospitals and provided a full range of services for women's health. During this time, an overabundance of physicians providing obstetrical care led to restrictions in nurse midwife practice through denial of hospital practice privileges, pressuring of physicians supportive of the midwifery model of care, and restricting midwife malpractice coverage (Varney & Thompson, 2016). Some OB/GYNs believed nurse midwives were no longer needed. The Federal Trade Commission became involved due to restraint-of-trade concerns. At the same time, healthcare costs were increasing while services by nurse midwives provided the same care and were more cost-effective. By 1984, nurse midwives were practicing in all 50 states. The legal practice of midwifery had gone from three states and one city to full legal status in all states plus the District of Columbia, Guam, Puerto Rico, and the Virgin Islands. This was a direct result of intense legislative efforts and by the ACNM and spawned the growth of out-of-hospital birth centers. Lay midwives organized and formed the Midwives Alliance of North American (MANA), which includes midwives in the United States, Canada, and Mexico (King et al., 2018).

Midwifery at the Turn of the 21st Century

Following an increased demand for nurse midwives and increase of nurse midwifery educational programs, nurse midwifery is currently recognized as safe and cost-effective. ACNM set the goal of having 10,000 midwives by the year 2001. By mid-2001, the total number of persons certified as midwives was 9,327 and 11,826 by 2017. The Accreditation Commission for Midwifery Education (ACME, 2020) identifies 39 accredited midwifery programs in the United States, although they note that this number may actually be higher given options for those entering with a graduate degree.

The American College of Obstetricians and Gynecologists (ACOG) anticipates a growing shortage of obstetricians and gynecologists with a shortfall of up to 22,000 practitioners by 2050 (Doximity, 2020). Public investment into the education of a single OB/GYN resident is approximately $127,000. Since nursing education is not publicly subsidized, CNMs represent a significantly effective option in terms of cost and high quality outcomes (ACNM, 2015). Coupled with excellent outcomes and high patient satisfaction, the decreased costs for nurse midwifery education make this role a viable solution to cost-effective, high-quality care (ACNM, 2012).

Legislative issues continue to be a priority in the 2000s. Legislation is focused on removing supervisory language in licensure laws, reimbursement, and liability insurance and removing barriers to practice and access to care. The most recent joint statement between ACOG and ACNM in 2011 highlights evidence-based practice and acknowledges that CNMs are licensed independent providers and should receive equivalent third-party reimbursement.

Role of the Midwife

The role of the midwife is varied. Midwives serve diverse populations requiring different services depending on regions or institutional setting. The midwife's role is also influenced by scope of practice as determined by legal jurisdictions, institutional policy, and individual education and training. At best, the laws support independent midwifery practice and collaboration. The most restrictive laws require direct physician supervision of midwives. Figure 9.2 presents 2019 employment data for nurse midwives.

Populations Served and Services Provided

Nurse midwives provide primary healthcare for women from adolescence through postmenopause and can also provide primary care for newborns. This care includes general health check-ups, screenings, and vaccinations; pregnancy, birth, and postpartum care; well-woman gynecologic care; treatment of sexually

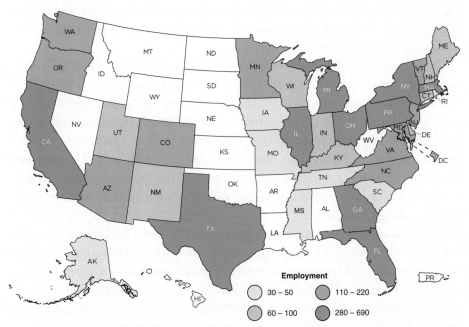

Figure 9.2. Employment of nurse midwives by state, May 2019. (From the U.S. Bureau of Labor and Statistics.)

transmitted infections; and prescription of medications. Care is provided any-where women are seeking healthcare, frequently providing care in rural or underserved populations as well as to those women who seek care with a holistic approach that is woman and family centered (see Figure 9.3). Care is provided

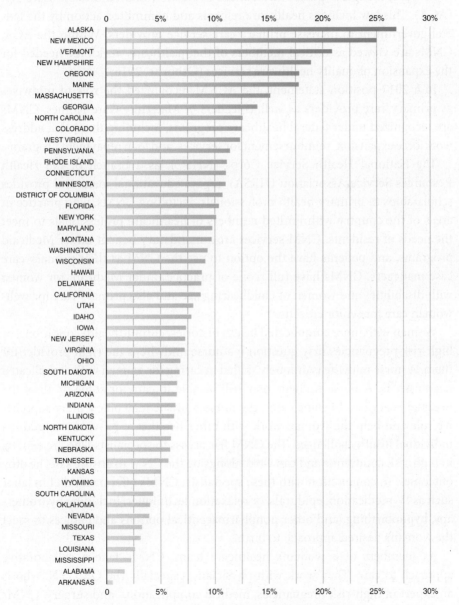

Figure 9.3. Percentage of births attended by midwives.

on a continuous and comprehensive basis to include wellness, preventive care, screening, and treatment for healthcare problems with a focus on the unique needs of various cultural, socioeconomic, and psychological factors that influence the health status of women.

In 2010, Congress passed the Patient Protection and Affordable Care Act (ACA). This law includes healthcare reforms and committed action by the federal government to increase primary care service providers. Within the ACA, CNMs are viewed as critical members of the healthcare workforce needed for the expansion of quality healthcare services (Osborne, 2016).

In a 2017 position statement, the ACNM recognized the role of midwives as primary care providers as well as leaders of Maternity Care Homes. CNMs are recognized under federal healthcare programs, including those that address workforce expansion, reimbursement for services, and loan repayment programs.

The National Health Service Corps (NHSC), as a branch of the Health Resources Service Association (HRSA), repays educational loans and provides scholarships to primary health professionals, including CNMs, who practice in areas of the country with limited numbers of healthcare professionals to meet the needs of residents. CNM services are a mandatory benefit under Medicaid programs, and patients have the option to use the CNM as their primary care case managers. CNMs have full scope of practice under Medicare for women with disabilities and women of childbearing age and also primary care for well-woman care for senior citizens.

Women with more complicated health histories, chronic health conditions, or high-risk pregnancies may question if a nurse midwife is the right provider for them. A nurse midwife is uniquely skilled in caring for women with complicated health needs. A nurse midwife may still be able to care for some or all of the necessary services. In some cases, the nurse midwife may play a more supportive role and help the woman work with other healthcare providers to address individual health challenges. The CNM has access to specialists who are experts in high-risk conditions and can work alongside the CNM to ensure safe, healthy outcomes. In conjunction with these specialists, CNMs offer pain relief in labor such as IV medication, epidurals, or relaxation techniques, including hydrotherapy, hypnobirthing, and other nonpharmaceutical options and choices to meet the woman's desired approach to birth.

As members of a woman's healthcare team, CNMs take a collaborative approach to care. They work with physicians, especially the OB/GYN, who is an expert in high-risk pregnancies, medical complications, and surgery. CNMs also work closely with doulas who provide emotional and physical support for women in labor, as well as advocating for and educating them. By working collaboratively with both OB/GYNs and doulas, CNMs help to ensure women have a full range of healthcare services available.

In Their Own Words

Kim Amsley-Camp, CNM, MS

The key points in understanding my role are… Midwife means, "with woman." Every woman deserves a midwife. What most do not know is that midwives are the primary care giver of women worldwide. CNMs in the United States are registered nurses with master's degrees in midwifery, licensed in every state and must pass a national certification exam. Many have PhDs or doctoral degrees. Ninety-five percent of births by midwives were in hospitals. The remaining 5% are done in birth centers or at home. We care for woman of all ages. We care for newborns from birth to 6 weeks of age and care for women from adolescence through menopause. We do well-woman gynecology, prescribe contraception, treat and screen for sexually transmitted diseases, provide obstetrical care through prenatal care and antepartum care, do deliveries, and provide postpartum care. Another common myth is that we don't provide pain medications. We offer all pain medications including epidurals and are expert in nonpharmaceutical pain management and can help develop a birth plan that best fits the woman's personal needs and desires. Even if a woman has a chronic health condition or is high-risk, midwives are able to provide some or all of the care needed. In some cases, the midwife may play more of a supportive role and help work with other healthcare professionals to coordinate and work alongside specialists who are experts in high-risk conditions to ensure safe, health outcomes. All women can be cared for by a midwife if she chooses.

What keeps me coming back every day is… I especially enjoy watching the woman change and grow over her lifespan. Women change when they become mothers. They become far more focused on their children and their families and their needs change. My goal is to empower the woman to have a safe, healthy, family-centered birth. Midwives "mother the mother" which models for her how to "mother" her children and feel confident in that role. For those women who do not have children, primary and gynecological needs change

(Continued)

over a lifetime. The goal is to assist the woman in living a healthy lifestyle through general health check-ups, screenings, and vaccinations. I am inspired by women and in awe of their strength. It is truly an honor and a privilege to have a front seat to birth and to spend just a moment of someone's life with them in one of the most important events in their life.

My greatest challenge is... Balance. To be sure to care for myself and take time for myself so I can care for others. We can never give all we have or we will have nothing left for ourselves and our families. We have to be able to maintain boundaries and rely on the team around us to coordinate care. It is truly a team approach between the midwife, the obstetrician, and the woman, and her family. We have to be flexible enough to care for the woman who has a healthy birth and go to the next examining room and share in a difficult experience such as a pregnancy with significant anomalies. Both women need us and deserve our skill and compassion. That having been said, this is the greatest career I could have ever chosen.

I wish someone had told me... Rest, eat, and use the rest room. Those are the downfalls of our work. Days can be long and tiring and we give of ourselves emotionally and intellectually. Our needs come after those we care for. So, I have learned to fuel up with good nutrition, before I go to the office or hospital, arrive well rested, stay hydrated, and empty my bladder when I get the chance.

I need to be a lifelong learner because... The one thing that is constant is change. Thank goodness. We learn new things, embrace new ways of doing things, discard those processes which are no longer effective in caring for women, and keep on reading and learning. We are required to complete continuing education every year to maintain our state licensure and our national certification. We read journal articles from both our *Journal of Midwifery* and the *Obstetrics & Gynecology* journal, to name a few.

Another point to understand is... Women are important. If their healthcare needs are ignored or not cared for adequately, the entire family suffers. It is women who are usually the gatekeeper for the family's healthcare needs. The woman has far more interaction with the healthcare system through her own care and that of her children. If she is happy with an institution, she can trust them to care for her family as well. Midwifery is vital to addressing the challenges of providing high-quality maternal and newborn care for women and newborns, through a proven track record of providing evidence-based care which improves lives.

Nurse midwives practice in hospitals, freestanding birth centers, clinics, private practices, homes, and medical offices. Many practice in more than one setting to ensure their clients have access to a range of desired services and to allow for specific health considerations. About 95% of CNMs work in hospitals, from community hospitals to tertiary and academic institutions. *Lancet* (2014) published a series of landmark articles declaring "Midwifery matters now more than ever." Despite the highest per capita spending on healthcare, the United States ranks higher in infant and maternal mortality and morbidity compared with other high-wealth countries (GBD 2015 Maternal Mortality Collaborators, 2016). The 2014 *Lancet* series on midwifery further recognizes the skilled and supportive care midwives provide for all women and infants, regardless of their socioeconomic status, education level, or health status. This framework of care promotes normalization of the birth process while providing highly skilled emergency care to the individual woman, which serves to strengthen her capabilities as a woman and a mother. Midwives in this role can change and strengthen the communities they serve by combining care and service to bring midwifery into the mainstream of the wider health system.

In *Varney's Midwifery* (2018), King and associates outline a review of obstetrical outcome measures, comparing care by CNMs and other providers including OB/GYNs. CNM-attended births consistently have better outcomes for moms and neonates.

Competencies and Scope of Practice

The *Core Competencies for Basic Midwifery Practice* is the basis of midwifery practice in the United States for midwives certified by the ACNM or the AMCB. This document, most recently reviewed in 2012, applies to all settings for midwifery care, including hospitals, ambulatory care settings, birth centers, and homes. It provides the framework for midwifery education and ultimately certification by the board. These competencies are based on the understanding of health sciences theory and clinical preparation that shapes knowledge, judgment, and skills. ACNM strongly believes that adherence to these standards in their entirety ensures the safety of women's care.

Competencies can be expanded based on additional skills and procedures necessary to provide primary healthcare management to women and newborns. Many nurse midwives are certified in ultrasound technology, serve as surgical first assistants, and perform colposcopies, endometrial biopsies, and newborn male circumcisions, if needed by their practice setting (American College of Nurse Midwives, 2016).

The midwife's scope of practice is determined by legal jurisdictions, institutional policy, and individual education and training. Laws support independent midwifery practice and collaborative management, but some states require direct supervision by physicians. Professional organizations such as ACNM and MANA outline state midwifery law summaries on their web sites. As these laws are constantly changing, knowing a reliable source for the most current information is essential (see Web Resources Box).

Midwives who attend births in hospitals and some birth centers are credentialed and granted privileges by the healthcare facility. Bylaws of the organization define the requirements of granting privileges and often specify the roles of the midwives in relation to their consulting physician and the responsibilities of the physician in relation to their collaborating midwives. Sometimes these institutional bylaws are more restrictive than state laws.

Most CNMs in the United States are also independent healthcare providers who operate with a collaborative agreement with a physician (Figures 9.3 and 9.4). Statutory or regulatory language that differentiates scope of practice or practice authority based on birth site or practice setting rather than credential is not supported by the ACNM, nor is physician supervision supported by ACNM (Osborne, 2015). Specifics of collaborative agreements also vary by state and can be restrictive. In general, the agreement outlines when a consultant or referral will be made. This is intended to be a critical safety mechanism that assures women and babies will be safe and provides for a complete continuum of care if healthcare needs change or become more complex.

Key provisions of the Affordable Care Act were aimed at increasing access to health insurance coverage. The 2010 report of the Institute of Medicine, *The Future of Nursing: Leading Change and Advancing Health,* identifies CNMs as one of the advanced practice registered nurses (APRNs) and highlights the crucial role they will play in meeting increasing demand for primary care providers. The report also references lifting "the constraints of outdated policies, regulations, and cultural barriers, including those related to scope of practice...most notably for APRNs" (p. 519).

Although regulations have been updated in some states, barriers still exist for full-practice authority for CNMs. Midwifery practice is regulated at the state level and must be changed one state at a time. This process of change is complex and challenging. To enact a statute, a bill must be first passed by the legislature and signed into law by the governor. Administrative rules must be written and adopted by a regulatory body. This regulatory body differs from state to state. Some regulatory bodies are assisted by advisory boards, but midwives may not be represented on these boards. Interpretation of legislation affecting midwives may fall to ancillary personnel, such as respiratory therapists, undertakers, or any nonphysician licensed person in the state. The presence of midwives at policymaking tables is essential to prevent policies that create barriers to practice or that limit the ability of midwives to increase access to comprehensive care.

Prescriptive Authority

Prescriptive authority is governed by regulatory boards and individual state agencies and varies widely across states. Inconsistent regulatory requirements often impose barriers to full-practice authority and limit patients' access to necessary services. Nurse midwives have prescriptive authority in all 50 states, as well as District of Columbia, American Samoa, Guam, and Puerto Rico. Despite improvements in regulatory environments, many states face statutory barriers to full-practice authority including barriers to autonomous prescribing privileges (see Figure 9.4). Most midwives can prescribe controlled substances and have Drug Enforcement Administration (DEA) licenses. More detailed information related to prescriptive authority is provided in Chapter 7.

Certification and Continuing Education

The AMCB is the national certifying body for candidates in nurse midwifery education who have received graduate-level education in programs accredited by the ACME. This certification is considered the gold standard of midwifery in all 50 states. The AMCB (2013) identifies the role of certification as the means of protecting "the public by ensuring that certified individual have met predetermined criteria for safety in practice" (para. 3). While state licensure provides the legal basis for practice, most states require AMCB certification for licensure, and many institutions require AMCB certification to grant practice privileges.

Independent practice—
Full prescriptive authority, and ability to practice independently:

- Alaska, Arizona, Colorado, Connecticut, Hawaii, Idaho, Iowa, Maine, Maryland, Massachusetts, Montana, New Hampshire, New Mexico, New York, North Dakota, Oregon, Rhode Island, Utah, Vermont, Washington, Washington D.C.

Restricted practice—
Prescriptive authority with collaborative agreement:

- Indiana, Kentucky, Michigan, Oklahoma, Tennessee, Texas, West Virginia

Not independent practice—
Collaborative practice agreement required:

- Alabama, Arkansas, California, Florida, Delaware, Georgia, Illinois, Kansas, Louisiana, Mississippi, Missouri, Nebraska, North Carolina, Ohio, Pennsylvania, South Carolina, South Dakota, Virginia, Wisconsin

Figure 9.4. Independent prescribing.

Certification is effective for 5 years. Modules in Antepartum and Primary Care of the Pregnant Woman, Intrapartum, Postpartum and Newborn, and Gynecology and Primary Care for the Well-Woman must be completed every 5 years. In addition, recertification requires completion of 20 contact hours of continuing education along with payment of annual fees and completion of a recertification application. Continuing education is a requirement for every certification cycle. In lieu of a portion of the contact hours, this requirement can be granted by one of the following nine alternative ways:

1. Graduate-level coursework
2. DNP- and PhD-level coursework in health-related field
3. Formal presentation on a topic that has contact hour approved from AMCB
4. Publication in a peer-referred journal as the primary author
5. Primary author of a chapter in a peer-reviewed textbook
6. Peer reviewer of an article for a referred journal or textbook chapter
7. Direct clinical supervision as a preceptor to a nursemidwifery student from an ACME accredited program
8. Participation in an ACNM or AMCB committee
9. Participation in an ACME Accreditation review

Summary

Midwives have long provided excellent primary care and are committed to improving health outcomes of women and babies. In many countries, midwives are the accepted standard for care during the birthing process including prenatal and postpartum support to the mother and infant. Midwives also specialize in primary care for women across their lifespan.

Competencies, standards of care, and a code of ethics are set by the ACNM. ACNM also oversees the accreditation of nurse midwifery educational programs and supports this education at the master's level. Certification as a nurse midwife is regulated through the AMCB.

Nurse midwives are highly educated and dedicated to the wellness of women and their children. Midwifery programs are rigorous and attract highly motivated individuals who are not only committed to the profession but to the clients they serve. Midwives dedicate themselves to advocate for woman and actively pursue legislative and regulatory challenges that threaten their autonomy or the commitment to science and evidence for the benefit of the women and families they serve. Every woman deserves a midwife.

Chapter Highlights

- Nurse midwifery has a rich heritage of providing maternity and primary care services to women and infants, particularly in areas where physician access is limited.
- Though nurse midwives provide necessary services to underserved populations, they remain challenged by legislation that hinders their licensure, reimbursement and liability insurance, and full-practice authority.
- Nurse midwives not only care for women experiencing a "normal" pregnancy, but they are well prepared to care for women with complicated and complex health needs.
- Nurse midwives take a collaborative approach to their rendering of patient care, working both with physicians and with doulas to ensure their patients have a full range of services.

Web Resources

The World Health Organization—Maternal Health: https://www.who.int/maternal-health/en/

The Maternal Health Task Force: https://www.mhtf.org/

UNICEF—Maternal Mortality: https://data.unicef.org/topic/maternal-health/maternal-mortality/

United Nations—Maternal Health: https://www.unfpa.org/maternal-health

Professional Organizations

Accreditation Commission for Midwifery Education: https://www.midwife.org/acme

American College of Nurse-Midwives (ACNM): http://www.midwife.org/

American Midwifery Certification Board: https://www.amcbmidwife.org/

Midwife Alliance of North America (MANA): https://mana.org/

References

Accreditation Commission for Midwifery Education (ACME). (2020). *Certified Nurse-Midwife (CNM) degree programs with ACME accreditation by degree.* https://www.midwifeschooling.com/accredited-nurse-midwife-programs/#:~:text=Although%20there%20are%20currently%2039,students%20with%20different%20educational%20backgrounds

American College of Nurse-Midwives. (2012). *Core competencies for basic midwifery practice.* http://www.midwife.org/ACNM/files/ACNMLibraryData/UPLOADFILENAME/000000000050/Core%20Comptencies%20Dec%202012.pdf

American College of Nurse-Midwives. (2015). *Midwives: The answer to the US maternity care provider shortage.* http://www.midwife.org/acnm/files/cclibraryfiles/filename/000000007474/DetailedTPsonMaternityCareWorkforce.pdf

American College of Nurse Midwives (ACNM). (2016). *Expansion of midwifery practice and skills beyond basic core competencies.* https://www.midwife.org/ACNM/files/ACNMLibraryData/UPLOADFILENAME/000000000066/Expansion-of-Midwifery-Practice-June-2015.pdf

American College of Nurse-Midwives. (2017). *Comparison of certified nurse-midwives, certified midwives, certified professional midwives clarifying the distinction among professional midwifery credential in the U.S.* http://www.midwife.org/acnm/files/ccLibraryFiles/FILENAME/000000006807/FINAL-ComparisonChart-Oct2017.pdf

American Midwifery Certification Board. (2013). *Purpose/objectives.* https://www.amcbmidwife.org/certificate-maintenance-program/purpose-objectives

American Midwifery Certification Board. (2018). *Candidate handbook.* https://www.amcbmidwife.org/amcb-certification/candidate-handbook

Centers for Disease Control and Prevention. (2018). *Wonder online databases.* https://wonder.cdc.gov

Davis-Floyd, R., & Johnson, C. B. (2006). *Mainstreaming midwives: The politics of change.* Routledge.

Doximity. (2020). *2018 OB-GYN workforce study: Looming physician shortages: A growing women's health crisis.* https://www.doximity.com/press/obgyn_report

Edmonds, J. K., Ivanof, J., & Kafulafula, U. (2020). Midwife led units: Transforming maternity care globally. *Annals of Global Health, 86*(1), 44. https://www.ncbi.nlm.nih.gov/pmc/articles/PMC7193683/

Global Burden of Disease (GBD) 2015 Maternal Mortality Collaborators. (2016). Global, regional, and national levels of maternal mortality, 1990–2015: A systematic analysis for the global burden of disease study 2015, *The Lancet, 388*(10053), 1775–1812.

International Confederation of Midwives. (2017). *Essential competencies for basic midwifery practice.* http://internationalmidwives.org/what-we-do/education-coredocuments/essential-competencies-basic-midwifery-practice/

King, T., Brucker, M., Jevitt, C. M., & Osborne, K. (2018). *Varney's midwifery* (6th ed.). Jones and Bartlett Publishers.

Mayer, R., Dingwall, A., Simon-Thomas, J., Sheikhnureldin, A., & Lewis, K. (2019). *The United States mortality rate will continue to increase without access to data.* https://www.healthaffairs.org/do/10.1377/hblog20190130.92512/full/

Osborne, K. (2015). Regulation of prescriptive authority for certified nurse-midwives and certified midwives: 2015 national overview. *Journal of Midwifery &Women's Health, 60*(5), 519–533. doi:10.1111/jmwh.12368

Osborne, K. (2016). Engaging in health policy: There's no time like the present. *Journal of Midwifery & Women's Health, 61*(3), 306–314.

Rooks, J. P. (1997). *Midwifery and childbirth in America.* Temple University Press.

The American College of Nurse Midwoves (ACNM). (2019). *Essential facts about midwives.* https://www.midwife.org/acnm/files/cclibraryfiles/filename/000000007531/EssentialFactsAboutMidwives-UPDATED.pdf

Varney, H., & Thompson, J. B. (2016). *The midwife said fear not: A history of midwifery in the United States.* Springer.

Vedam, S., Stoll, K., MacDorman, M., Declercq, E., Cramer, R., Cheyney, M., Fisher, T., Butt, E., Yang, Y. T., & Kennedy, H. P. (2018). Mapping integration of midwives across the United States: Impact on access, equity, and outcomes. *PLoS One, 13*(2), e0192523. doi:10.1371/journal.pone.0192523

Veteto, K. J. (2015). *Certified professional midwife vs. certified nurse midwife.* http://www.kristaveteto.com/certified-professional-midwife-vs-certified-nurse-midwife-cpm-vs-cnm/

10

Certified Registered Nurse Anesthetists

Tony Umadhay · John McFadden

LEARNING OBJECTIVES

After completing this chapter, you will be able to:

1. Trace the development of anesthesiology as a specialty within the field of nursing.

2. Describe the practice settings and populations served by CRNAs.

3. Defend the role and scope of the CRNA against a changing healthcare system.

4. Compare and contrast the educational, certification, and recertification requirements for CRNAs to other advanced practice nursing specialties.

5. Operationalize the AANA Standards of Practice for the CRNA in real-life and case-study scenarios.

KEY TERMS

American Association of Nurse Anesthetists (AANA): The professional organization that disseminates practice standards and guidelines for CRNA practice and supports CRNAs through education and research grants to students, faculty, and practicing CRNAs.

Anesthesia services: Also known as anesthesia-related care, services that anesthesia professionals provide upon request, assignment, and referral by the patient's healthcare provider authorized by law, most often to facilitate diagnostic, therapeutic, and surgical procedures, or for pain management (COA Standards for Accreditation of Nurse Anesthesia Programs—Practice Doctorate, Glossary, 2018). For a description of the full scope of practice of a CRNA, see the AANA Scope of Nurse Anesthesia Practice (2013a, 2013b).

Anesthesiology: The study and practice of the science and art of anesthesia delivery, which is a recognized specialty of both nursing and medicine, unified by the same standard of care (AANA Scope of Nurse Anesthesia Practice, 2013a, 2013b).

Certified registered nurse anesthetist (CRNA): An advanced practice registered nurse (APRN) who, in collaboration with a variety of healthcare providers on the interprofessional team, delivers high-quality, holistic, and evidence-based anesthesia and pain care services for patients at all acuity levels across the lifespan in a variety of settings (AANA Scope of Nurse Anesthesia Practice, 2013a; 2013b).

Continued Professional Certification: The process approved by the National Board of Certification and Recertification for Nurse Anesthetists for recertification as a CRNA. CPC was implemented in 2016 and is built around 8-year cycles (from https://www.nbcrna.com/continued-certification).

Council on Accreditation of Nurse Anesthesia Educational Programs (COA): The agency that accredits nurse anesthesia programs within the United States and Puerto Rico that awards post-master's certificates, master's or doctoral degrees, or postgraduate CRNA fellowships, including programs offering distance education (from https://www.coacrna.org/about/Pages/default.aspx).

National Board of Certification and Recertification for Nurse Anesthetists (NBCRNA): The agency that administers the National Certification Examination (NCE) for initial certification as a CRNA and administers the CPC process for recertification as a CRNA (from https://www.nbcrna.com/about-us).

Nurse anesthesia: Also known as nurse anesthesiology, an advanced practice specialty of nursing that encompasses the delivery of anesthesia services and anesthesia-related care by a CRNA (AANA Scope of Nurse Anesthesia Practice, 2013a; 2013b).

Introduction

Certified registered nurse anesthetists (CRNAs) are registered nurses with advanced education in the specialty of anesthesiology. More than 50,000 CRNAs and student registered nurse anesthetists (SRNAs) within the United States administer roughly 45 million anesthetics annually (AANA, 2018). CRNAs practice throughout the country in every setting in which anesthesia is delivered. They are the primary providers of anesthesia services in rural locations. In their roles, CRNAs collaborate with all members of the healthcare team, particularly surgeons, anesthesiologists, dentists, podiatrists, other physician specialists, nurses, and other qualified healthcare professionals.

History and Evolution

Surgery, as a medical specialty, continues to develop along with the evolving understanding of diseases and how the human body adapts. The 19th century, in particular, produced many strides for modern surgery. In her 1991 article, "The History of Nurse Anesthesia Education: Highlights and Influences," Gunn identified many of the inhibiting and facilitating factors related to this development. The discovery of germ theory and the practices that controlled the development and spread of infection addressed one major obstacle to a positive surgical outcome. The cultivation of trained, professional nurses and the formation of hospitals as safe places for healing also supported the advancement of surgery. A third major contributor was the discovery of surgical anesthesia. An array of anesthesia experiments by many individuals occurred over a protracted period. The successful public demonstration of surgical anesthesia by dentist William T. G. Morton at Massachusetts General Hospital on October 16, 1846, delineated the start of a new field of practice in the delivery of healthcare (Fenster, 2001). Morton's demonstration also established the need for refinement in the techniques of administration of anesthesia: the years following Morton's demonstration were filled with haphazard, if not rogue and dangerous, anesthetics administered by unskilled "anesthetizers." Frequently, an untrained hospital attendant or inexperienced medical intern with the least skills was given the role of an anesthetizer. The result was often suffocation, pneumonia, and death.

Anesthesiology as a Practice of Nursing

Some surgeons gained the assistance of religious nuns or "sisters," whose religious orders opened and serviced many hospitals in the United States during the 19th century. In her work, *The History of Anesthesia with an Emphasis on the Nurse Specialist*, Virginia Thatcher (1953) provided a detailed accounting of the contributions of these religious sister-nurses to the advancement of anesthesia. Thatcher, in her scholarly writings, identified many orders that prepared trained nurse anesthetists. They include the Order of the Hospital Sisters of St. Francis, the Order of the Sisters of Mercy, the Sisters of Charity, the Daughters of Charity of St. Vincent de Paul, the Sisters of Mercy of Wilkes-Barre, the Sisters of St. Joseph, the Franciscan Sisters of the Sacred Heart, and the Lutheran Diaconate. Two of the earliest sister-nurse anesthetists known by students of nurse anesthesia history include Sr. Mary Bernard, who within her first year of entering St. Vincent's hospital in 1877 began administering anesthesia, and Sister Secundina Mindrup of the Third Order of St. Francis. Thatcher writes, "Sister Secundina devised her own method for judging when more ether or chloroform or alcohol-chloroform-ether mixture should be given—a decade of prayers on her rosary and it was time to give a little more." (pp. 54–55).

In 1889, the Sisters of St. Francis established St. Mary's Hospital in Rochester, Minnesota, under the medical direction of Dr. William Worrell Mayo. Here two nurses who graduated from the School of Nursing at the Women's Hospital in Chicago, Dinah and Edith Graham, served as the Mayo Clinic's first nurse anesthetists. Although Dinah Graham stopped practicing early, Edith Graham continued to practice anesthesia until her marriage to Dr. Charles Mayo in 1893. Alice Magaw, another graduate from the same school of nursing, took over for Edith (Figure 10.1). Magaw's article, "*Observations in Anesthesia*," published in the *Northwestern Lancet* in 1899, reported on the successful delivery of more than 3,000 anesthetics. By 1906, she authored "*Review of Over Fourteen Thousand Surgical Anesthesias*" published in *Surgery, Gynecology and Obstetrics*. Not a single death was attributed to the anesthesia or the practice of Mayo's nurse anesthetists. Magaw's commitment to perfecting the administration of anesthesia led Dr. Charles Mayo to bestow upon her the title "Mother of Anesthesia."

The techniques of these early nurse anesthetists using open drop ether spread throughout the Midwest. More and more nurses were trained as nurse anesthetists, even as far east as the Gynecean Hospital in Philadelphia, Pennsylvania. As early as 1893, nurse educator Isabel Adams Hampton Robb included a chapter on the

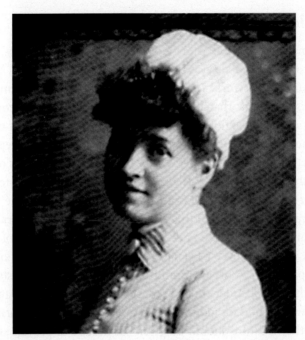

Figure 10.1. Alice Magaw, circa 1899. (Reprinted with permission from American Association of Nurse Anesthetists (AANA) Archives.)

administration of anesthesia in her textbook, *Nursing: Its Principles and Practices for Hospital and Private Use*. The practice of anesthesia by nurses, dating back to the latter half of the 19th century, became the first advanced practice nursing specialty.

In the early 1900s, surgeon George W. Crile practiced at the Lakeside Hospital in Cleveland, Ohio. Crile, a renowned expert on shock, favored the use of a nitrous oxide-oxygen mixture over the Mayo Clinic's use of open drop ether. Crile hired nurse Agatha Hodgins, someone he considered to have the best personal and professional qualities to administer anesthesia, as his nurse anesthetist in 1908 (Figure 10.2). Hodgins originally trained at the Boston City Hospital Training School for Nurses and chose to work at the Lakeside Hospital upon graduation. She learned anesthesia under Crile and also visited the Mayo Clinic to learn their techniques of administration.

Visiting surgeons soon began sending their nurses to learn the techniques of Crile and Hodgins. By the time World War I began, Crile and Hodgins had established the Lakeside Hospital School of Anesthesia. This program joined the ranks of other formal anesthesia training programs, including St. Vincent's Hospital in Portland, Oregon (1909), St. John's Hospital in Springfield, Illinois

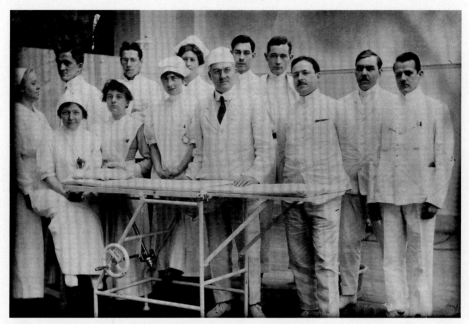

Figure 10.2. George Crile and Agatha Hodgins. (Reprinted with permission from American Association of Nurse Anesthetists (AANA) Archives.)

(1912), the New York Post-Graduate Hospital in New York City (1912), and the Long Island College Hospital in Brooklyn, New York (1914).

Crile and Hodgins were early responders to the call for medical assistance during the start of World War I. In December 1914, they departed for Neuilly, France, to serve in the Lakeside Unit at the American Ambulance Hospital. Along with two other nurse anesthetists, they taught others how to provide a nitrous oxide-oxygen anesthetic (see Figure 10.2). Crile returned to the United States after 2 months abroad to help promote the creation of other hospital units to serve in the war. Hodgins stayed on to provide care and train others—including physicians—in her techniques of anesthesia administration. Nurses were also trained stateside as anesthesia providers at St. Mary's Hospital in Rochester, Minnesota, and Pennsylvania Hospital in Philadelphia, Pennsylvania, through the U.S. Army and Navy to assist with the war effort (Gunn, 1991).

In 1915, nurse Mary J. Roche-Stevenson replaced Hodgins as the Lakeside Unit's Chief Anesthetist in France. Hodgins, back in Cleveland, graduated the first class of anesthetists from the Lakeside School consisting of 11 nurses, 6 physicians, and 2 dentists in 1916. Hodgins and many other nurses were instrumental in teaching physicians the art and science of anesthesia care.

The service of Agatha Hodgins and Mary J. Roche-Stevenson, along with nurse anesthetists Sophie Gran Winton, Anne Penland, and countless other nurses and nurse anesthetists, denotes a remarkable history of the heroic contributions of the nursing profession to battlefield healthcare. Unfortunately, while American nurse anesthetists voluntarily risked their lives in World War I, World War II, the Korean War, the Vietnam War, and recent conflicts and wars in the Middle East, some members of organized medical groups brought forth their own wars against nurses administering anesthesia. In 1916, physicians attempted to close the Lakeside School by petitioning a resolution to the Ohio Medical Board denouncing the administration of anesthesia by nurses. Physicians were determined to make the specialty of anesthesia a physician-only practice. Legal challenges were also brought forth in Kentucky (*Frank v. South*, 1917) and California (*Nelson v. Chalmers-Frances*, 1936) to the right of nurses to administer anesthesia. All cases were upheld in favor of nurse anesthesia. In present times, some organized medical groups continue to promote restrictions by external agencies or legal actions that restrict nurse anesthetists' practice.

Birth of the Professional Association

In 1923, Hodgins organized the alum of the Lakeside School into the Alumnae Association of the Lakeside School of Anesthesia. This was the start of what would initially be the National Association of Nurse Anesthetists. In 1931, Hodgins invited her alumnae and other nurse anesthetists from around the country to meet at Western Reserve University to discuss the creation of a national organization. Hodgins's focus was on creating clear standards for the education of nurse anesthetists. The original plan was to affiliate with the American Nurses Association (ANA). After a series of miscommunications and perhaps head-strong wills, it became apparent that a relationship with the ANA would not be possible. Instead, Hodgins's successor and the second President of the Association, Gertrude Fife, helped create an alliance with the American Hospital Association (AHA) (Figure 10.3). The AHA became an incubator for the young profession and its strong advocate. The first meeting of the new National Association of Nurse Anesthetists was held in conjunction with the meeting of the AHA from September 12 to 15, 1933.

Fife and her colleagues set a few goals for the immediate future of the professional association. These included advancing the art and science of anesthesiology,

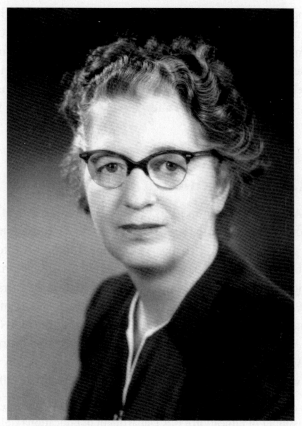

Figure 10.3. Gertrude Fife. (Reprinted with permission from American Association of Nurse Anesthetists (AANA) Archives.)

promoting cooperation between nurse anesthetists and the medical profession, developing educational standards and accreditation processes for anesthesia schools, establishing national board examinations for nurse anesthetists, and promoting public awareness about the profession.

The hardworking, volunteer leaders of the association made steady strides during the early years of the association. An education committee was formed in 1933. By May of 1937, education committee chairman Helen Lamb and her committee members had constructed and promoted a recommended cur-riculum for all nurse anesthesia schools. This document set forth required hours of classroom and operating room instruction, as well as a set number of required anesthetic cases. The name of the association changed in 1939 to the **American Association of Nurse Anesthetists (AANA)**. On June 4, 1945, the first qualifying examination for membership in the AANA was held. The first Institute for Instructors of Anesthesiology, the start of a formal faculty development program, was held the week of October 8, 1945. A program for the accreditation of nurse anesthetist programs was implemented in January 1952. By 1956, the CRNA credential was officially adopted. Sadly, Agatha Hodgins passed away on March 24, 1945, witnessing only a few of her visions become a reality.

Accreditation of Educational Programs

In 1955, the AANA was recognized by the U.S. Commissioner of Education as the sole agency for the accreditation of nurse anesthesia educational schools. In 1975, several political and legal challenges prompted the AANA to transfer this function to a body that was separate from the members' association. This resulted in the formation of the AANA's Council on Accreditation of Nurse Anesthesia Educational Programs/Schools (COA). The COA functioned as an autonomous, multidisciplinary body under the corporate structure of the AANA until 2009, when the COA separately incorporated. The COA has a proud history of national recognition. According to a detailed history provided in the COA Standards for Accreditation of Nurse Anesthesia Programs—Practice Doctorate (2018), the COA:

> has been continuously recognized by the US Secretary of Education (formerly the U.S. Commissioner of Education), U.S. Department of Education (USDE) since 1975, as well as by the Council on Postsecondary Accreditation (COPA) or its successor, the Commission on Recognition of Postsecondary Accreditation (CORPA), since 1985. The Council for Higher Education Accreditation (CHEA) assumed CORPA's recognition functions in 1997. COA maintains USDE recognition under the legislative mandate that calls for the US Secretary of Education to identify reliable authorities for the quality of training that is offered by programs. COA maintains CHEA recognition to demonstrate its effectiveness in assessing and encouraging improvement and quality in programmatic accreditation. COA also subscribes to the Code of Good Practice for accrediting organizations through membership in the Association of Specialized and Professional Accreditors (ASPA) (p. 42).

In its initial years, the focus of the educational guidelines was on hospital-based schools of anesthesia. In 1970, schools were encouraged to pursue college credit for the coursework offered. The first COA requirement for degree programs was published in the 1990 standards for all nurse anesthesia programs to transition from awarding certificates to awarding master's degrees. All accredited nurse anesthesia programs offered master's level education as of October 1, 1998, and all programs must offer doctoral degrees by 2022. All entry-into-practice graduates from nurse anesthesia educational programs will be required to possess a doctoral degree as of January 1, 2025. A CRNA must complete an accredited nurse anesthesia program that prepares the graduate for the full scope of nurse anesthesia practice. Likewise, the clinical curriculum must also provide the student nurse anesthetist with unrestricted experiences that cover the full scope of current practice in a variety of work settings (COA, 2018).

The COA remains the only accreditor for nurse anesthesia educational programs in the United States. An individual who wishes to sit for the NCE in order to become a CRNA, meet state licensing requirements to be a nurse anesthetist, or become employed as a CRNA must graduate from a COA-accredited program.

In Their Own Words

Jacqueline S. Rowles, DNP, MBA, MA, CRNA, ANP-BC, FNAP, DAIPM, FAAN
Director, DNP Nurse Anesthesia Program
President, International Federation of Nurse Anesthetists

The key points in understanding my role are... The specialty of anesthesia was started by nurses during the Civil War era as physicians wanted to be surgeons and the role of anesthesia was seen as lesser than that of the surgeon. While there are differences in educational preparation for the anesthesia role, there is one standard of care for the provision of anesthesia services, so practice competencies remain the same regardless of provider type. A nurse anesthetist is expected to provide the same quality of care as a physician, and multiple scientific studies validate that there is no difference in quality of anesthesia care between a physician and a certified registered nurse anesthetist.

What keeps me coming back every day is... First and foremost, the patients. I enjoy the opportunity to provide one-on-one, individualized, and focused care to my patients. Anesthetized patients are unable to advocate for themselves. They put their trust in us and their lives in our hands. Each and every day, I have the opportunity to make a difference in the lives of my patients and

(Continued)

their families. It is a responsibility I don't take lightly. Moreover, I enjoy being a part of the perioperative team, working alongside my colleagues in an effort to achieve the best outcome possible for each patient.

My greatest challenge is... Finding an effective way to bring the nursing profession together—to raise visibility of our collective actions and work for the good of the profession. Often, I find there is a lack of understanding of various nursing roles and responsibilities coupled with too much criticism of one another. Nurses are the largest group within the healthcare workforce, and if we would come together in full support of each other, we would be unstoppable. Further, I am constantly advocating that each nurse must find a way to identify his or her contributions and worth. As a whole, we are not very good about promoting the positive effects and outcomes directly related to the care we provide.

I wish someone had told me... How much I would love being a nurse, especially a nurse anesthetist, and the number of hours I would spend as a volunteer leader in giving back to my profession. I should have warned my husband and family, so they would have been better prepared for all the life events I was late to or missed. Still, I am extremely blessed to have had the opportunity to serve my patients and to be a servant leader. I wouldn't want to change my journey as it has molded me into the person I am today.

I need to be a lifelong learner because... Technological and pharmacological advances occur constantly! In order to provide the best care, I need to continually be aware of new research and evidence-based practice, new equipment, new medications or changes in medication protocols, treatment guidelines, as well as simulation-based training opportunities, enhanced communication techniques... the list is never ending. The one thing that is constant in healthcare is change. We need to have the knowledge, skills, and competencies to move forward as our specialty, and others, progress. Continual learning keeps us engaged, challenged, and humble and enhances our expertise. I believe it also keeps us active and in a younger state of mind.

Another point to understand is... Taking time for ourselves and our friends/families is important. Advanced practice nursing careers are stressful. We don't have jobs; we are the job. Our steadfast commitment is to serve and help others. Sometimes we get lost along the way. Understanding the need to incorporate wellness activities into our lives is an important part of happiness, health, and success.

Reimbursement of Services

Reimbursement for nurse anesthesia services has a complex history. In the beginning, some nurse anesthetists were paid a wage through their employing hospital or surgeon. As healthcare insurance evolved and government-sponsored programs, such as Medicare, Medicaid, TRICARE/TRICARE for Life, the State Children's Health Insurance Program (SCHIP), the Veterans Health Administration (VHA) program, and the Indian Health Service (IHS) program, were established, anesthesiologist-led practice groups employed CRNAs. This arrangement allowed anesthesiologists to oversee multiple CRNAs, sometimes in different facilities, providing anesthesia simultaneously. The anesthesiologist, in turn, billed for each anesthetic and paid a wage to the CRNA. The working relationship between the anesthesiologist and the CRNA and the responsibilities of the anesthesiologist were nebulous at best. The central issue has involved such concepts as oversight, direction, and supervision that have been debated by professional associations, state licensing and regulatory bodies, hospital and ambulatory surgery center licensing statutes and rules, and even the courts, resulting in conflicting information (Blumenreich, 1997).

The creation of the Medicare program in 1965 led to the development of a set of requirements for healthcare facilities to meet in order to participate in and receive reimbursement from the program. These federal requirements, published in the Code of Federal Regulations, are called Conditions of Participation (CoPs) and have evolved over time. The CoPs require CRNAs work under the supervision of a physician who may or may not be an anesthesiologist.

In 1982, Medicare began to set conditions for anesthesiologist reimbursement during those times that they "directed" nurse anesthetists. These Tax Equity and Fiscal Responsibility Act (TEFRA) requirements must be met in order for a physician anesthesiologist to be reimbursed for participating in an anesthetic with a CRNA (Blumenreich, 1997). In 1986, Congress passed legislation providing CRNAs direct reimbursement under Medicare Part B. Thus, nurse anesthesia became the first nursing specialty to gain direct reimbursement rights under Medicare.

In 2001, the Centers for Medicare and Medicaid Services (CMS) published a rule in the Federal Register (66 FR 35395-99) that permits state governors to request from the Secretary of Health and Human Services a waiver or "opt-out" from the federal physician supervision requirement of CRNAs. This changed the federal physician supervision rule for nurse anesthetists (AANA, 2018). To date, 17 states have opted out of the federal physician supervision requirement, including Iowa, Nebraska, Idaho, Minnesota, New Hampshire, New Mexico, Kansas, North Dakota, Washington, Alaska, Oregon, Montana, South Dakota, Wisconsin, California, Colorado, and Kentucky. Additionally, other states have no physician supervision laws. Anesthesia services, therefore, may be delivered in several different models. If state law permits, CRNAs may provide anesthesia services without physician supervision. Alternatively, CRNAs may provide anesthesia services under physician direction or supervision, depending on the anesthesiologist-to-CRNA ratio. There are expense and revenue implications for each delivery model, but study after study has found no difference in patient care outcomes (Dulisse & Cromwell, 2010; Hogan et al., 2010; Negrusa et al., 2016; Quraishi et al., 2017; The Lewin Group, 2016).

The contributions of nurse anesthetists to the early development of the safe administration of anesthetics are sadly discounted by some of the medical profession and many medical publications. Fortunately, Thatcher (1953) chronicled some of the early history of nurses in anesthesia in her book, *History of Anesthesia, with Emphasis on the Nurse Specialist*. Ira Gunn (1991) reported many important details of the beginning of the nurse anesthesia specialty in her seminal work. Marianne Bankert (1993) furthered the historical accounting of nurses in the delivery of anesthesia through her inspirational historical research study, *Watchful Care—A History of America's Nurse Anesthetist*. These works have proven invaluable in capturing additional insights on the history of nurse anesthesia through the early 1990s and were a major source of reference for this chapter.

Questions to Ask Yourself

1. What are the foundational nursing skills a CRNA builds upon to engage in advanced practice? In which of these skills do you profess proficiency?
2. Which skills do you need to develop?
3. How do the challenges to the CRNA specialty by other organized professional groups compare with the challenges experienced by other advanced practice nursing specialties? Why?

Professional Role

CRNAs are advanced practice registered nurses (APRNs) licensed as independent practitioners. CRNAs practice both autonomously and in collaboration with a variety of healthcare providers on the interprofessional team to deliver high-quality, holistic, evidence-based anesthesia and pain care services. Nurse anesthetists care for patients at all acuity levels across the lifespan in a variety of settings for procedures including, but not limited to, surgical, obstetrical, diagnostic, therapeutic, and pain management. CRNAs serve as clinicians, researchers, educators, mentors, advocates, and administrators.

Role Specifics

CRNAs provide anesthesia care wherever anesthesia services are needed. Settings include, but are not limited to, surgical, obstetrical, diagnostic, therapeutic, and pain management locations. Many nurse anesthetists provide anesthesia services in battlefield makeshift hospitals overseas. The population foci are not limited by age; CRNAs care for patients across the lifespan regardless of acuity level (AANA Scope of Nurse Anesthesia Practice, 2013a; 2013b).

Scope of Practice

The history of nurses delivering anesthesia extends more than 150 years. The practice of anesthesia, therefore, has been a recognized nursing specialty for more than a century. When anesthesia is delivered by a nurse anesthetist, it is the practice of nursing; when anesthesia is delivered by a physician, it is the practice of medicine (AANA, 2017). The standard of care is the same for both professionals. Courts have affirmed that anesthesia is a specialty within the field of nursing from as early as 1917 (Blumenreich, 1998).

Multiple influencers govern the scope of practice of a CRNA: formal and continuing education, experiences, state and federal laws, and institutional policies and privileges. Box 10.1 presents the CRNA scope of practice as published by the AANA in its 2013 document.

BOX 10.1

▶ AANA SCOPE OF NURSING PRACTICE

The practice of anesthesia is a recognized nursing and medical specialty unified by the same standard of care. Nurse anesthesia practice may include, but is not limited to, these elements: performing a comprehensive history and physical; conducting a preanesthesia evaluation; obtaining informed consent for anesthesia; developing and initiating a patient-specific plan of care; selecting, ordering, prescribing and administering drugs and controlled substances; and selecting and inserting invasive and noninvasive monitoring modalities. CRNAs provide acute, chronic and interventional pain management services, as well as critical care and resuscitation services; order and evaluate diagnostic tests; request consultations; and perform point-of-care testing. CRNAs plan and initiate anesthetic techniques, including general, regional, local, and sedation. Anesthetic techniques may include the use of ultrasound, fluoroscopy and other technologies for diagnosis and care delivery, and to improve patient safety and comfort. Nurse anesthetists respond to emergency situations using airway management and other techniques; facilitate emergence and recovery from anesthesia; and provide post-anesthesia care, including medication management, conducting a post-anesthesia evaluation, and discharge from the post-anesthesia care area or facility.

From *AANA Scope of Nursing Practice*, The Standards for Office Based Anesthesia Practice were adopted by the AANA Board of Directors in 1999 and revised in 2001, 2002, November 2005, and January 2013. Upon the February 2019 revision of the Standards of Nurse Anesthesia Practice, the Standards for Office Based Anesthesia Practice were archived, as they are subsumed within the Standards for Nurse Anesthesia Practice. The supplemental resources from the Standards for Office Based Anesthesia Practice were transitioned to resource documents on the AANA website. © Copyright 2019.

CRNAs are inherently also engaged in pain management services. This includes acute, chronic, and interventional pain management services. Pain management, like most other areas of nurse anesthesia practice, has been challenged by organized medical groups. Louisiana remains the only state in which the court has issued a declaratory statement that interventional pain management is exclusively the practice of medicine and involved procedures are not delegable (Louisiana State Board of Medical Examiners, 2006). In contrast, the Iowa Supreme Court in 2013 issued a final decision that explicitly permits APRNs, including CRNAs, to use fluoroscopy for interventional pain management (Iowa Supreme Court, 2013). This area of practice will no doubt be a continued area of conflict between nursing and medicine. As society, healthcare, and technology evolve and new research evidence is formed, the scope of practice will undoubtedly also change.

Prescriptive Authority

CRNAs directly administer pharmacologic agents, including controlled substances, intraoperatively. In addition, CRNAs are often involved in ordering and/or directly administering pharmacologic agents, including controlled substances, throughout the perioperative continuum. Neither of these scenarios meets the definition of "prescribing" under federal law. The U.S. Department of Justice Drug Enforcement Administration (DEA) defines a prescription as "an order for medication which is dispensed to or for an ultimate user. A prescription is not an order for medication which is dispensed for immediate administration to the ultimate user" (DEA, 2018). Most CRNAs do not traditionally prescribe drugs, including controlled substances; most CRNAs, therefore, have not had to register with the DEA.

All APRNs, including CRNAs, are permitted to prescribe controlled substances, some as licensed independent practitioners and others under existing supervision and protocol requirements. Many states continue to make changes to existing laws that regulate the scope of practice for APRNs. Wide variability and disparities exist among states with respect to prescriptive authority. In addition, as a national response to the worsening opioid crisis, many states have also adopted new rules or regulations that relate to opioid prescriptions and pain management. Like other APRNs, CRNA prescriptive authority continues to evolve and vary depending on state law. Figure 10.4 depicts the geographic variability of CRNA prescriptive authority laws.

Professionalism

Since its early beginnings, the nurse anesthetist professional association sought to describe and define the outcomes desired at the end of the specialty's educational pathway. Statements about the development of competence in nurse anesthesia practice have evolved over time and experiences. The authors suspect these observable and measurable abilities will adapt as new perspectives are gained.

A significant move to further promote the recognition of nurse anesthetists as APRNs who are experts in the art and science of anesthesiology was

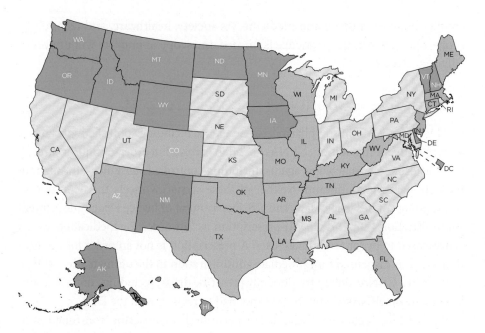

Prescriptive Authority

█ Independent prescriptive authority meaning states where CRNAs are eligible for prescriptive authority without physician involvement, and that includes all controlled substances schedules

░ States that grant some prescriptive authority to CRNAs, but that authority either includes physician involvement, does not include all controlled substance schedules, or both

Figure 10.4. Certified registered nurse anesthetist (CRNA) prescriptive authority map.

the adoption by the AANA Board of Directors of the "nurse anesthesiologist" descriptor. Upon the recommendation of a nurse anesthesiologist descriptor task force formed to evaluate utilization of the "nurse anesthesiologist" title and explore legal and regulatory implications, the following statement concerning use of titles was adopted on July 2018:

The practice of anesthesia has been a recognized nursing specialty for more than 100 years. The AANA presents this statement in an effort to clarify for the public the many ways someone may refer to a CRNA.

The AANA recognizes the following titles:

Certified Registered Nurse Anesthetist
CRNA
Nurse Anesthetist

The AANA acknowledges additional descriptors for nurse anesthetists which could include, but are not limited to, the following:

Advanced Practice Registered Nurse (APRN)
Licensed Nurse Practitioner (LNP)
Licensed Independent Practitioner (LIP)
Advanced Practice Provider (APP)
advanced practice professional
nurse anesthesiologist

Regardless of the title or the descriptor being used, as a profession we believe it is time for the focus to be on the quality of the healthcare provided and not the title of the healthcare provider.

American Association of Nurse Anesthetists (AANA). 2019. *AANA Board Approves Statement of titles and descriptors for CRNAs. AANA Anesthesia E-ssential* [newsletter for AANA members]. January 10, 2019. https://www.aana.com/publications/anesthesia-e-ssential/anesthesia-e-ssential-january-10-2019

The Certified Registered Nurse Anesthetist (CRNA) credential came into existence in 1956. The title "nurse anesthesiologist," which is synonymous with the title "nurse anesthetist," is currently being used by some CRNAs.

Competencies

Both the AANA and the COA have provided foundational frameworks to guide educators in structuring curricula and support practitioners in professional practice and research. Table 10.1 lists the AANA Standards of Nurse Anesthesia Practice. Table 10.2 lists the COA Graduate Student Standards.

CRNAs begin their anesthesia careers as registered nurses entering nurse anesthesia education programs and transition into various practice roles as clinicians, educators, researchers, and administrators over a career. Nurse anesthetists continue to improve professionally through self-assessment and peer review of clinical and nonclinical skills to effectively transition to new practice roles and evolve in their careers.

Additionally, the AANA constructed a Code of Ethics for the CRNA (2020) and a set of Professional Attributes of the Nurse Anesthetist (2016). The description of nonclinical attributes provides a framework for the professional CRNA

Table 10.1. Standards for Nurse Anesthesia Practice

Standard	Description
I	Perform and document a thorough preanesthesia assessment and evaluation.
II	Obtain and document informed consent for the planned anesthetic intervention from the patient or legal guardian, or verify that informed consent has been obtained and documented by a qualified professional.
III	Formulate a patient-specific plan for anesthesia care.
IV	Implement and adjust the anesthesia care plan based on the patient's physiologic status. Continuously assess the patient's response to the anesthetic, surgical intervention, or procedure. Intervene as required to maintain the patient in optimal physiologic condition.
V	Monitor, evaluate, and document the patient's physiologic condition as appropriate for the type of anesthesia and specific patient needs. When any physiological monitoring device is used, variable pitch and threshold alarms shall be turned on and audible. The CRNA should attend to the patient continuously until the responsibility of care has been accepted by another anesthesia professional. **Va. Oxygenation**: Continuously monitor oxygenation by clinical observation and pulse oximetry. If indicated, continually monitor oxygenation by arterial blood gas analysis. **Vb. Ventilation:** Continuously monitor ventilation. Verify intubation of the trachea or placement of other artificial airway devices by auscultation, chest excursion, and confirmation of expired carbon dioxide. Use ventilatory pressure monitors as indicated. Continuously monitor end-tidal carbon dioxide during controlled or assisted ventilation and any anesthesia or sedation technique requiring artificial airway support. During moderate or deep sedation, continuously monitor for the presence of expired carbon dioxide. **Vc. Cardiovascular:** Continuously monitor cardiovascular status via electrocardiogram. Perform auscultation of heart sounds as needed. Evaluate and document blood pressure and heart rate at least every 5 min.

Table 10.1.	Standards for Nurse Anesthesia Practice (continued)	
Standard	**Description**	
	Vd. Thermoregulation: When clinically significant changes in body temperature are intended, anticipated, or suspected, monitor body temperature in order to facilitate the maintenance of normothermia. **Ve. Neuromuscular:** When neuromuscular blocking agents are administered, monitor neuromuscular response to assess depth of blockade and degree of recovery. **Vf. Positioning:** Monitor and assess patient positioning and protective measures, except for those aspects that are performed exclusively by one or more other providers. **Interpretation of Standard V** Continuous clinical observation and vigilance are the basis of safe anesthesia care. Consistent with the CRNA's professional judgment, additional means of monitoring the patient's status may be used depending on the needs of the patient, the anesthesia being administered, or the surgical technique or procedure being performed.	
VI	Document pertinent anesthesia-related information on the patient's medical record in an accurate, complete, legible, and timely manner.	
VII	Evaluate the patient's status and determine when it is safe to transfer the responsibility of care. Accurately report the patient's condition, including all essential information, and transfer the responsibility of care to another qualified healthcare provider in a manner that assures continuity of care and patient safety.	
VIII	Adhere to appropriate safety precautions as established within the practice setting to minimize the risks of fire, explosion, electrical shock, and equipment malfunction. Based on the patient, surgical intervention, or procedure, ensure that the equipment reasonably expected to be necessary for the administration of anesthesia has been checked for proper functionality and document compliance. When the patient is ventilated by an automatic mechanical ventilator, monitor the integrity of the breathing system with a device capable of detecting a disconnection by emitting an audible alarm. When the breathing system of an anesthesia machine is being used to deliver oxygen, the CRNA should monitor inspired oxygen concentration continuously with an oxygen analyzer with a low-concentration audible alarm turned on and in use.	

(continued)

Table 10.1.	Standards for Nurse Anesthesia Practice (continued)	
Standard	**Description**
IX	Verify that infection control policies and procedures for personnel and equipment exist within the practice setting. Adhere to infection control policies and procedures as established within the practice setting to minimize the risk of infection to the patient, the CRNA, and other healthcare providers.
X	Participate in the ongoing review and evaluation of anesthesia care to assess quality and appropriateness.
XI	Respect and maintain the basic rights of patients.

Adapted from American Association of Nurse Anesthetists (AANA). (2019). *Standards for nurse anesthesia practice*. https://www.aana.com/docs/default-source/practice-aana-com-web-documents-(all)/standards-for-nurse-anesthesia-practice.pdf

Table 10.2.	Standards of Accreditation of Nurse Anesthesia Programs, Practice Doctorate (COA, 2018)	
Domains	**Competencies**
Patient safety	The graduate must demonstrate the ability to • Be vigilant in the delivery of patient care. • Refrain from engaging in extraneous activities that abandon or minimize vigilance while providing direct patient care. • Conduct a comprehensive equipment check. • Protect patients from iatrogenic complications.
Perianesthesia	The graduate must demonstrate the ability to • Provide individualized care throughout the perianesthesia continuum. • Deliver culturally competent perianesthesia care. • Provide anesthesia services to all patients across the lifespan. • Perform a comprehensive history and physical assessment. • Administer general anesthesia to patients with a variety of physical conditions. • Administer and manage a variety of regional anesthetics. • Maintain current certification in ACLS and PALS.

Table 10.2. Standards of Accreditation of Nurse Anesthesia Programs, Practice Doctorate (COA, 2018)   (continued)

Domains	Competencies
Critical thinking	The graduate must demonstrate the ability to • Apply knowledge to practice in decision-making and problem-solving. • Provide nurse anesthesia services based on evidence-based principles. • Perform a preanesthetic assessment before providing anesthesia services. • Assume responsibility and accountability for diagnosis. • Formulate an anesthesia plan of care before providing anesthesia services. • Identify and take appropriate action when confronted with anesthetic equipment-related malfunctions. • Interpret and utilize data obtained from noninvasive and invasive monitoring modalities. • Calculate, initiate, and manage fluid and blood component therapy. • Recognize, evaluate, and manage the physiological responses coincident to the provision of anesthesia services. • Recognize and appropriately manage complications that occur during the provision of anesthesia services. • Use science-based theories and concepts to analyze new practice approaches. • Pass the National Certification Examination (NCE) administered by the National Board of Certification and Recertification of Nurse Anesthetists (NBCRNA).
Communication	The graduate must demonstrate the ability to • Utilize interpersonal and communication skills that result in the effective exchange of information and collaboration with patients and their families.

(continued)

Table 10.2.	Standards of Accreditation of Nurse Anesthesia Programs, Practice Doctorate (COA, 2018) (continued)
Domains	**Competencies**
	• Utilize interpersonal and communication skills that result in the effective interprofessional exchange of information and collaboration with other healthcare professionals. Respect the dignity and privacy of patients while maintaining confidentiality in the delivery of interprofessional care. • Maintain comprehensive, timely, accurate, and legible healthcare records. • Transfer the responsibility for care of the patient to other qualified providers in a manner that assures continuity of care and patient safety. • Teach others.
Leadership	The graduate must demonstrate the ability to • Integrate critical and reflective thinking in his or her leadership approach. • Provide leadership that facilitates intraprofessional and interprofessional collaboration.
Professional role	The graduate must demonstrate the ability to • Adhere to the Code of Ethics for the Certified Registered Nurse Anesthetist. • Interact on a professional level with integrity. • Apply ethically sound decision-making processes. • Function within legal and regulatory requirements. • Accept responsibility and accountability for his or her practice. • Provide anesthesia services to patients in a cost-effective manner. • Demonstrate knowledge of wellness and substance use disorder in the anesthesia profession through completion of content in wellness and substance use disorder. • Inform the public of the role and practice of the CRNA. • Evaluate how public policy-making strategies impact the financing and delivery of healthcare.

in successful role transitions. All of these resources help support a unified vision of the 21st-century nurse anesthetist and the specialty's desire to meet the ever-changing needs of the public and the healthcare system.

Professional Attributes

Professional attributes are the nonclinical knowledge, skills, attitudes, and judgments that are fundamental for success (Figure 10.5). In addition to formal nurse

I. Collaborative:
- The nurse anesthetists works with others to develop shared solutions.

II. Culturally competent:
- The nurse anesthetist respectfully interacts with others, regardless of their culture, to achieve a shared vision.

III. Evidence-based practice:
- The nurse anesthetist evaluates and integrates scientific research, expert opinion, patient preferences, and other metrics to improve processes and outcomes.

IV. Leader:
- The nurse anesthetist creates and articulates clear direction and vision to engage others to accomplish shared goals.

V. Professionally engaged:
- The nurse anesthetist advances and advocates for the nurse anesthesia specialty.

VI. Situationally aware:
- The nurse anesthetist uses knowledge, experience, and perception to identify critical elements to make a decision.

VII. Teacher:
- The nurse anesthetist fosters an environment that encourages successful learning and understanding of information for patients and others.

VIII. Well:
- The nurse anesthetist makes lifestyle choices that promote the positive and healthy balance of personal and professional environments.

Figure 10.5. Professional attributes. (Adapted from American Association of Nurse Anesthetists. (2016). *Professional attributes.* https://www.aana.com/docs/default-source/practice-aana-com-web-documents-(all)/professional-attributes-of-the-nurse-anesthetist.pdf)

anesthesia education and practice experience, these professional attributes serve as the foundation for ongoing professional development, personal satisfaction, and career engagement. CRNAs and SRNAs are devoted to professional excellence and acquire additional skills and attributes specific to their area of interest.

Certification

The **National Board of Certification and Recertification of Nurse Anesthetists (NBCRNA)** regulates the certification and recertification of nurse anesthetists. It also provides an accredited nonsurgical pain management (NSPM) program. Through the development and implementation of credentialing programs that support the lifelong learning of nurse anesthetists, the NBCRNA seeks to promote patient safety by enhancing the quality of providers in the field of anesthesia (NBCRNA, 2018a; 2018b). The NBCRNA collaborates with the AANA, which sets the standards of practice for nurse anesthetists, as well as the COA, which sets the standards for all nurse anesthesia educational programs. The National Commission for Certifying Agencies (NCCA) granted initial accreditation to the NBCRNA in 1984. It also was one of the first national certification bodies accredited by the Accreditation Board for Specialty Nursing Certification, Inc. (ABSNC). Only graduates of COA-accredited nurse anesthesia educational programs may apply to sit for the NCE administered by the NBCRNA. Certification by the NBCRNA is required for state licensure and the right to practice.

Questions to Ask Yourself

1. CRNAs became the first nursing specialty to gain direct reimbursement rights under Medicare. How does reimbursement influence the delivery of care?
2. Reflect on the nonclinical professional attributes of the CRNA. Identify which attributes you possess and which attributes would need further improvement.
3. What new insights about the CRNA role have you gained after reading this chapter?

Continued Professional Certification

The recertification process for CRNAs was formerly based on demonstrating continuing education every 2 years. The NBCRNA began a revision to the process for recertification in 2011 to reflect the growing trend of emphasizing continuing competency and current best practices in credentialing. The revised process, called the Continued Professional Certification (CPC) program, was approved and implemented in 2016.

The CPC program is built around 8-year cycles of recertification, comprising two 4-year cycles. The program consists of earning 60 Class A and 40 Class B credits and completing four educational core modules every 4-year cycle. The core modules address the four areas of anesthesia practice, which apply to all nurse anesthetists regardless of practice focus: airway management, applied clinical pharmacology, human physiology and pathophysiology, and anesthesia equipment and technology. These core modules are optional for the first 4-year cycle. Class A credits are anesthesia continuing education (CE) credits that are provided preapproved and include some type of assessment. Class B credits may include a wide range of professional activities that enhance knowledge of anesthesia practice to support patient safety and/or foster an understanding of the healthcare environment. Prior approval and assessments are not required for Class B credits. A CPC assessment based on the four anesthesia areas of practice derived from a professional practice analysis of CRNAs must be taken to meet performance and passing standards. The authors anticipate that the CPC program will evolve as improved assessment technologies develop and new research on demonstration of professional proficiencies become available. Figure 10.6 is a pictorial representation of the CPC program.

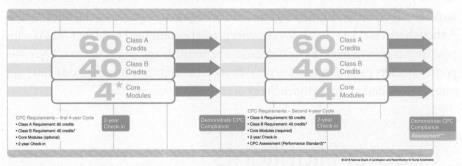

Figure 10.6. Pictorial representation of the Continued Professional Certification (CPC) Program. (Reprinted with permission of National Board of Certification & Recertification for Nurse Anesthetists (NBCRNA). (2020). *The Continued Professional Certification (CPC) Program.* https://www.nbcrna.com/continued-certification)

Summary

Nurses have been administering anesthesia since its early development in the mid-19th century, positioning nurse anesthetists as the first advanced practice nursing specialists. The development of a volunteer professional association, which in 1939 became the AANA, led to the creation of a curriculum of study, a qualifying examination, formal faculty development programs, and an educational program accreditation process. The CRNA credential was officially adopted in 1956.

Beginning with the Civil War and continuing today with the ongoing conflict in the Middle East, nurses have been actively serving in the military. Nurses helped train French and British nurses and physicians in anesthesia techniques during World War I. Many nurse anesthetists volunteered for service during World War II and the Korean and Vietnam wars and continue serving today. It is not unusual to find CRNAs providing anesthesia care independently on the front line, on navy ships, and in field hospitals.

The evolution of the specialty has been met with many legal and professional challenges due to the high risk of the practice, the overlapping practice with physicians, and reimbursement. Yet CRNAs continue to practice in every setting in which anesthesia is needed throughout the United States. CRNAs are the primary providers of anesthesia services in rural America, offering surgical, obstetrical, trauma, and pain management services.

Approximately 90% of all U.S. nurse anesthetists are members of the AANA, making it one of the most represented and engaged professional associations in the United States. Beginning in January 2025, all entry-into-practice graduates from nurse anesthesia educational programs will be required to possess a doctoral degree. Although speculative at best, all indicators predict a continued need for CRNAs with positive job growth over the next decade. The breadth and depth of the CRNA role positively affect patient outcomes, provide access to high-quality anesthesia and pain care services, and promote the delivery of cost-effective healthcare.

Chapter Highlights

- CRNAs with a practice of administering anesthesia since the profession's early development in the mid-19th century positioning CRNAs as the first advanced practice nursing specialists.

- Though titles have varied, the CRNA credential was officially adopted in 1956.
- The development of anesthesia techniques during World War I placed nurses in key position to help train French and British nurses and physicians.
- Nurse anesthetists have a long history of serving the military. They volunteered for service during World War II and the Korean and Vietnam wars and continue serving independently today on the front lines, navy ships, and in field hospitals.
- The CRNA role has faced numerous legal and professional challenges throughout their evolution as a profession, including the high risk of the practice, the overlapping practice with physicians, and reimbursement.
- As primary providers, CRNAs have administered anesthesia services in rural America, offering surgical, obstetrical, trauma, and pain management services.
- Almost all CRNAs (about 90%) in the US are members of the AANA, making it one of the most represented and engaged professional associations in the United States.
- CRNAs will soon (by January 2025) be required to graduate from nurse anesthesia educational programs with doctoral degrees for entry-into-practice.
- CRNAs provide access to high-quality anesthesia and pain care services and promote the delivery of cost-effective healthcare. The CRNA role has proven to positively affect patient outcomes.

Web Resources

American Association of Nurse Anesthetists (AANA): https://www.aana.com/about-us
Association of Veteran Affairs Nurse Anesthetists (VACRNA): https://www.vacrna.com/
Council on Accreditation of Nurse Anesthesia Programs (COA): https://www.coacrna.org/Pages/default.aspx
National Board of Certification and Recertification for Nurse Anesthetists (NBCRNA): https://www.nbcrna.com/about-us/affiliated-organizations
Center for Medicare & Medicaid Services (CMS): https://www.cms.gov/
International Federation of Nurse Anesthetists (IFNA): https://ifna.site/
The Global Alliance for Surgical, Obstetric, Trauma and Anaesthesia Care: http://www.theg4alliance.org/

Professional Organizations

American Association of Nurse Anesthetists: https://www.aana.com/
National Board of Certification and Recertification for Nurse Anesthetists: https://www.
nbcrna.com/
Nurse Anesthetist: http://nurseanesthetist.org/

References

American Association of Nurse Anesthetists. (2013a). *Scope of nurse anesthesia practice.* www.aana.com/docs/default-source/practice-aana-com-web-documents-(all)/scope-of-nurse-anesthesia-practice.pdf?sfvrsn=250049b1_2

American Association of Nurse Anesthetists. (2013b). *Scope of practice.* https://www.aana.com/practice

American Association of Nurse Anesthetists. (2017). *The practice of anesthesia position statement.* https://www.aana.com/practice/practice-manual

American Association of Nurse Anesthetists. (2018). *Certified registered nurse anesthetists fact sheet, from the 2018 member profile survey.* https://www.aana.com/membership/become-a-crna/crna-fact-sheet

American Association of Nurse Anesthetists (AANA). (2019). *AANA board approves statement of titles and descriptors for CRNAs.* AANA Anesthesia E-ssential. [newsletter for AANA members]. January 10, 2019. https://www.aana.com/publications/anesthesia-e-ssential/anesthesia-e-ssential-january-10-2019

American Association of Nurse Anesthetists. (2020). *Code of ethics for the CRNA: Overview and resources.* https://www.aana.com/practice/clinical-practice-resources/code-of-ethics-for-the-CRNA

Bankert, M. (1993). *Watchful care: A history of America's nurse anesthetists.* Continuum Publishing Company.

Blumenreich, G. A. (1997). The nature of supervision. *American Association of Nurse Anesthetists, 65*(3), 208–211. https://www.aana.com/publications/aana-journal/legal-briefs

Blumenreich, G. A. (1998). The overlap between the practice of medicine and the practice of nursing. *AANA Journal, 66*(1), 11–15. https://www.aana.com/publications/aana-journal/legal-briefs

Council on Accreditation of Nurse Anesthesia Educational Programs. (2018). *Standards for accreditation of nurse anesthesia programs – practice doctorate.* www.coacrna.org/accreditation/Documents/Standards%20for%20Accreditation%20of%20Nurse%20Anesthesia%20Programs%20-%20Practice%20Doctorate,%20rev%20May%202018.pdf

Drug Enforcement Administration (DEA). (2018). *Part 1300 definitions.* https://www.deadiversion.usdoj.gov/21cfr/cfr/1300/1300_01.htm

Dulisse, B., & Cromwell, J. (2010). No harm found when nurse anesthetists work without supervision by physicians. *Health Affairs, 29*(8), 1469–1475.

Fenster, J. M. (2001). *Ether day: The strange tale of America's greatest medical discovery and the haunted men who made it.* HarperCollins.

Gunn, I. P. (1991). The history of nurse anesthesia education: Highlights and influences. *AANA Journal, 39*(1), 53–61. https://www.aana.com/search?keyword=History%20nurse%20anesthesia%20education%20highlights%20gunn

Hogan, P. F., Seifert, R. F., Moore, C. S., & Simonson, B. E. (2010). Cost effectiveness analysis of anesthesia providers. *Nurse Economics, 28*(3), 159–169.

Iowa Board of Nursing. (2013). *Iowa Supreme court decision - fluoroscopy.* https://nursing.iowa.gov/document/iowa-supreme-court-decision-fluoroscopy

Louisiana State Board of Medical Examiners. (2006). *Statement of position.* https://www.lsbme.la.gov/sites/default/files/documents/Statements%20of%20Position/Interventional%20Pain%20Management.pdf

Negrusa, B., Hogan, P. F., Warner, J. T., Schroeder, C. H., & Pang, B. (2016). Scope of practice laws and anesthesia complications: No measurable impact of certified registered nurse anesthetist expanded scope of practice on anesthesia-related complications. *Medical Care, 54*(10), 913–920.

Quraishi, J. A., Jordan, L. M., & Hoyem, R. (2017). Anesthesia Medicare trend analysis shows increased utilization of CRNA services. *AANA Journal, 85*(5), 375–383.

Thatcher, V. S. (1953). *The history of anesthesia with an emphasis on the nurse specialist.* JB Lippincott.

The Lewin Group, prepared for the American Association of Nurse Anesthetists. (2016). *Update of cost effectiveness of anesthesia providers: Final report.* http://www.lewin.com/content/dam/Lewin/Resources/AANA-CEA-May2016.pdf

The National Board of Certification and Recertification of Nurse Anesthetists. (2018a). *About the NBCRNA.* https://www.nbcrna.com/about-us

The National Board of Certification and Recertification of Nurse Anesthetists. (2018b). *Initial certification.* https://www.nbcrna.com/initial-certification .

11

Clinical Nurse Specialists

Jennifer L. Embree

LEARNING OBJECTIVES

After completing this chapter, you will be able to:

1. Identify how the clinical nurse specialist (CNS) role evolved.

2. Describe patient populations that CNSs serve.

3. Discuss CNS competencies.

4. Identify certification opportunities for CNS.

5. Discuss implications of prescriptive authority for clinical nurse specialists.

KEY TERMS

At-risk population: Refers to populations with a risk factor from the social determinants of health; for example, the poor, economically disadvantaged, homeless, racial and ethnic minorities, or victims of abuse.

Change agents: A person who helps an institution to improve effectiveness or quality of services.

Clinical nurse specialist (CNS): An advanced practice registered nurse with specialized graduate-level preparation in nursing.

Collaborative practice (collaboration or supervision required): Advanced practice registered nurse (APRN) practice in a state requiring a written agreement specifying scope of practice and medical acts allowed with or without a general supervision requirement by a medical doctor (MD), Doctor of Osteopathic Medicine (DO), Doctor of Dental Surgery (DDS) or podiatrist; or direct supervision required in the presence of a licensed, MD, DO, DDS, or podiatrist with or without a written practice agreement.

Full scope of practice: Nurses working in states that have no requirement for a written collaborative agreement, no supervision, and no conditions for practice are considered to be allowed to practice to the full scope of their education and training.

Independent licensed provider (independent authority): Defined by the Joint Commission as individuals permitted by law, regulation, and the institution to provide services within their scope of practice without direction or supervision.

Limited scope of practice: CNSs have no advanced practice authority.

No Prescribing Authority: An APRN is not authorized to prescribe pharmacologic and nonpharmacologic therapies beyond the perioperative and periprocedural periods.

Synergy Model: The American Association of Colleges of Nursing Synergy Model for Patient Care is a conceptual framework that aligns patient needs with nurse competencies.

Introduction

The **clinical nurse specialist** (CNS) is an advanced practice registered nurse (APRN) with specialized graduate-level preparation in nursing (master's or doctorate). Unique and advanced-level competencies of the CNS meet the needs of improving quality and reducing costs within the healthcare system. The scope of CNS practice meets needs through direct care of complex patients, including assessment, diagnosis, and management which may include prescriptive authority. As **change agents**, CNSs lead health organizations and develop scientific evidence-based programs to prevent avoidable complications and improve quality. CNSs are facilitators of interprofessional teams across the continuum of care and improve quality and safety, including, but not limited to, preventing hospital-acquired infections, reducing length of stays, and preventing hospital readmissions.

The CNS is prepared to provide care to **at-risk populations** with increasingly complex health needs, such as our aging populations, and supports a nursing workforce that will have fewer seasoned nurses taking direct care of those complex patients. The CNS serves as a resource to the novice through expert nurses in our healthcare workforce.

Consistent with recommendations to practice to the fullest extent of education and training and function as full partners with physicians, the 2010 Institute of Medicine (IOM) report, *The Future of Nursing: Leading Change, Advancing Health*, along with CNS research and demonstration projects continue to validate the unique ability of the CNS to lead evidence-based quality improvement across the healthcare continuum. CNS leadership has been demonstrated in the areas of prenatal care, prevention and wellness care, behavioral healthcare, care to those with chronic conditions, and care transitions (IOM, 2011; NACNS, 2020a).

As APRNs, CNSs optimize patient outcomes, implement evidence-based practice, close the gap in access to care, and enhance quality cost-effectively and creatively. Strengthened by the availability of health information technology, CNSs have heightened analytic capabilities, mobile- and cloud-based service integration, and access to numerous databases to demonstrate impact on outcomes. Patients can access care across the continuum from CNSs. CNSs are further impacting healthcare systems through health information technology (NACNS, 2020b).

Many federal and state policy barriers impair the ability of CNSs to practice to the full extent of their education (NACNS, 2020b), despite increased demands for cost-effective, high-quality healthcare. CNSs lead and diffuse quality improvement outcomes and cost savings across all models of care and are integral members of interprofessional teams.

State laws and administrative rules for CNS practice vary from state to state. Eight states have granted CNSs the authority to practice without a physician's supervision. Six states have granted CNSs independent authority to prescribe drugs and durable medical equipment. These permissions represent 32% and 40% increases, respectively, in the number of states that grant such authority; CNSs can practice independently in 28 states and prescribe independently in 19 states (Figure 11.1). In addition to the 28 states in which CNSs have independent practice authority, 13 states recognize CNSs as APRNs but require them to have a **collaborative practice** agreement with a physician (Figure 11.2). There are 19 states that require a CNS to have a

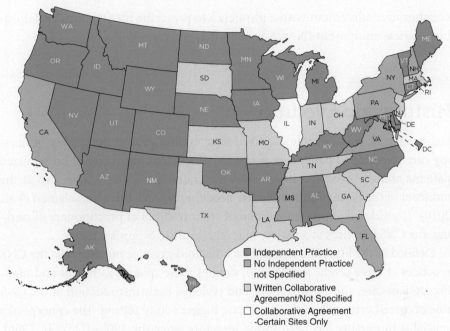

Figure 11.1. CNS Independent Prescriptive Authority. (Reprinted with permission from the National Association of Clinical Nurse Specialist (NACNS). (2020). https://nacns.org/advocacy-policy/policies-affecting-cnss/scope-of-practice/)

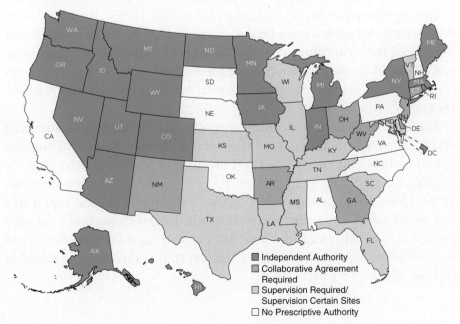

Figure 11.2. CNS Independent Prescriptive Authority. (Reprinted with permission from the National Association of Clinical Nurse Specialist (NACNS). (2020). https://nacns.org/advocacy-policy/policies-affecting-cnss/scope-of-practice/)

collaborative agreement with a physician to prescribe medications and durable medical equipment (NACNS, 2020c).

History and Evolution

Delineation of the CNS role occurred after finding gaps in the quality of nursing care provided to patients in hospitals. The increasing acuity of hospitalized patients and the need for a higher level of nursing expertise were also at the forefront of the discussion around the need for the CNS role (Kaasalainen et al., 2010). Considered appreciably different from traditional practitioners of nursing, the CNS practices at a variety of levels (Hamric & Spross, 1989).

Defined in the literature as a critical advanced practice nursing role, the CNS practices at three levels. Reed (2020) defines these spheres as nurses and nursing, patient care, and organizations and systems. Early introduction of the CNS role occurred primarily in the acute care higher acuity setting. The concept of a specialist in nursing has been in the literature since the 1900s (DeWitt, 1900). Nurse specialists were first identified in 1910 and defined as being proficient in a specific area of nursing, a completer of a postgraduate nursing course, or a nurse who was technically savvy (Gordon et al., 2012).

First mentioned by Peplau as dating back to 1938 (1965), the CNS date of origin is not well agreed upon (Hamric & Spross, 1989). In the 1940s, Reiter introduced the term "nurse clinician" as a nurse with advanced knowledge and clinical skills prepared to provide higher levels of care to patients with complex needs (Hamric, Spross, & Hanson, 2009; Montemuro, 1987; Reiter, 1966).

The concept of having a clinical specialist was elevated to an advanced practice nursing role through the work of the National League for Nursing (NLN) in 1944 (Norris, 1977). The University of Minnesota advanced the concept of a CNS role as a reality in a formal conference setting (Smoyak, 1976). These early nursing leaders crafted a vision of a clinical expert role that would address the need for highly skilled nurses who could not only provide care but also lead care provided by others and decrease barriers to the delivery of high-quality care (Fulton, 2014). It is this vision that lead to creation of the CNS role.

Given that current opportunities for nurses wishing to receive advanced academic preparation were limited, nurse faculty questioned how they could expand academic education to accommodate additional nurses interested in becoming CNSs. Nurses returning from World War II were eligible for advanced education, but there was no room in the existing academic programs to accommodate the number of nurses who were interested in achieving advanced academic preparation (Critchley, 1985).

In response to identifying mental health nursing as a core mental health discipline, nurses had the opportunity to receive federal funds from the 1946 National Mental Health Act research and training funds for undergraduate and graduate nursing education (Critchley, 1985). The initial advanced psychiatric nursing program was developed in 1954 by Peplau at Rutgers University (Critchley, 1985). The funding for and the work of this first advanced psychiatric nursing program was the driving force for the preparation of clinical specialists at the graduate level. Peplau's program was a prerequisite to the establishment of the CNS role (Sills, 1983). Beginning as a graduate cancer nursing course in 1947, the Oncology Nursing Society founded a cancer nursing specialty and contributed to the CNS oncology role (Sills, 1983).

Brown's *Future of Nursing* (1948) continued to speak of the gap in nursing clinical content, teaching, and the newer development of nurse collaborators in care, public health, and medicine. Brown contended that nursing students needed enhanced judgment and leadership abilities. This report focused on the prevention and treatment of illness, nursing skill improvement and growth, teaching and leading others, and interprofessional collaboration from local to international levels (Allen et al., 1948).

Faculty recognized that previous curricula focused on preparing teaching and learning experiences for nurses. Additional focus would be required to develop curricula aimed to facilitate clinical expert preparation. Studies were then funded to create teaching and learning experiences for nurses (Hiestand, 2006). The first dean of the Graduate School of Nursing at New York Medical College, Frances Reiter, called for development of education programs that would prepare a variety of specialists as advanced clinical experts (Hiestand, 2006). The first CNS master's program was initiated by Hilda Peplau in 1954 as a psychiatric CNS program at Rutgers University (Bignee & Amidi-Nouri, 2000). In 2003, the number of CNS programs had grown to 157 programs at 139 different schools with the majority of those programs focused on adult health (53%) (Walker et al., 2003).

As nursing education drove the curriculum guiding the knowledge and skills of the nurse, the assumption was that prior nursing education for nursing practice stopped at the diploma level (Norris, 1977). Into the 1950s, education for nurses in baccalaureate and master's level courses occurred in the same classroom, and both levels of students received the same instruction (Smoyak, 1976). With both levels of students receiving the same instruction, nurses seeking master's level content and assignments were not expected to expand their thinking to an advanced level. Specialty hospitals offered supervised postgraduate on-the-job training experiences meant to enhance the necessary skills developed by students in the undergraduate programs, but the on-the-job experiences were unavailable in academic programs (Norris, 1977).

As nursing faculty attention increased for the clinical specialist graduate-level preparation, the NLN sponsored a national working conference in 1956 to deliberate the need for a psychiatric clinical nurse expert (NLN, 1958). Meeting participants at the NLN working conference identified the need for a new psychiatric clinical nurse expert role and labeled the role as the "clinical specialist" (NLN, 1958).

The CNS role was intended to advance the art and science of psychiatric nursing and endorse new knowledge and techniques in the care of patients (NLN, 1958/1973). Graduate preparation for this clinical specialist was required of nurses aspiring to be CNSs. A need was identified to delineate clinical competencies for the new role of the CNS. Essential elements of a graduate-level curriculum were developed to provide a foundation for the CNS role (NLN, 1958/1973).

A previous focus in nursing education had been on training faculty and administrators vs. teaching and expanding the clinical role of nurses. The earlier emphasis was to provide education to prepare those who would be faculty and administrators, responding to the need for leaders responsible for developing programs at the undergraduate level and teaching undergraduate nurses. Driven by the hospitals' needs for nurses, early specialists in nursing were private duty nurses (Hamric & Spross, 1989). Specialization in graduate nursing education first focused on functional roles instead of clinical preparation of nurses and was related to the need to enhance hospitals' organizational structures for the supervisory model vs. the private duty model of nursing care (Smoyak, 1976).

Through the 1960s, multiple journal articles helped define and establish the CNS role core competencies for practice (Fulton, 2014; Table 11.1). The

Table 11.1. CNS Core Competency Categories	
Direct Care Competency	Direct interaction with patients, families, and groups of patients to promote health or well-being and improve quality of life. Characterized by a holistic perspective in the advanced nursing management of health, illness, and disease states.
Consultation Competency	Patient-, staff-, or system-focused interaction between professionals in which the consultant is recognized as having specialized expertise and assists the consultee with problem-solving.
Systems Leadership Competency	The ability to manage, change, and empower others to influence clinical practice and political processes both within and across systems.
Collaboration Competency	Working jointly with others to optimize clinical outcomes. The CNS collaborates at an advanced level by committing to authentic engagement and constructive patient, family, system, and population-focused problem-solving.
Coaching Competency	Skillful guidance and teaching to advance the care of patients, families, groups of patients, and the profession of nursing.
Research Competency	The work of thorough and systematic inquiry. Includes the search for, interpretation, and use of evidence in clinical practice and quality improvement, as well as active participation in the conduct of research.
Ethical Decision-Making, Moral Agency, and Advocacy Competency	Identifying, articulating, and acting on ethical concerns at the patient, family, healthcare provider, system, community, and public policy levels.

CNS, clinical nurse specialist.

Professional Nurse Traineeship Program added CNS education in 1963 and provided funding to advance clinical nursing specialists (National League for Nursing, 1984).

In 1966, as this extra funding was available, Reiter insisted that additional importance be placed on preparing expert clinical nurses (1966). These nurses would be master practitioners for all dimensions of nursing practice—basic, technical, accelerated assessment capabilities, prioritization of care, and implementation of interventions to achieve positive outcomes. An expert clinical nurse's practice was grounded in theory, scientific evidence, clinical practice, mentoring, quality, and collaborative expertise. The clinical expert's knowledge included sound basic science and principles foundational to care, promotion of care quality, and mitigation of system-level obstacles to high-quality care (Reiter, 1966, p. 6). The clinical expert would possess the talent to directly and indirectly influence care at the level of the patient, nurse, and system (Reiter, 1966).

In the 1970s, MacPhail summarized the CNS role competencies as a science synthesizer, role model, change agent, educator, and facilitator of quality and performance improvement intended to enhance outcomes (1971). As CNS competencies were identified, further work was needed around CNS academic preparation. Riehl and McVay (1973) recognized a need for clinical nursing practice experts and recognized curricular standards, pedagogical knowledge, and instruction in translating science and theory into practice (Bullough & Bullough, 1979; Ellis & Hartley, 2004). As a result of these needs, nurse educators and clinical leaders emphasized curricula, scientific quality, and clinical educational experiences (Fulton, 2014).

In Their Own Words

Sean M. Reed, PhD, APN, ACNS-BC, ACHPN

The key point in understanding my role is… Being a clinical nurse specialist (CNS) means mixing science and art. The science of being a CNS is multifaceted: as an expert clinician, I assess, prescribe, and manage care for individuals and populations; as a consultant, I contribute to interdisciplinary think tanks and participate on interprofessional policy panels; as a researcher, I design/conduct studies to make discoveries and publish findings to expand the knowledge base; and as an educator, I challenge paradigms and inculcate evidence-based practices. So, then, what is the art of being a CNS? The art is to harmonize all of those roles and use all that I am. The art is to influence stakeholders and drive

(Continued)

optimal outcomes for patients, nurses, and healthcare organizations and systems. In other words, the art of being a CNS is to lead. I have diverse, essential skill set, and I am a leader. I am a CNS.

What keeps me coming back every day is… Knowing that, as a CNS, I am the most versatile of all APRNs. No other APRN is focused on impacting the three spheres of healthcare: nurses and nursing, patient care, and organizations and systems. I collaborate with my fellow APRNs (NPs, CRNAs, and CNMs), and my education and skill set allow me to function in various different roles within the changing healthcare system. I take great pride in working with stakeholders to achieve the highest possible outcome for my patient population. For me, being a CNS is more than just a job—it is an ethic in caring for the seriously ill.

My greatest challenge is… Having 10 plates in the air and asking someone to toss me another…knowing when and how to say "No" is a challenge, as is sharing as much as I can with those whose wants exceed my limits and boundaries…all in all, overextending myself is probably one of my greatest CNS-related challenges. Yet I continue to learn that, despite my good intentions, I am human and cannot be all things to all people.

I wish someone had told me… The "imposter phenomenon" is an expected lived experience as a new CNS. Because the CNS is not a well-understood role, we are always on stage. We are constantly having to reaffirm our specific contribution to healthcare and remind stakeholders who we are and what we do. As leaders in healthcare innovation and change, we are VERY visible, and therefore, we need to ensure that we maintain our balance of passion, drive, excellence, and emotional intelligence. Anyone who innovates should expect to be questioned and challenged, and realize those moments engaged with questions and challenges indicate curiosity rather than hostility.

I need to be a lifelong learner because… Being a "Master Student" is integral to being a CNS. A CNS constantly learns about relationships, leadership, the human experience, humility, and role modeling. Absorbing information helps me understand the why, what, when, and how of events; as a result, I try to take each event in my life and professional career as raw learning material. Then, I use the infrastructure provided by my training and history to process the incoming materials into value-added products. After that, I share the products with my students, mentees, and colleagues to help elevate their professional practice. To be such a factory and produce beneficial output, I always need more and different and higher quality input. This entails being a Master Student, which entails lifelong learning.

(Continued)

> **Another point to understand is...** It is critical to codify and disseminate the value proposition of your role. Develop SMART goals around each area of the value equation: Value = Quality + Safety + Service/Cost or Resources. CNSs should consistently collect data as evidence of our impact on the three spheres of healthcare; CNSs must do this via metrics that capture our contributions to quality, safety, service, and cost/resources. We need to report our outcomes on a routine basis (e.g., quarterly). Finally, it is imperative that we give voice to our work, disseminating our outcomes through presentations that evolve into peer-reviewed publications.

Defining the Clinical Nurse Specialist Role

The public believed that nurses should expand their direct care practice. Expansion of direct care practice included activities that were previously reserved for the physician's practice (ANA, 1974). The American Nurses Association (ANA) Congress of Nursing Practice described CNS and nurse practitioner (NP) roles and began defining the increasing nursing scope of practice.

At the same time, the need for foundational preparation was under development, the number of baccalaureate-prepared nurses had grown, and by 1984, the number of accredited academic programs preparing CNSs increased to 129 (NLN, 1984). CNS academic programs grew in the 1980s. In the 1990s, CNS roles shifted away from being expert clinicians to administrative or educator roles (Hamric et al., 2009). This shift contributed to clouding of the CNS role and the need to further clarify the CNS's value to organizations and the nursing profession.

The acceptance of the CNS role was discussed in 1983 at the Task Force on Nursing Practice in Hospitals (Mcclure et al., 1983). At the National Commission on Nursing (1983), and within the American Nurses Association (1986), concerns were expressed regarding the future and viability of the CNS role in the face of pressures of healthcare systems to decrease costs (Hamric, 1983).The early vision of the CNS was a nurse expert capable of facilitating direct patient care, leading the development of nurses, and influencing delivery of care at the systems level (Fulton, 2014).

Based on the concerns about clarity and conservation of the CNS role, a group of CNSs from three states—California, Indiana, and Ohio—met at conferences in the 1980s and 1990s to ensure that the Council of Nurses in Advanced

Practice continued to support the CNS role. These nurses founded the National Association of Clinical Nurse Specialists (NACNS). The goal of NACNS was to advance and preserve the CNS role in healthcare (NACNS, 2020b). NACNS also provided a national forum for legislative and other activity that helped support the subsequent CNS Medicare reimbursement eligibility in 1997 (Hamric et al., 2009) and the continuation of the CNS role as a critical role for advanced practice nursing at the patient, nurse, and system level. The NACNS gives voice to more than 70,000 CNSs. NACNS exists to enhance and promote the unique, high-value contribution of the CNS to the health and well-being of individuals, families, groups, and communities, and to promote and advance the practice of nursing (NACNS, 2020b).

The representation of CNSs in NACNS has grown to more than 2,000 members. NACNS launched a peer-reviewed journal, created numerous task forces to address the crucial CNS role, generated policy papers, and increased legislator, health professional, and public awareness of the importance of the CNS role in ensuring that evidence-based care improved patient outcomes and reduced healthcare costs (NACNS, 2020b).

As the CNS role was central to quality improvement, patient safety, and improved healthcare outcomes, CNSs continued to support the IOM report for increased quality and safety in healthcare in the United States (IOM, 2011). The NACNS's statement on practice and education clearly defined the role as having subroles that were divided into direct patient care provider, consultant, educator, researcher, collaborator, and clinical leader (Goudreau et al., 2007; NACNS, 2004). CNSs were the first group of APRNs to be recognized as advanced practice nurses with a unique body of knowledge and competencies based on education at the graduate level (Mick & Ackerman, 2002). Despite their early beginnings, the breadth of the CNS role continued to cloud the ability of the public to distinguish the CNS from other advanced nursing roles (Fulton et al., 2020).

While the clouding of the CNS role made it difficult to distinguish the CNS from other advanced nursing roles, CNSs continued to expand their influence through roles in consulting, education, research, and executive-level administration. The value of the CNS role and the expertise developed from academic and practice preparation have been highlighted through CNSs leading a variety of systems, national organizations, and associations, including Dr. Michelle Janney, CNS, past president of the American Organization of Nurse Executives (Thompson, Anderson, Bradley, & Herrin-Griffith, 2017); Dr. Janet Fulton, past president of NACNS (Antai-Otong, 2003); and Dr. Pam Cipriano, CNS, current president of the ANA and one of the 100 most influential people in American healthcare by *Modern Healthcare Magazine* (Modern Healthcare, 2018).

To identify CNS demographics in the United States, NACNS conducted a 2014 CNS census survey of more than 72,000 CNSs working in hospitals, private practice, clinics, and other healthcare settings. Eighty-five percent of these CNSs worked full-time with 66% working in hospital settings. More than 44% of CNSs responding to the survey had responsibility across entire hospital systems. Results of the survey indicate that the CNS role typically encompasses time in a variety of responsibilities, including (1) providing direct patient care of complex patients (25%); (2) consulting with nurses, staff, and others (20%); (3) teaching nurses and staff (19%); and (4) facilitating evidence-based practice projects (14%) (NACNS, 2015a).

In 2016, the NACNS census captured data from over 3,000 CNSs in the United States. The majority of these CNSs (80%) worked full-time in hospital settings. More than half of those CNSs (58%) had hospital system or system-wide responsibility. Other CNSs span of influence was over one or two nursing service areas. While the majority of CNSs in 2016 were white women, the CNS census was completed by more men and minorities in 2016 than in 2014. The survey also revealed that two in three CNSs were nationally certified and more than 1 in 10 held a doctorate (NACNS, 2016).

Questions to Ask Yourself

1. What is appealing to you about CNS practice?
2. How might CNSs collaborate to increase the number of states with independent CNS practice?
3. As a future CNS, how might you enhance others' understanding of the complex CNS role?

Role Specifics

CNSs have been defined as expert clinicians with advanced education and training in a specialized area of nursing practice who work in a wide variety of healthcare settings. A CNS's specialty is defined by the population, setting, disease, medical subspecialty, or type of care or problems they address. While the breadth of CNS specialty practice is extensive, CNS talent is transferable across patients/people, nurses/staff, and systems/organizations.

In Their Own Words

Katie Swafford, DNP, RN, CNS-BC, CCRN
Clinical Nurse Specialist and Critical Care Manager
Eskenazi Health, Indianapolis, IN

The key points in understanding my role are... I was fortunate to transition into an Adult Health Clinical Nurse Specialist role in the same critical care department where I was a staff nurse. Ultimately, the position was new, so I molded the CNS position into what I determined the department needed the most. My focus in my role as a CNS in critical care has been departmental quality and performance improvement. I am a nursing advocate in multiple interprofessional committees and shared governance councils in my healthcare system. Thus, I tend to seek out projects and opportunities in which the department staff nurses can become involved. I centered my attention toward maintaining quality measures and adjusting nursing practice to new guidelines and recommendations based on the evidence. I am a resource to staff for clinical skills that they may be unfamiliar with and assist with developing and providing staff education. Over the past 3 to 4 years, our department has initiated new skill sets for the bedside caregivers, including intra-aortic balloon pumps and continuous electroencephalograms. I assisted with the implementation and sustainability of these two programs specifically. Another role that I cherish is that of encouraging staff development. I guide staff nurses in obtaining the next level in the facility's clinical ladder program. I firmly believe and the metrics support that developing staff to become engaged in performance initiatives of the department increased patient safety and patient care. Last year, I transitioned into a dual role of a Clinical Nurse Specialist and Clinical Manager. The dual purpose of this role has allowed me to enhance my leadership skills but maintain my focus on quality improvement and staff development.

What keeps me coming back every day is... Throughout my career, I never questioned why I became a nurse. I initially decided to become a nurse after I had cardiac surgery as a child. I realized at the age of 9 years what a positive

(Continued)

influence nurses made in my recovery. I chose to become a nurse to make a difference in the lives of my patients and families. As I have transitioned in my career and stepped away from the bedside, the ability to support the bedside nurse has become my goal. I am passionate about staff development and love seeing new nurses grow and develop new skills that were once foreign to them. The success of my colleagues and the difference that the nursing profession makes as a whole keep me coming back to work every day. Furthering my academic education in conjunction with increasing my role responsibilities assists me in growing in all spheres of the CNS role.

My greatest challenge is... As my career trajectory has changed over the years, so have my objectives. One of the most challenging aspects of my current position is transitioning care to accommodate revised guidelines and documentation requirements of the bedside nurse. While the recommendations adjust, so do the care and education of the staff nurses providing the care. As a nurse leader, specializing in quality improvement, the stressors of regulatory guidelines and maintaining outcomes can be overwhelming. Being prepared as a CNS provides me with talent at the patient, nurse, and system levels. This preparation helps me be successful in both my CNS and Clinical Manager roles. Optimal care and patient outcomes are the ultimate goals of both roles. However, many patients have traumatic injuries, comorbidities, and socioeconomic challenges leading to revisions of care and challenges for the nursing profession. I must be diligent with my leadership, role modeling, and clinical care to enhance the outcomes for the patients. I work every day to streamline the care of the bedside nurse and try to decrease barriers to excellent care.

I wish someone had told me... I wish someone would have told me that the ability to effectively communicate would be as important as the expertise with clinical skills. As healthcare has evolved, the emphasis on patient satisfaction and patient-centered care has increased. The basis for both of these concepts is communication. As I have matured and worked on my communication skills over my career, I now thoroughly understand the impact of good vs. poor communication skills. I also wish someone would have told me that it was okay to express emotion. I am not a very emotional person, but I frequently hide my feelings, especially when at work. I work in a critical care department, which has a lot of anxiety, stress, and devastation, which affects the nurse as well. Continually hiding my emotions is not healthy, and part of my personal development is to find ways to ensure that I am appropriately dealing with my feelings, as I know that this is helpful to me as well as for the staff that I lead.

(Continued)

I need to be a lifelong learner because… Healthcare is dynamic and continually changing. To be successful, I must be willing to adapt and learn new recommendations and evidence-based practice. As a nurse leader, I must understand the latest findings to help bedside caregivers practice at the highest level. I am currently enrolled in the Doctorate of Nursing Practice (DNP) program at Indiana University. My goal is to become a nursing professor and aid in the education and development of future nurses at the academic level, like I have done in my roles as a CNS and Clinical Manager. I believe furthering my education will provide me with the tools to continue my success in the nursing profession.

Another point to understand is… Nurses must become engaged in their profession. Far too often, nurses take a back seat to other disciplines. This cannot happen. We must be at the table and advocate for the profession of nursing. Many times, nurses become frustrated with changes in healthcare, but are unwilling to join a professional nursing organization to support the cause. The best way we can support nurses is to become informed and join the professional nursing organizations that work collectively to support and advance nursing and the care of our patients.

The CNS role is a functional nursing role that is represented through professional practice competencies. The CNS roles include **independent licensed provider**; clinical expert in primary, secondary, and tertiary care; as well as nurse educator, coach, and mentor. Working at patient, nurse, and system levels, the CNS monitors and improves quality of care and educates others. Leading interprofessional teams, CNSs address complex clinical patient, nurse, and system issues that impact healthcare (Gordon et al., 2012; NACNS, 2020a). While the specialist title emerged in the early 1900s, the ANA officially recognized the CNS role, obtained through master's education, in 1974 (Gordon et al., 2012; Hamric et al., 2009).

The CNS has been a recognized leader in the complex healthcare system in the United States for more than 60 years. From its rich history, based on the need for a multitalented clinical expert, the role of the CNS profession is widely accepted in healthcare systems. As a standardized, licensed, and fully regulated healthcare occupation, the CNS profession impacts patients, nurses, and systems by facilitating and providing safe, quality, evidence-based healthcare services (NACNS, 2020b).

Populations Served

Populations that CNSs serve may include the following: pediatrics, geriatrics, women's health/gender-specific, adult health, gerontology, family/individual across the lifespan, psychiatric/mental health, and neonatal (NACNS, 2020b). CNSs can be found in inpatient nursing settings such as critical care, emergency departments, medical-surgical, psychiatry, women and family, perioperative, burn, or trauma. CNSs are well suited for quality and performance improvement across all healthcare settings. CNSs also work in private practice, clinics, accountable care organizations, informatics and technology, and rehabilitation, and as entrepreneurs (Fulton et al., 2020).

Three of four CNSs specialize in adult health or gerontology (NACNS, 2016-Survey). The majority of CNSs work in acute care hospitals that have American Nurses Credentialing Center's (ANCC) Magnet Designation or are seeking Magnet Designation. Approximately half of all CNSs are responsible for clinical nursing care at the systems level; however, only one in five CNSs is authorized to prescribe medications.

Professionalism

The context of CNS practice is exhibiting influence across the continuum of care. Typically lacking line authority, essential characteristics drive CNS success. *Influence* is defined as "the power to produce outcomes by shifting others into action" (Merriam Webster's Learner Dictionary, 2018). Since the impact of CNS practice is so broad, exhibiting essential professional attributes is necessary for successful CNS outcomes. Figure 11.3 presents the essential CNS characteristics or talents as identified by the NACNS (2004).

Eight characteristics represent emotional competence: self-awareness, social awareness, the ability to verbalize emotion and expression, the capacity for

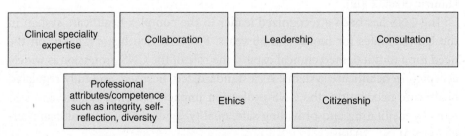

Figure 11.3. Clinical nurse specialist (CNS) skills.

empathetic involvement, the ability to differentiate subjective emotional experience from external emotional expression, adaptive coping, the awareness of emotional relationship communication, and emotional self-efficacy capacity (Saarni, 1999). The success of the CNS is dependent upon exhibiting the components of emotional intelligence, self-awareness, self-management, social awareness, and relationship management (Raghubir, 2018). Thoughtful analysis of ethical dilemmas and mindfully modeling leadership behavior that is representative of all CNSs help solidify CNS community impact (Bingle & Davidson, 2014). CNS emotional competence is a critical prerequisite to accomplishing clinical and fiscal outcomes and sustainability (Bingle & Davidson, 2014).

Services Provided

Practicing at three levels, CNSs provide diagnoses, treatment, and ongoing management of patients. CNSs also provide expertise and mentoring to guide nurses caring for patients at the bedside, facilitate practice and organizational changes, and ensure best practice and evidence-based care. Outcome-focused, CNS attention is on achieving the best possible patient outcomes (NACNS, 2020b). Expertly identifying healthcare gaps, CNSs guide designing and implementing interventions, assessments, and evaluations to improve healthcare outcomes.

Outcomes achieved by CNSs and their teams include reduced healthcare expenses, length of stay, and unnecessary emergency room visits. Care improvement outcomes include improved pain management practices, patient experiences, and complications related to hospitalized patients (NACNS, 2020b).

Disease or Medical Subspecialty

The CNS is a self-directed practitioner. CNS practice flexes to meet patients, nurses, and systems where they are and where the need is the greatest (Hamric & Spross, 1983; Reed, 2020). CNS practice is grounded in principles of population-based analysis at the following perspectives: community, clinical epidemiologic, prevention, and outcome measurement (Ibrahim et al., 2001). The list of disease-specific work by CNSs is exhaustive but may include diabetes, oncology, cardiovascular, neurology, orthopedics, pediatrics, psychiatry, or pulmonology. CNSs serve as direct care providers, consultants, system leaders, collaborators, mentors, researchers, ethical decision-makers, moral agents, and advocates (Hamric, 1983). The work of a CNS also includes identification of barriers to care, problems related to process breakdowns, and types of problems such as pain, wounds, and stress

(NACNS, 2020b). The breadth of the abilities of the CNS has contributed to role confusion by those outside the specialty. National and international CNSs continue to expand the CNS footprint and clarify the importance of the CNS role across the continuum of care and at all levels of practice (NACNS, 2020b).

Competencies

Core competencies for the CNS were first published in 1998 (Fulton, 2014). The organizing framework for CNSs and the core competencies for practice were generated through rigorous content analysis, an extensive literature review, and interviewing practicing CNSs and administrators (Fulton, 2014). The final CNS competency list was validated by a national external review panel (Baldwin et al., 2007). CNS core competencies were updated and validated through evidence in 2004 (Baldwin et al., 2009). The CNS framework was organized into domains or spheres of influence of patient/client, nurses/nursing practice, and organizations/systems (NACNS, 1998) as presented in Figure 11.4.

CNS practice is conceptualized into three interacting spheres. The spheres are represented in specialty practice and directed by specialty knowledge and standards. The spheres of CNS influence portray the scope or practice reach of activities that distinguish the CNS scope or practice and target outcomes (Fulton, 2020). Central to the CNS organizing framework is the CNS as a clinical expert in the patient/client sphere. The nurses and nursing practice domain are indicative of how CNSs influence nursing practice and care delivery. At the organization/system level, the CNS facilitates elimination of barriers, quality of care, and enhanced patient outcomes (Fulton, 2014; NACNS, 2004).

The revised CNS core competencies were published in 2010. At the 2010 publication time, three different models existed for CNS practice: (1) the three spheres of influence as defined by NACNS; (2) the seven advanced practice nursing competencies as defined by Hamric and Spross; and (3) the nurse characteristics identified in the American Association of Colleges of Nursing (AACN) Synergy Model. The organizing framework for CNSs reflected a synthesis of the above three models. In the model, the three spheres of influence define the foundation for CNS practice. The nine advanced practice competencies identified by Hamric and Spross (direct care provider, consultant, system leader, collaborator, coach, researcher, ethical decision-maker, moral agent, advocate) provide the context for the specific, measurable behavioral statements listed below each overarching competency

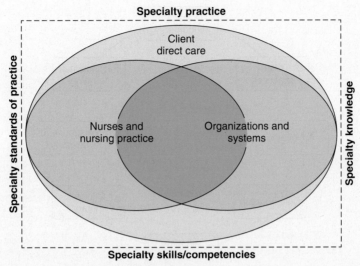

Figure 11.4. Clinical nurse specialist (CNS) practice conceptualized as core competencies in three interacting spheres actualized in specialty practice and guided by specialty knowledge and specialty standards. (From Fulton, J. S. (2004). *Statement on clinical nurse practice and education*. NACNS, used with permission.)

and were imbedded in the CNS practice foundation (NACNS, 2008). The eight nurse characteristics identified in the AACN Synergy Model, presented in Figure 11.5, were also imbedded within the model. Patients and families were the focus of the model, linking the framework together (National NACNS Competency Task Force, 2006-2008). The CNS core competencies include the expected behaviors, the spheres of influence, and the nurse characteristics (NACNS, 2020b).

After the 2010 published core competencies, specialty competencies for adult/ gerontology and women's health were identified. In 2019, NACNS published the third edition of the Statement on Clinical Nurse Specialist Practice and Education. This document combines all components of the original Statement and adds the following (NACNS, 2019):

- An updated conceptual model of the CNS;
- A change in terminology from spheres of influence, to spheres of impact;
- A refined approach to the presentation of the CNS competencies that consolidates and refines the competencies under the three spheres of impact;
- An enhanced discussion of the social mandate of the CNS;
- A discussion of the Consensus Model for APRN Licensure, Accreditation, Certification, and Education.

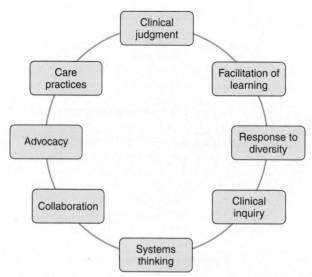

Figure 11.5. American Association of Colleges of Nursing (AACN) nurse characteristics. (From Fulton J. S. (2004). *Statement on clinical nurse practice and education.* NACNS, used with permission.)

In 2009, NACNS released the *Core Practice Doctorate Clinical Nurse Specialist Competencies* for CNSs. Practice doctorate programs for CNSs provided broader and more in-depth preparation for the APRN role. The preparation for CNSs at the doctoral level included an expanded theoretical and scientific foundation for practice; knowledge synthesis and translation into practice; system-level issue analysis, solution-design, and organization-wide change; interprofessional collaboration; use of information technology to improve systems of care; and influencing and shaping health policy (NACNS, 2020b).

The CNS spheres of influence were the organizing framework for the CNS practice doctorate competencies. The client sphere of influence is represented as conducting evidence-based, comprehensive assessments, integrating multiple source data. The CNS implements client assessment strategies based on psychometric properties analysis, clinical fit, feasibility, and utility. The CNS uses advanced clinical judgment to diagnose conditions related to disease, health, and illness within other contexts. Designing, implementing, and evaluating a broad range of evidence-based interventions could include prescribing and administering a variety of therapeutic interventions. The CNS directs analysis and dissemination of outcomes of client care programs based on multiple considerations. The CNS advocates for the integration of preferences and rights in healthcare decision-making across the profession. CNSs apply teaching/learning and health literacy principles to facilitate design, provision, and evaluation of client education. The CNS is a practice specialist, translating and generating evidence. Expert consultation also occurs at this level for the CNS.

At the nurse and nursing practice sphere of influence, the CNS leads the interprofessional team in incorporating ethical principles in healthcare planning and delivery. The CNS influences facilitation of interprofessional practice outcomes through knowledge translation. The CNS supports development of others' professional growth, fosters effective team functioning, and facilitates healthcare team process improvements to enhance clinical and fiscal outcomes.

At the organization/system sphere of influence, the CNS uses organizational and system theory to facilitate evidence-based, outcome-focused, collaborative, cost-effective, and ethical care delivery. The CNS influences informatics and technology development, integration, management, and evaluation to promote safety, quality, and resource management. The CNS synthesizes and applies evidence to advance healthcare delivery. As an entrepreneur, the CNS facilitates development of products, resulting in improved fiscal and clinical outcomes. Talent for making the business case for securing resources allows the CNS to advocate for products, programs, and services at this level of influence. As a healthcare policy advocate, the CNS guides others at local, regional, and national levels to optimize resources to enhance healthcare outcomes. The CNS leads, advocates, and mentors nurses through leadership on boards and task forces at all levels (NACNS, 2020b).

In Their Own Words

Francesca C. Levitt, MSN, RN-BC, ACNS-BC
Clinical Nurse Specialist

The key points in understanding my role are… A CNS is an advanced practice registered nurse who has earned a master's or a doctorate degree in nursing. CNSs are clinical experts and specialize in a particular area of practice (e.g., patient population, unit/department, disease, or type of problem). The CNS serves as a leader, consultant, and mentor to advance the practice of nursing within three spheres of influence for patients and families, for nurses, and at the organization/system level. Through developing relationships and partnerships with clients and stakeholders, the CNS helps to ensure quality care and optimal outcomes. The CNS works to bridge the gap between

(Continued)

what is known through research and current practice. The CNS prepares and educates nurses and then helps to implement evidence-based changes into practice when needed.

What keeps me coming back every day is... The varied work of the CNS is stimulating, challenging, and joy filled. Connecting with patients, nurses, and other colleagues to enhance the experience and support healing is at the core of my work. My focus as a CNS Is to become the best, most authentic version of myself so that I can support others to continuously improve outcomes. As a CNS, one of the most important attributes is to build relationships and influence others to deliver evidence-based quality care. Inspiring others to cultivate their full potential and profoundly impact patients is what motivates me and brings joy into my personal and professional life.

My greatest challenge is... One of my greatest challenges is saying no when someone asks me to work on a project or address an issue. I have had to learn to say that I can work on something within a certain time frame. I tend to take on too much at one time because I want to be supportive and responsive to the needs of others. Setting clear expectations is an important skill of an effective CNS.

I wish someone had told me... Territorial issues can be challenging for a new CNS. The first goal of a CNS should be to build trusting relationships that focus on seeking to understand well before goal-setting occurs. Recognizing conflict and addressing role confusion are skills that a CNS develops as one becomes more self- and socially aware and enhances their emotional intelligence. Developing a good working relationship with nursing directors, managers, and educators is essential to the collaborative skills needed by a CNS to guide evidence-based practice.

I need to be a lifelong learner because... I am intrinsically curious and want to stay abreast of the current best available evidence. I seek to challenge myself to learn more every day. If I don't seek new knowledge, I am standing still. I am motivated by and enjoy optimizing patient outcomes across the entire continuum. I enjoy lifelong learning and challenging myself as a clinician and informal nursing leader.

Another point to understand is... Nursing is a perfect blend of people skills and science. The success of the CNS is dependent on the establishment of respectful relationships and collaboration. Everyone has gifts and talents; the key is how to capitalize on those strengths and collectively innovate and grow both personally and professionally. As a CNS, I am outcome oriented, persistent, and, as my colleague recently stated, able to find evidence hidden under rocks. My approach to CNS practice is strategic, comprehensive, knowledge seeking, empathetic, collaborative, detail oriented, compassionate, and always patient-focused.

Certification

Defined by the American Board of Nursing Specialties (ABNS), certification is the formal recognition of specialized knowledge, skills, and experience demonstrated by meeting standards of a nursing specialty (ABNS, 2015). The public recognizes quality nursing care designated by national specialty certification (ABNS, 2015; Duffy, 2016). The 2012 APRN Consensus Model indicates that CNSs who practice in the majority of states must obtain certification based on a population area (NACNS, 2020d). Current certification examinations based on population include adult/gerontology, pediatrics, and neonatal. Current certification examinations based on population include adult/gerontology, pediatrics, and neonatal.

Certification for CNS practice was complicated given the vast number of existing certification examinations for undergraduate-prepared nurses. Advanced-level CNS certification emerged slowly. Not all states recognized examinations for APRN regulatory purposes (Cockerham & Keeling, 2014). For CNSs, certification is available through the ANCC or through specialty organizations such as the Oncology Nursing Society or the American Association of Critical Care Nurses. Certification examinations are not obtainable for many CNS specialties, such as cardiovascular, neuroscience, or perinatal nursing (Chan & Cartwright, 2014; Hamric et al., 2014). Previously offered certification examinations, such as the focus of the family and individual across the lifespan, were suspended. As certifying bodies experience declines in nurses needing certifications, other examinations may be affected. Table 11.2 lists sample certification examinations for CNSs.

Prescriptive Authority

The CNS and the other licensed APRNs are authorized to diagnose, prescribe, institute therapy, or refer patients to healthcare agencies, healthcare providers, and community resources as outlined in the Consensus Model (NACNS, 2020b). The CNS is authorized to prescribe, procure, administer, and dispense over-the-counter, legend, and controlled substances. The CNS is also authorized to plan and initiate therapeutic regimens including ordering and prescribing medical

Table 11.2. CNS Certification Options

Organization	Title	Credential	Website
American Nurses Credentialing Center	Adult-Gerontology CNS-Board Certified	AGCNS-BC	www.nurse-credentialing.org/cert
American Association of Critical-Care Nurses Certification Corporation	Adult-Gerontology CNS (appropriate for Adult-Gerontology, Pediatric, and Neonatal populations)	AGCNS (AGCNS-AG, AGCNS-P, AGCNS-N)	www.cert-corp.org
Oncology Nursing Certification Corporation	Advanced Oncology CNS	AOCNS	www.oncc.org

CNS, clinical nurse specialist.

devices and equipment and providing nutrition, diagnostic, and supportive services. The CNS's authority includes, but is not limited to, home healthcare, hospice, and physical and occupational therapy (NACNS, 2020b).

The NACNS developed a statement on prescriptive authority for CNSs. This statement designates support of CNS autonomous prescribing and ordering privileges. The Consensus Model allowed state boards of nursing to grant prescribing and ordering authority through the APRN licensure (NACNS, 2020b). NACNS supported grandfathering prescriptive authority for CNSs who graduated before the APRN regulation implementation and had prescribing and ordering authority in the state in which they practiced. The CNS who did not have prescribing authority at that time needed to meet current requirements in order to be granted prescriptive authority (NACNS, 2020b).

The CNS specializes in providing direct and indirect care to complex and vulnerable populations across the continuum of healthcare. The CNS assesses, diagnoses, and creates individual plans of care. The CNS-developed plans of care include prescriptive authority, equipment, and consultative, rehabilitative, and supportive services.

Results from the NACNS 2016 CNS census revealed issues around title protection and prescriptive authority, as these vary in the United States. Twenty-one percent of CNSs who responded to the survey were authorized to prescribe medications. Only 16% of CNSs at that time were authorized to prescribe durable medical equipment. A 2015 analysis of states in conjunction with the National Council of State Boards of Nursing indicated that CNSs have independent authority to prescribe in 19 states (NACNS, 20b). As with other advanced practice nurses, the CNS needs a collaborative agreement with a physician to legally prescribe in another 19 states. CNSs are eligible to prescribe in 38 states (NACNS, 2015b).

In Their Own Words

Kathleen E. Hubner, MSN, APRN, ACNS-BC, ANVP, CNRN
Acute Neurovascular Clinical Nurse Specialist and Stroke Coordinator
St. Vincent Neuroscience Institute
Indianapolis, IN

The key points in understanding my role are… (1) The CNS is the link between what is known and what is practiced. CNSs bring evidence to the bedside, and if there is no evidence, we perform the research. We bring the science to nursing. (2) CNSs are change agents, which go along with evidence-based practice. (3) As experts in our specialty areas, CNSs serve as resources for nurses caring for complex patients.

What keeps me coming back every day is… (1) I find great satisfaction in meeting the needs of the nurse when they say, "what do I do, or how do I do this, or why do I do this." I like to help them think through their questions and help them find the answer to their questions. (2) When we meet the needs of the nurses and bring the evidence to them at the bedside I know our patients' outcomes can be improved and they can reach their optimal level of wellness. (3) My favorite reaction from nurses is when they have experienced the "aha" moment. The look on their faces is rewarding to me at the time when something finally clicks in their brain and they understand the why behind the actions that need to occur.

My greatest challenge is… (1) Our greatest challenge is when people do not understand the role of the CNS. Everyone automatically thinks that CNSs are

(Continued)

educators, but education is just one small piece of the CNS role, and our education is just-in-time education to change a nurse's behavior and actions. (2) It is even more difficult for CNSs when administrators do not understand the CNS role. Even though we do not always generate revenue as a nurse practitioner does, we validate our salary with cost avoidance related to improved nurse-sensitive quality issues, decreased length of stay, and decreased readmissions. All of these cost avoidance factors lead to better reimbursements and less financial penalties that impact the financial health of the organization. We also generate revenue with research projects and outcomes. (3) Assessing organizational readiness to change helps us deal with the resistance to change, which is a universal challenge to CNSs in the role of change agent.

I wish someone had told me… That some of the biggest challenges we face are within our own nursing profession. Emotional intelligence to assist us with self-awareness, social awareness, and relationship management is crucial for nurses and can help CNSs address challenges within the nursing profession.

I need to be a lifelong learner because… The science of medicine and nursing is dynamic. The only constant is change, and we must maintain our nursing specialties and nursing practice. Also, our multigenerational nursing workforce requires all of us to exhibit leadership skills so that we can be successful with the different learning needs and demands of each generation.

Another point to understand is… CNSs advance the practice of nursing by continuing to practice nursing at an advanced level to escalated nursing practice. We are here to support nurses and provide what nurses need to achieve an even higher level of critical thinking to promote optimal wellness. Nursing must evolve in alignment with other healthcare professions.

Reimbursement

Another issue highlighted by the NACNS 2016 survey findings was reimbursement for care provided. CNSs in independent ambulatory care practice or those granted hospital advanced practice privileges were able to bill insurance companies directly for their services, decreasing insurance costs. According to the 2016 survey findings, only 6% of CNSs directly billed a third-party payor, as in a private insurance company, or an individual patient for provided services (NACNS, 2016).

Summary

This chapter presents the CNS scope of practice. The history and evolution of the CNS role furthers an understanding of how the complexity of the role has inceased as the role of the advanced practice nurse has evolved.

The CNS role was defined, emphasizing the complexity of the practice of the CNS at three levels and over the continuum of care, meeting patients, nurses, and systems where they exist. The specifics of CNS roles as well as the populations served continue to add to this complex advanced practice role. Essential professional CNS characteristics include (1) clinical specialty expertise; (2) collaboration; (3) leadership; (4) consultation; (5) professional attributes/competence that encompasses but is not limited to honesty, integrity, emotions, self-reflection, diversity; (6) ethics; and (7) citizenship (NACNS, 2004).

The revised CNS competencies have been vetted by a rigorous process and are expected to be released to the public in 2019 (NACNS, 2020c). The APRN Consensus Model states that CNSs who practice in the majority of states must obtain certification based on a population area. For CNSs, certification is available through the ANCC or through specialty organizations such as the Oncology Nursing Society or the American Association of Critical Care Nurses.

The CNS and the other licensed APRNs are authorized to diagnose, prescribe, institute therapy, or refer patients to healthcare agencies, healthcare providers, and community resources as outlined in the Consensus Model (NACNS, 2020b). Although authorized for prescriptive authority, only 6% of CNSs directly billed a third-party payor, as in a private insurance company, or an individual patient for provided services (NACNS, 2016).

Chapter Highlights

- CNS role evolution

The CNS role is defined as a graduate-level-prepared registered nurse with a defined area of knowledge and practice in a specific clinical nursing area (ANA, 1980). Defined in the literature as a critical advanced practice nursing role, the CNS practices at three levels: nurse and nursing, patient care, and organizations and systems. Early introduction of the CNS role occurred primarily in the acute care higher acuity setting (DeWitt, 1900).

● Populations served

Populations that CNSs serve may include the following: pediatrics, geriatrics, women's health, adult health, gerontology, family/individual across the lifespan, psychiatric/mental health, women's health/gender-specific, and neonatal (NACNS, 2020b). CNSs are well suited for quality and performance improvement across all healthcare settings. CNSs also work in private practice, clinics, accountable care organizations, informatics and technology, rehabilitation, and as entrepreneurs (Fulton et al., 2020).

● CNS competencies

Unique and advanced-level competencies of the CNS meet the needs of improving quality and reducing costs within the healthcare system. The CNS core competencies included the expected behaviors, the spheres of influence, and the nurse characteristics (NACNS, 2020c).

● CNS credentialing

Certification for CNS practice was complicated given the vast number of existing certification examinations for undergraduate prepared nurses. Advanced-level CNS certification emerged slowly. The public recognizes quality nursing care designated by national specialty certification (ABNS, 2015; Duffy, 2016).

● Prescriptive authority for the CNS

The scope of CNS practice meets need through direct care of complex patients, including assessment, diagnosis, and management which may include prescriptive authority. CNSs can practice independently in 28 states and prescribe independently in 19 states (NACNS, 2020c).

Professional Organizations

American Nurses Association (ANA): https://www.nursingworld.org/ana/
American Nurses Credentialing Center (ANCC): https://www.nursingworld.org/ancc/
National Association of Clinical Nurse Specialists (NACNS): https://nacns.org/
National League for Nursing (NLN): http://www.nln.org/
Sigma Theta Tau International (Sigma): https://www.sigmanursing.org/

Web Resources

Centers for Disease Control and Prevention (CDC): https://www.cdc.gov/
Healthy People 2020: https://www.healthypeople.gov/
World Health Organization (WHO): https://www.who.int/

References

Allen, R. B., Koos, E. L., Bradley, F. R., & Wolf, L. K. (1948). The Brown report. *The American Journal of Nursing, 48,* 736–742. https://journals.lww.com/ajnonline/citation/1948/48120/the_brown_report.9.aspx

American Board of Nursing Specialties (ABNS). (2015). *ABNS vision, mission, valued.* http://nursingcertification.org

American Nurses Association. (1980). *Nursing: A social policy statement.*

American Nurses Association. (2004). *Nursing: Scope and standards of practice.*

American Nurses Association (ANA). (1974). *Historical review.* https://www.nursingworld.org/~48de6f/globalassets/docs/ana/ana-expandedhistoricalreview.pdf

American Nurses Association (ANA), Council of Clinical Nurse Specialists. (1986). *The role of the clinical nurse specialist.*

Antai-Otong, D. (2003). Notes from the board. *Clinical Nurse Specialist, 17*(5), 229–231.

Baldwin, K. M., Clark, A. P., Fulton, J., & Mayo, A. (2009). National validation of the NACNS clinical nurse specialist core competencies. *Journal of Nursing Scholarship, 41*(2), 193–201.

Baldwin, K. M., Lyon, B. L., Clark, A. P., Fulton, J., Davidson, S., & Dayhoff, N. (2007). Developing clinical nurse specialist practice competencies. *Clinical Nurse Specialist, 21*(6), 297–302.

Bignee, J. L., & Amidi-Nouri, A. (2000). History and evolution of advanced nursing practice. In A. B. Hamric, J. A. Spross, & C. M. Hanson (Eds.), *Advanced nursing practice. An integrative approach* (2nd ed., pp. 3–32). Saunder.

Bingle, J. M., & Davidson, S. B. (2014). Professional attributes in the context of emotional intelligence, ethical conduct, and citizenship of the clinical nurse specialist. In J. S. Fulton, B. L. Lyon, & K. A. Goudreau (Eds.), *Foundations of clinical nurse specialist practice.* Springer.

Bullough, B., Bullough, V. L., & Elias, J. (Eds.). (1979). *Gender blending.* Prometheus Books.

Chan, G. K., & Cartwright, C. C. (2014). In A. B. Hamric, C. M. Hanson, M. F. Tracy, & E. T. O'Grady (Eds.), *Advanced practice nursing a holistic approach* (pp. 359–391). Elsevier Saunders.

Cockerham, A. Z., & Keeling, A. W. (2014). In A. B. Hamric, C. M. Hanson, M. F. Tracy, & E. T. O'Grady (Eds.), *Advanced practice nursing a holistic approach* (pp. 1–21). Elsevier Saunders.

Critchley, D. L. (1985). Evolution of the role. In D. L. Critchely & J. T. Maurin (Eds.), *The clinical specialist in psychiatric mental health nursing* (pp. 5–22). John Wiley.

DeWitt, K. (1900). Specialties in nursing. *American Journal of Nursing, 1*(1), 14–17.

Duffy, M. (2016). Obtaining certification: Considering the options. In M. Duffy, M. Dresser, & J. S. Fulton (Eds.), *Clinical nurse specialist toolkit: A guide for the new clinical nurse specialist.* Springer Publishing Company.

Ellis, J. R., & Hartley, C. L. (2004). *Nursing in today's world: Trends, issues & management.* Lippincott Williams & Wilkins.

Fulton, J. (2014). Evolution of the clinical nurse specialist role and practice in the United States. In J. S. Fulton, B. L. Lyon, & K. A. Goudreau (Eds.), *Foundations of clinical nurse specialist practice* (2nd ed., pp. 1–16). Springer Publishers.

Fulton, J. S. (2020). Evolution of the clinical nurse specialist role and practice in the United States. In J. S. Fulton, K. A. Goudreau, & K. L. Swartzell (Eds.). *Foundations of clinical nurse specialist practice* (3rd ed., pp. 1–20). Springer Publishing Company.

Fulton, J. S., Goudreau, K. A., & Swartzell, K. L. (Eds.), (2020). *Foundations of clinical nurse specialist practice* (3rd ed.). Springer Publishing Company.

Gordon, J. M., Lorilla, J. D., & Lehman, C. A. (2012). The role of the clinical nurse specialist in the future of health care in the United States. *Perioperative Nursing Clinics, 7*(3), 343–353.

Goudreau, K. A., Baldwin, K., Clark, A., Fulton, J., Lyon, B., Murray, T., Rust, J. E., Sendelbach, S., & National Association of Clinical Nurse Specialists. (2007). A vision of the future for clinical nurse specialists: Prepared by the national association of clinical nurse specialists, July 2007. *Clinical Nurse Specialist, 21*(6), 310–320.

Hamric, A. B. (1983). Role development and functions. In A. B. Hamric & J. A. Spross (Eds.), *The clinical nurse specialist in theory and practice* (pp. 39–56). Grune & Stratton.

Hamric, A. B., Hanson, C. M., Tracy, M. F., & O'Grady, E. T. (2014). *Advanced practice nursing-e-book: An integrative approach.* Elsevier Health Sciences.

Hamric, A. B., & Spross, J. A. (1983). *The clinical nurse specialist in theory and practice* (pp. 39–56). Grune & Stratton.

Hamric, A. B., & Spross, J. A. (Eds.). (1989). *The clinical nurse specialist in theory and practice.* W.B. Saunders Company.

Hamric, A. B., Spross, J. A., Hanson, C. M. (2009). *Advanced practice nursing: an integrative approach* (4th ed.) Saunders Elsevier.

Hiestand, W. C. (2006). Frances reiter and the graduate school of nursing at the New York medical College, 1960-1973. *Nursing History Review, 14*, 216–226.

Ibrahim, M. A., Savitz, L. A., Carey, T. S., & Wagner, E. H. (2001). Population-based health principles in medical and public health practice. *Journal of Public Health Management and Practice, 7*(3), 75–81.

Institute of Medicine. (2011). *The future of nursing: Leading change, advancing health.* The National Academies Press.

Kaasalainen, S., Martin-Misener, R., Kilpatrick, K., Harbman, P., Bryant-Lukosius, D., Donald, F., Carter, N., & DiCenso, A. (2010). A historical overview of the development of advanced practice nursing roles in Canada. *Nursing Leadership (Toronto, Ont), 23*, 35–60.

Mcclure, M. L., Poulin, M. A., Sovie, M. D., & Wandelt, M. A. (1983). Magnet hospitals: Attraction and retention of professional nurses. American academy of nursing. Task Force on nursing practice in hospitals. American nurses association. *American Nurse association Publication, (G-160)*, 1–135.

Merriam Webster's Learner's Dictionary. (2018). *Learner's dictionary.* http://www.learnersdictionary.com/definition/influence

Mick, D. J., & Ackerman, M. H. (2002). Deconstructing the myth of the advanced practice blended role: Support for role divergence. *Heart and Lung, 31*(6), 393–398.

Modern Healthcare. (2018). *100 most influential people in healthcare—2018.* https://www.modernhealthcare.com/awards/100-most-influential-people-healthcare-2018

Montemuro, M. A. (1987). The evolution of the clinical nurse specialist: Response to the challenge of professional nursing practice. *Clinical Nurse Specialist, 1*(3), 106–110.

National Association of Clinical Nurse Specialists. (1998). *Statement on clinical nurse specialist practice and education.*

National Association of Clinical Nurse Specialists. (2008). *Clinical nurse specialist core competencies.* http://www.nacns.org/wp-content/uploads/2017/01/CNSCoreCompetenciesBroch.pdf

National Association of Clinical Nurse Specialists. (2019). *Statement on CNS practice and education.* https://nacns.org/professional-resources/practice-and-cns-role/cns-competencies/

National Association of Clinical Nurse Specialists. (2020a). *Impact of the clinical nurse specialist role on the costs and quality of health care.* https://nacns.org/advocacy-policy/position-statements/impact-of-the-clinical-nurse-specialist-role-on-the-costs-and-quality-of-health-care/

National Association of Clinical Nurse Specialists. (2020b). 2018-*2020 public policy agenda.* https://nacns.org/advocacy-policy/public-policy-agenda/

National Association of Clinical Nurse Specialists. (2020c). *Scope of practice.* https://nacns.org/advocacy-policy/policies-affecting-cnss/scope-of-practice/

National Association of Clinical Nurse Specialists. (2020d). *National association of clinical nurse specialist's statement on the APRN consensus model implementation.* https://nacns.org/advocacy-policy/position-statements/national-association-of-clinical-nurse-specialists-statement-on-the-aprn-consensus-model-implementation/

National Association of Clinical Nurse Specialists (NACNS). (2004). *Statement on clinical nurse specialist practice and education.*

National Association of Clinical Nurse Specialists (NACNS). (2015a). *CNS census.* http://nacns.org/professional-resources/practice-and-cns-role/cns-census/

National Association of Clinical Nurse Specialists (NACNS). (2015b). *CNS prescriptive authority by state.* http://www.nacns.org/wp-content/uploads/2016/11/5-AuthorityTable.pdf

National Association of Clinical Nurse Specialists (NACNS). (2016). *CNS census.* http://nacns.org/professional-resources/practice-and-cns-role/cns-census/

National League for Nursing (NLN). (1958). *Report of the national working conference: Education of the clinical specialist in psychiatric nursing.*

National League for Nursing (NLN). (1958/1973). Report of the national working conference: Education of the clinical specialist in psychiatric nursing. In J. P. Riehl & J. W. McVay (Eds.), *The clinical nurse specialist: Interpretations* (p. 8). Appleton-Century-Crofts.

National League for Nursing, (NLN). (1984). *Master's education in nursing: Route to opportunities in contemporary nursing.* Author.

Norris, C. M. (1977). One perspective on the nurse practitioner movement. In A. Jacox & C. Norris (Eds). *Organizing for independent nursing practice* (pp. 21–33). Appleton-Century-Crofts.

Peplau, H. (1965). Specialization in professional nursing. *Nursing Science, 3,* 268–287.

Raghubir, A. E. (2018). Emotional intelligence in professional nursing practice: A concept review using rodgers's evolutionary analysis approach. *Advanced Practice Nursing, 5*(2), 126–130.

Reed, S. M. (2020). President's Message: Three health care spheres, one role. *Clinical Nurse Specialist, 34*(3), 89-91.

Reiter, F. (1966). The nurse-clinician. *American Journal of Nursing, 66,* 274–280.

Riehl, J. P., & McVay, J. W. (1973). *The clinical nurse specialist: Interpretations.* Appleton-Century-Crofts.

Saarni, C. (1999). *The development of emotional competence.* Guilford Press.

Sills, G. M. (1983). The role and function of the clinical nurse specialist. In N. L. Chaska (Ed.), *The nursing profession: A time to speak* (pp. 563–579). McGraw-Hill.

Smoyak, S. A. (1976). Specialization in nursing: From then to now. *Nursing Outlook, 24*(11), 565–681.

Thompson, P. A., Anderson, R., Bradley, C., & Herrin-Griffith, D. (2017). Leaders of the American organization of nurse executives. The first fifty years. *Nurse Leader, 15*(2), 110–116. http://doi.org/10.1016/j.mnl.2016.11.011

Walker, J., Gerard, P. S., Bayley, E. W., Coeling, H., Clark, A. P., Dayhoff, N., & Goudreau, K. (2003). A description of clinical nurse specialist programs in the United States. *Clinical Nurse Specialist, 17*(1), 50–57.

PART FOUR

The Leadership Journey

12

Leadership Preparation

Omar Ali · Nagia Ali

LEARNING OBJECTIVES

After completing this chapter, you will be able to:

1. Explain the relevance of Benner's "Novice to Expert" theory to the leadership development for the advanced practice nurse (APN).

2. Use two leadership self-assessment tools for developing leaders.

3. Apply interpersonal communication techniques for leaders.

4. Describe the characteristics and benefits of effective teams.

5. Assess methods of conflict resolution.

6. Evaluate reflective strategies for leaders.

7. Develop methods for finding a mentor.

8. Assess methods to find emotional balance.

KEY TERMS

Conflict Management: The process of utilizing strategies to find common ground between two or more parties.

Emotional Balance: The ability to maintain stability during unpleasant states including negative thoughts and emotions.

Interpersonal Communication: The process of communicating with one or more individuals.

Leadership Development: The process of attaining the knowledge and skills necessary to lead.

Maxim: A maxim is a brief statement that contains a piece of wisdom or a general rule of behavior that packs much meaning. Example: Actions speak louder than words.

Mentorship: The relationship in which an experienced individual promotes the development of another less seasoned.

Novice to Expert: A theory of skill-acquisition during which an individual attains knowledge and skills through five levels of proficiency: novice, advanced beginner, competent, proficient, and expert.

Reflective Practice: The intellectual and affective processes where previous experiences are explored for new understanding.

Self-Assessment: The reflective process of evaluating one's preferences, values, and aptitudes in order to gain a better understanding of self.

Team building: The process of organizing and motivating individuals to accomplish goals.

Introduction

This chapter explores the nature and experience of the Advanced Practice Nurse's (APN) leadership development. The professional development of direct-care nurses informs the science of nurse leadership development. Benner's Novice to Expert theory is surveyed then conceptualized to describe how nurse leaders acquire the skills necessary to lead. Self-assessment tools are used to identify a leader's traits, preferences, and talents. The importance of self-awareness, communication, and team building is highlighted and discussed. The chapter concludes with practical strategies to facilitate one's leadership journey.

Novice to Expert: Benner's Steps of Skill Acquisition

Dreyfus and Dreyfus (1980) developed a model of skill acquisition in which a learner progresses through five levels of proficiency. The learner transitions from relying on context-free rules to utilizing intuition to solve problems. This model of learning values experience and the ability to reflect and learn from one's experiences.

Patricia Benner (1982) conceptualized this model to the nursing profession with her Novice to Expert theory. Benner identified five stages through which nurses and nursing students progress while acquiring the skills necessary for practice: novice, advanced beginner, competent, proficient, and expert. Benner reported that this progression is informed by the nurse's experience, educational level, and past successes and failures.

Benner (1984) asserted three principles guide nurses through these five stages of proficiency. First, the nurse moves away from abstract conceptualization to the use of past and specific experiences. Lessons learned from previous successes and failures drive the decision-making process. Next, the nurse transitions from viewing situations as separate pieces to perceiving them in context. Situational patterns and relationships emerge from seemingly disparate events. The third principle involves the separation from the detached observer to the engaged performer. The nurse begins to recognize how his or her actions affect the patient experience and expected outcomes.

Novice

The novice nurse is expected to apply safe care using general principles learned in school. New nurses rely on objective measurable data including weight, temperature, blood pressure, and pulse (Benner, 1982). Without prior experience, the novice nurse applies context-free rules to patient parameters. This rule-governed behavior is rigid and inflexible, and the nurse is unable to predict what may happen next. Patient care is comprised of task completion without discretionary judgment to prioritize these tasks in response to unique patient situations (Benner, 1984).

Advanced Beginner

The advanced beginner performs at a marginally acceptable level where some previous experience and events are recognized and brought to the situation at hand (Benner, 1984). The advanced beginner begins to recognize the meaning of different events and indicators for their recurrence in different clinical situations. Like the novice, the advanced beginner focuses on recalling rules learned in school and is still unable to prioritize important tasks in unique situations.

The advanced beginner can identify *aspects*, which are recurrent meaningful situational components (Benner, 1982). Aspects are not completely objective and require previous experience to recognize. The advanced beginner is only beginning to identify patterns and may feel overwhelmed by the effort to notice relevant elements. Thus, a mentor can mitigate this tension and assist them in identifying aspects and relevant information through guided reflection of previous similar situations (Benner, 1982).

Competent

A competent nurse has been on the job for 2 or 3 years where observation of similar clinical situations has taken place. In this stage, the nurse begins to master, manage, and cope with different clinical situations. The nurse starts to identify plans and perceive specific long-term patient goals. The nurse's actions become more conscious and deliberate (Benner, 1982).

The competent nurse begins to feel more responsible for the outcomes of their actions. Necessity and uncertainty remove the competent nurse from the role of the observer to the accountable actor (Benner et al., 2009). Successful situations are deeply satisfying while negative patient outcomes are not soon forgotten. Although the competent nurse is capable of correctly perceiving the outcomes of their actions, he/she lacks speed and flexibility of a proficient nurse (Benner, 1984).

Proficient

The proficient nurse perceives a situation as whole rather than individual aspects (Benner, 1982). Maxims guide practice as the proficient nurse considers less options and can better hone in on an appropriate course of action. Maxims allow the proficient nurse to recognize when a normal situation does not materialize.

Decisions are based upon a deep understanding of context and the interacting forces within a designated situation. The proficient nurse relates situations to previous ones and can recognize which course of action will lead to a positive outcome (Benner et al., 2009).

Expert

The expert nurse no longer uses rigid protocols or maxims to guide practice (Benner, 1982). Intuition guides practice as the expert nurse can focus on the most relevant aspect(s) of the problem without wasteful consideration of irrelevant pieces that can be distracting to less experienced nurses. Although intuition guides practice, the expert nurse continues to use analytical thinking during new situations where events and behaviors are different from their expectations, and/or when the expert nurse takes the wrong route to resolve a clinical problem (Benner, 1982) (Table 12.1).

Table 12.1. Going to Computed Tomography (CT)

Level of Proficiency	Perception	Focus
Novice	I had to go to CT today	Internally focused; task driven
Advanced beginner	I have taken these sort of patients to CT	Internally focused; recognizes patterns
Competent	Patient education enhanced my patient's CT experience	Internally and externally focused; actions and their consequences are recognized
Proficient	Ensuring patient comfort during their CT enhances image quality	Externally focused; past experience informs future goals
Expert	Promoting an interdisciplinary approach between nurses and imaging professionals can enhance patient safety during diagnostic tests	Externally focused; long-term goals are planned

Leadership Skill Acquisition

Benner's skill acquisition model can be applied to the leadership development of nurse leaders. Shirey (2007) reported that nurses acquire leadership skills much like direct care nurses gain clinical competence. Like the direct-care nurse, nurse leader's transition from relying on context-free rules to recognizing patterns and the consequences of their actions to eventually understanding the "bigger picture" and their role in it. Several leadership programs that help build leadership skills are presented in Box 12.1.

BOX 12.1

▶ LEADERSHIP DEVELOPMENT PROGRAMS

1. Sigma Theta Tau International (Sigma) (https://www.sigmanursing.org/learn-grow/sigma-academies):
   a. Nurse Educator Development Academy
   b. New Academic Leadership Academy
   c. Experienced Academic Leadership Academy
   d. Nurse Leadership Academy for Practice

2. National League for Nursing (www.nln.org)
   a. LEAD
   b. Leadership Development Program for Simulation Educators

3. American Organization of Nurse Executives (AONE) (http://www.aone.org/)
   a. Emerging Leader Institute (ENL)
   b. Nurse Manager Institute
   c. Nurse Manager Fellowship
   d. Nurse Director Fellowship
   e. Executive Fellowship in Innovation Health Leadership

4. American Association of Colleges of Nursing (AACN) (http://www.aacnnursing.org/)
   a. Leadership for Academic Nursing Program (LANP)

The novice nurse leader has no experience and relies on concepts learned in school and/or previous leadership training. This leader completes role-associated tasks and may struggle with prioritization. The new leader is internally focused and relies on rule-governed task completion. The novice leader focuses on how events affect his or her own experience.

After 1 or 2 years of practice, nurse leaders have encountered a variety of leadership situations. Patterns emerge but the leader is unable to recognize context and the consequences of his or her actions. Mentors are essential to aid new leaders learn from successes and failures. Mentors can also help leaders identify the organization vision, goals, and policies and introduce the mentee to other nurses who are performing similar roles (Dracup & Bryan-Brown, 2004; Mazzoccoli & Wolf, 2016).

The competent leader has been in a leadership role for several years. In this stage, the leader begins to recognize how their actions affect others. The leader demonstrates abstract and analytical decision-making. A deeper understanding of the issues allows the leader to cope with deviations from an expected outcome. The leader becomes externally focused and begins to recognize the importance of communication and interpersonal relationships. Reflections of past experiences transform memories into lessons learned.

The proficient leader uses a holistic approach to decision-making. The leader can identify critical aspects of a situation and make decisions accordingly. The leader has a better understanding of context and the perspectives of different stakeholders. They can assess the overall picture and extract the most salient aspects. The proficient leader utilizes maxims, abstract reasoning, and indicative processes to guide decision-making (Shirey, 2007). The consequences of the past decisions are considered during the decision-making process.

The expert leader's actions are informed by years of experience. The decision-making process is fluid and flexible, independent of rigid rules and guidelines. Intuition allows the expert leader to anticipate the long-term consequences of his or her actions. Leaders being to see the "big picture" and identify long-term goals. Generativity, legacy, and the desire to develop others often defines the final stage of the leadership journey.

A comparison of professional development with leadership development is provided in Table 12.2. The comparison notes the leader's reliance on personal strengths as leadership skills are developed.

Questions to Ask Yourself

1. Where do I see myself as a professional nurse?
2. Am I prepared to be a novice advanced practice nurse?
3. Where do I see myself as a leader?
4. Am I prepared to make more difficult decisions as a leader?

Self-Assessment

Self-awareness is the quintessential attribute of a leader. A deep self-knowledge promotes a natural confidence that draws others to leaders. Self-assessment is the reflective process of evaluating one's preferences, values, and aptitudes in order to gain a better understanding of self. Recognizing follower's traits, preferences, and strengths allows leaders to better understand their team and what influences them. The ability to influence others through reason and emotion is the main competency of a leader (Grenny et al., 2013). The Myers-Briggs Type Indicator

Table 12.2. Nurse Professional vs. Leadership Development

	Novice	Advanced Beginner	Competent	Proficient	Expert
Nurse Professional Development	Relies on objective measurable data using inflexible rules	Identifies the meaning of different events and factors for their recurrence	Transitions from the role of the observer to actor	Considers less options to quickly identify an appropriate course of action	Utilizes intuition and no longer bound by rigid guidelines
Nurse Leadership Development	Reflects on personal strengths and areas for opportunities	Recognizes patterns in different situations	Acts considering previous success and failures	Considers less options in decision-making	Examines the role in a larger context

(MBTI), the Keirsey Bates Temperament Sorter (KTS), and StrengthsFinder are self-assessment tools that assist individuals gain a deep understanding of one's traits, preferences, and strengths.

Myers-Briggs Type Indicator

The MBTI is a 93-question tool that helps individuals identify their psychological preferences in how they perceive the world and how these views shape their actions. This tool focuses on an individual's normal psyche without judging one's preferences as "good" or "bad."

Individuals identify four personality preferences: how one directs and receives energy, processes information, makes decisions, and approaches the outside world (Consulting Psychologists Press, 2018).

Keirsey Bates Temperament Sorter

The KTS is a modified assessment tool based on the MBTI (Keirsey & Bates, 1984). The main distinction is the MBTI focuses on psychological preferences, while the KTS focuses on observable behavior.

The KTS is a free tool that can be accessed at http://www.lifeconnectionson-line.org/wp-content/uploads/2014/12/Keirsey-Temperament-Sorter.pdf. It is a 70-item questionnaire that identifies one's observable personality traits, including habits of communication, patterns of actions, attitudes, values, and talents (Keirsey & Bates, 1984).

These traits are categorized into four categories producing 16 personality traits. The first category is how one interacts with others: Extraversion (E) or Introversion (I). Extroverts enjoy being around people and are generally outgoing, while Introverts are more reserved and prefer being around fewer people. The second addresses how one makes decisions: Intuitive (N) or Sensing (S). The Intuitive individual tends to focus on relationships with others, while the Sensor would rather work with objective facts. The third category addresses how one bases their judgments: Thinker (T) or Feeler (F). The Thinker tends to base judgments on logic, while the Feeler makes decisions on personal values. And finally, the fourth category addresses one's preferences in planning: Judging (J) or Perceptive (P). The Judge prefers a planned and orderly way of life, while the Perceiver is more flexible and spontaneous.

Questions to Ask Yourself

1. How have my personality traits/preferences helped me in the workplace?
2. How have my personality traits/preferences hindered me in the workplace?
3. Can I recognize personality traits in others that make it easier for me to work with them?
4. Can I recognize personality traits in others that make it more challenging to work with them?
5. How can I use this understanding of myself and others to improve work relations?

Application of MBTI and KTS

The MBTI and KTS provide the leader insight into the nature of self. Leaders gain a deeper understanding of how their preferences inform their communication style, interactions with others, and decision-making process (Bower, 2015). With this knowledge, leaders can seek appropriate resources to transform his or her preferences into assets. For example, an extroverted nurse leader can seek professional development opportunities to refine and adapt his or her communication skills for different stakeholders. A flexible leader can implement unconventional team building activities tailored toward the unique makeup of their team. An empathic leader can engage followers' emotions and passions to connect on a deeper level. An overview of the 16 personality traits is presented in Table 12.3.

StrengthsFinder

StrengthsFinder is a 177-item tool that identifies 34 talents individuals innately possess. Talent is the ability to perform certain tasks with greater ease and effectiveness than others (Rath, 2007). Dr. Donald Clifton (the father of Positive Psychology) developed this tool in 1998 to help individuals identify what they do the best. StrengthsFinder encourages individuals to invest time in nurturing the strengths they already possess. A CliftonStrengths version was released in 2017, noting the name change from StrengthFinder assessment to CliftonStrengths (Gallup, 2020b). The book provides an overview of the 34 talents.

Individuals can gain more when they expend effort on building upon strengths instead of attempting to remedy weaknesses. Attempting to fix weaknesses prevents failure, while focusing on strengths promotes success (Rath,

Table 12.3. Personality Traits

Temperaments	Overview		Keywords	
Artisan	Promoter	Crafter	Optimist	Daring
	ESTP	ISTP	Impulsive	Playful
	Performer	Composer	Adaptable	Persuasive
	ESFP	ISFP		
Guardian	Supervisor	Inspector	Factual	Cautious
	ESTJ	ISTJ	Dependable	Law-abiding
	Provider	Protector	Concerned	Steady
	ESFJ	ISFJ	Respectable	Detailed
Idealist	Teacher	Counselor	Imaginative	Intuitive
	ENFJ	INFJ	Relational	Empathetic
	Champion	Healer	Diplomatic	Kindhearted
	ENFP	INFP	Romantic	Sensitive
Rational	Field Marshal	Mastermind	Ingenious	Logical
	ENTJ	INTJ	Pragmatic	Curious
	Inventor	Architect	Strategic	Innovative
	ENTP	INTP	Calm	Independent

Adapted from Keirsey.com (n.d.). https://www.keirsey.com/

2007). Team members who spend more hours a day believing they use their strengths report having more energy, being happy, and feeling well-rested (Rigoni & Asplund, 2016).

Leaders are tasked with aligning the strengths of his or her team members with organizational goals and objectives. Leaders delegate tasks to individuals who will excel at them. For instance, an introverted team member who enjoys writing can be tasked with developing a unit policy. An extroverted artistically inclined employee can lead a team responsible for unit holiday or event decorations. A future-oriented team member can serve

---

BOX 12.2

▶ SELF-ASSESSMENT RESOURCES AND WEBSITES

Myers-Briggs	https://www.cpp.com/
The Keirsey Bates Temperament Sorter (KTS)	http://www.lifeconnectionsonline.org/wp-content/uploads/2014/12/Keirsey-Temperament-Sorter.pdf
StrengthsFinder	https://www.gallup.com/press/176429/strengthsfinder.aspx

---

on an organizational planning committee tasked with planning and implementing long-term goals and initiatives. An individual who recognizes how his or her unique skills benefit the team is more likely to be engaged at work (Rath, 2007).

Questions to Ask Yourself

1. What are my strengths and opportunities for improvement?
2. How do these strengths inform my leadership development?
3. How do these strengths inform my choice of advanced practice role?
4. What strengths would I need from other team members to be a successful leader?

StrengthsFinder talents can be categorized into four leadership domains: influencing, executing, strategic thinking, and relationship building (Gallup, 2020a). Each domain contains seven to eight related talents. The influencing domain contains talents such as communication, self-assurance, command, and woo. Leaders with several identified talents in this domain are skilled at inspiring and motivating others. The executing domain includes talents such as deliberative, discipline, focus, and responsibility. Leaders with several talents in this domain are "doers" who make things happen. These leaders take charge and complete initiatives. The strategic thinking domain contains talents of the future-orientated leader. Talents such as futuristic, context, analytical, and intellection describe a leader who aids teams in considering what could be. Finally, the relationship building domain contains strengths such as empathy, harmony, realtor, and includer. These leaders connect with followers by displaying empathy and creating space for followers to share their emotions. Table 12.4 provides an overview of the four leadership domains.

Table 12.4. Clifton StrengthsFinder Domains of Leadership		
Strength Domain	**Strengths**	**Overview**
Influencing	Activator, command, communication, competition, maximizer, self-assurance, significance, woo	How an individual moves others to action; interpersonal strengths that enable a person to impact or influence others in powerful ways by taking charge, speaking up, and making sure ideas are heard, inside and outside a group
Executing	Achiever, arranger, belief, consistency, deliberative, discipline, focus, responsibility, restorative	What pushes an individual toward results; motivational strengths that generate and focus energy to achieve and accomplish a lot, for themselves and their teams.
Strategic thinking	Analytical, context, futuristic, ideation, input, intellection, learner, strategic	How a person analyzes the world; strengths of perception, organization, and information, and processing that produce lifelong learners and help teams make better decision. Helps us focus on what could be, stretching our thinking for the future.
Relationship building	Adaptability, connectedness, developer, empathy, harmony, includer, individualization, positivity, relator	How a person builds connections with others including interpersonal bonding, forming deeply meaningful and close personal relationship. In teams, these themes are the essential glue that holds a team together—creating groups that are greater than the sum of their parts

Adapted from Gallup (2020). *The 34 Clifton strengths themes explain your talent DNA.* https://www.gallup.com/cliftonstrengths/en/253715/34-cliftonstrengths-themes.aspx

In Their Own Words

Holly Ma, MS, RN, BSN, CRN

Director of Nursing Professional Development and Education
Adult Academic Health Center at Indiana University Health

The key points in understanding my role are… I am responsible for the oversight of general new hire orientation and any nursing and support staff educational initiatives, school of nursing clinical placements, transitions to practice program (residency), and unit-based educators. I also provide direction and vision for our clinical education team. I make connections with other departments and build relationships. I advocate for my team and demonstrate the value we provide to the organization. I challenge my team to grow and innovate. My role helps with breaking down barriers my team encounters.

What keeps me coming back every day is… I know I can make a positive impact for patients and staff. I have the ability to create change and improve the environment and care of staff and patients. I enjoy change and find it exciting and sometimes challenging. My ability to adapt and be flexible in the environment and be willing to take calculated risks has helped me in my career. A positive perspective on new initiatives helps me see possibilities and solutions and sustain my energy in a fast paced, ever-changing environment. Life is 10% of what happens to you and 90% of how you choose to respond.

My greatest challenge is… My greatest challenge is dealing with silos and ability to get individuals to work well with one another. We may have a common goal, but I often encounter individuals doing their "own thing." This results in inefficiencies, inconsistencies, and a product that is not as optimal.

I wish someone had told me… You do not have to be the smartest, a formal leader, or the most experienced in the room to accomplish things and influence others. Often, individuals who have persistence follow through and have the ability to see the possibilities rather than the problems; they are the ones who succeed.

I need to be a lifelong learner because… I equate lifelong learning with continually improving and evolving myself professionally and personally. I will never

(Continued)

know everything or be an expert on every situation I encounter. Continual growth helps ensure I do not grow stagnant and I am better equipped to handle the challenges of a leadership role. If I feel like I am not growing, I often become restless in a role and feel unchallenged.

Another point to understand is... My advice would be to not take anything personal. People may not always agree with you or even like you. I have noticed other leaders fall into the trap of wanting to be their employees' friend. It is nice if you can have a friendly relationship, but as a leader, it is most important they respect you rather than like you. Do not be afraid to take risks and potentially fail. Usually, there is some success within trying something new, and nothing will ever be perfect when you start.

Interpersonal Communication

Words matter. The ability to communicate effectively is the definitive skill of a successful leader (Huston, 2018). **Interpersonal communication** is the process of communicating with one or more individuals. It facilitates the exchange of information, thoughts, and feelings. It is an integral part of nursing care and a function of education and experience (Kourkouta & Papathanasiou, 2014). Effective communication among nurses is associated with improved patient outcomes, increased staff satisfaction, and reduced burnout leading to increased retention (Miller et al., 2018). Skilled communicators are active listeners who convey their interest and attention to what is being said.

Active listening is pivotal to successful communication. Active listeners engage others with eye contact, head nodding, and reflection. This contrasts with passive listening, which is essentially hearing what others are saying but not concentrating on the message or delivery. Table 12.5 demonstrates the difference in active and passive listening.

Awdish and Berry (2017) stress the importance of active listening to convey respect for patient's self-knowledge and build trust. There are serious consequences for patients when health professionals fail to engage in active listening. Treatments can be ineffective or undesired if information is missed or not clarified. This can result in human and financial costs. The patient's voice must be valued.

Table 12.5. Active vs. Passive Listening

	Active	Passive
Activity	Fully engaged and listening	Hearing but no reaction to ideas
Who/Whom?	Two-way communication with individuals	One-way communication with individuals, TV, music, podcasts, etc.
Interaction	Listener reacts Eye contact, head nod, reflecting, paraphrasing, and asking questions Focused on individual	Listener does not react Noncommittal phrases (i.e., "Oh yeah") Able to multitask

Adapted from Gillespie, C (2019). *Difference between active listening and passive listening.* https://www.theclassroom.com/strengths-weaknesses-auditory-learner-11372616.html

Team members choose to follow leaders whom they believe to be genuine and authentic. Thus, leaders must articulate a clear message they themselves believe in. Choosing the right words, tone, and delivery method is an essential consideration when communicating with team members. The APN is required to effectively communicate with a variety of audiences, including patients, families, and others in the interdisciplinary team. The main routes of interpersonal communication include written, verbal, and social media (SM) exchanges.

Written Interprofessional Communication

Written communication encompasses email, written reports, and employee or program evaluations. It can also include legal documentation of patient records including electronic and paper medical records. When writing in the professional setting, two important maxims to remember are *know thy audience* and *know thy subject* (Pietrucha, 2014). The effective nurse leader judiciously chooses the proper words for the appropriate audience and context. A document written for staff will differ from one being addressed to one's superiors. Notes in a patient's record may be less formal and contain more subjective narrative observations.

Verbal Interprofessional Communication

A nurse leader's speech should be articulate, relevant, and concise. Proper verbal communication can convey respect and empathy which are essential for nurses and nurse leaders. The ability to modify tone, volume, and speed when communicating with followers, colleagues, and superiors is essential in a leadership role.

Nurses must also be mindful of using abbreviations and lingo, which can mean different things to others. For instance, LOC can mean "level of consciousness" for the critical care nurse, "level of care" for the emergency room nurse, and "laxative of choice" for the rehabilitation nurse. A "high-risk patient" among direct care nurses can mean a patient has a transmittable disease, while in an interdisciplinary meeting, it may refer to a patient who is likely to fall or develop certain infections.

Social Media Communication

SM has revolutionized how people connect, communicate, and share information. SM includes LinkedIn, Facebook, Twitter, YouTube, and Instagram and can serve as a convenient method of communication and networking among patients, healthcare providers, researchers, funders, and health policy makers (Burton et al., 2016). Breach of patient confidentiality and unprofessional postings are significant considerations for nurse leaders. Nurse leaders should be aware of the benefits and risks of SM use, identify employer's policies regarding the use of SM, and follow institution guidelines.

Team Building

Leaders produce results by motivating and inspiring team members to work toward a shared purpose (Huston, 2018). Team building is the process of organizing and motivating individuals to accomplish group goals. Effective team building is an essential competency of a leader. As the APN assumes a leadership role, he or she must engage employees to create a collaborative work environment to accomplish professional, departmental, and organizational goals.

Effective leaders motivate, engage, and empower employees to achieve shared goals (Bergstedt & Wei, 2020). Employee engagement is a product of autonomy, empowerment, job satisfaction, and commitment to the organization

(Sherman, 2020). Organizations that promote employee engagement have more satisfied employees, experience increased retention, and have better patient outcomes (Kutney-Lee et al., 2016). Successful employee engagement has significant financial implications as nurse turnover costs hospitals billions of dollars a year and Medicare reimbursements are affected by patient satisfaction scores (Dempsey & Reilly, 2016; Kutney-Lee et al., 2016)

Effective communication is the foundation of a high-functioning team. Facilitating the interpersonal communication skills of employees enhances teamwork and promotes group cohesion (Vertino, 2014). Effective teams are comprised of individuals who can assume roles where he or she can have the greatest contribution (Sherman, 2020). High-functioning teams share a sense of "collective activism" where team members are empowered to work independently and assume additional tasks born out of empathy and compassion for others (Thusini & Mingay, 2019).

Emotions play a pivotal role in team building. Emotional intelligence (EI) is the ability to recognize ones' emotions, the emotions of others, and how emotions influence interpersonal communication (Bradberry & Greaves, 2009). EI is a function of self-awareness, social awareness, self-management, and relationship management (Sherrod et al., 2019). Emotionally intelligent leaders acknowledge and engage the emotions of their followers (Mansel & Einion, 2019). Employees who feel understood, respected, and valued are more engaged and thus more successful in their role (Dempsey & Reilly, 2016). Successful leaders possess a genuine interest in the emotions of team members and how these emotions affect team dynamics.

Team members are evaluated on their ability to think critically, offer new ideas, and implement their strengths to promote team goals (Valiga, 2019). Leaders can further empower followers by devoting time, during formal and informal employee evaluation, to discuss how to nurture and adapt team member's talents in order to benefit the team. It is a leader's responsibility to recognize and engage team members' traits and talents to influence a positive change (Valiga, 2019).

Conflict Resolution

Conflict exists in every part of life; it is an inevitable part of the work environment (Johansen, 2012). It can be described as a process involving two or more individuals where one perceives opposition from another (Ylitormanen et al., 2015). As a leader, one must address not only conflict with others but also between others. One maxim to remember is *"everyone wants to be heard."* Active listening and demonstrating empathy are essential in managing conflict. Validating one's feelings promotes de-escalation.

Thomas-Kilmann Conflict Mode Instrument

The Thomas-Kilmann Conflict Mode Instrument (TKI) (https://takethetki. com/) identifies the most common methods of dealing with conflict. It is a 30-item tool designed to measure how individuals prefer to deal with conflict. It identifies five conflict resolution modes: competing, accommodating, avoiding, collaborating, and compromising. The results are arranged by a raw and percentile score. The raw score is the number of times one chooses a statement for a specific mode, while the percentile shows how the raw score compares to previous assessment takers (Consulting Psychologists Press, 2017).

Competing

The first mode is competing which is a power-oriented strategy. Individuals who score high in this category are assertive and can be uncooperative. It should be used when a quick and decisive action is required or when an important or unpopular course of action must be taken (i.e., budget cuts). Signs that a leader is overusing this strategy include having coworkers or direct reports hesitate to ask questions or provide input. Other signs of underuse include being perceived as passive or unable to make difficult decisions. Leaders should use this mode sparingly as staff's "buy-in" is essential to moving projects and initiatives forward (Consulting Psychologists Press, 2017).

Accommodating

Accommodating is the opposite of competing. With this mode, an individual is willing to appease others and is often cooperative and unassertive (Consulting Psychologists Press, 2017). This often involves one party neglecting their concerns to satisfy the concerns of others. This is useful in leadership when a short-term resolution is needed or when conflict does not warrant confrontation. This strategy can also be used if one is simply wrong or the issue is more important to the other individual and the implications do not significantly affect the department or others. Signs of underuse include being unwilling to admit mistakes or being perceived as unreasonable. Signs of overuse include being perceived as being too passive or indecisive. Sometimes leaders need to preserve harmony, admit when they are wrong, or simply wait to "fight" another day.

Avoiding

Conflict is uncomfortable, and thus, avoiding is a commonly used strategy (Patterson et al., 2012). Avoiders are often uncooperative and unassertive (Consulting Psychologists Press, 2017). For leaders, avoiding conflict can be helpful when gathering information is more useful than immediate action. Also, it is wise to avoid conflict in a threatening situation when escalation can bring harm to the individual or others.

Collaborating

Collaborating is the opposite of avoiding. Collaborators are assertive and cooperative. They are problem solvers who believe in the power of consensus and information sharing (Consulting Psychologists Press, 2017). Individuals who use this mode are skilled at "digging deeper" to find the underlying concerns of the involved parties. Collaborating can be a resource-intensive strategy and sometimes common ground cannot be reached between the individuals experiencing conflict. If collaborating is not possible, a leader may have to take a competing approach.

Compromising

The final mode is compromising. Compromisers can find common ground between balancing assertiveness and cooperation (Kilmann Diagnostics, 2018). They do not avoid conflict or neglect their concerns or those of others. Like collaborators, compromisers look for a mutually acceptable solution, but unlike collaborators, they do not spend as much time exploring the situation in depth and are more likely to seek a quick middle ground.

Unresolved conflict can result in an uncomfortable work environment, stress among staff, decrease in productivity, and reduction in one's loyalty to their work (Patterson et al., 2012). Unresolved conflict can also lead to adverse patient outcomes including medication errors, falls, and reduced quality and efficacy of care (Johansen, 2012). Leaders must understand their conflict management preferences and those of their staff. This understanding will facilitate the effective management of conflict and mitigate its negative effects on staff and patients.

Questions to Ask Yourself

1. How do I manage conflict?
2. What effect does that have on the team?
3. What are the disadvantages/advantages of my mode of resolving conflict?
4. How can I improve my conflict management skills?

Using Reflective Practice

The ability to reflect and learn from past events is essential to the professional development of nurses (Benner, 1984) and the experienced-based development of leaders (Knipfer et al., 2016). Reflection is the active, deliberate, and cognitive process where events are examined from different perspectives, allowing the individual to gain new knowledge from past experiences (Jacobs, 2016). Reflective practice encompasses the intellectual and effective activities individuals utilize to explore previous experiences to gain a new understanding and appreciation of those experiences (Walsh & Mann, 2015). Replaying events and interactions allows leaders the time and space to extract the nuanced elements of those situations.

Invariably in leadership, as in nursing practice, there will be certain experiences that will forever transform one's career such as assuming a leadership role or losing a job. An effective leader recognizes the gravity of these formative events and "digs deeper." The leader reflects on the event, the emotions involved, and why he or she made certain decisions. This insight informs future actions and promotes a deeper understanding of past events. The Schon's Reflection Model, Gibbs' Reflective Cycle, and Kolb's Experiential Learning Theory are useful in describing methods that facilitate the reflective practice.

Schon's Reflection Model

Schon's model is comprised of two steps: reflection-in-action and reflection-on-action (Schon, 1983). The former refers to doing and thinking simultaneously *during* the event. That is, noticing and analyzing one's actions and environment without interrupting the interaction. It involves pausing and noticing while remaining engaged in the situation. In other words, reflection-in-action involves "tuning in" to the cognitive, intuitive, and sensory information to better understand the experiences in the moment, while reflection-on-action refers to the retrospective process used to learn from the information gathered and actions taken during the event. In this step, the individual challenges the assumptions and actions used during the event. This is used to inform how one modifies behaviors during future similar events.

Gibbs' Reflective Cycle

Gibbs' (1988) Reflective Cycle outlines six steps (Table 12.6) in the reflective process: *description* (what happened?), *feelings* (what were one's thoughts and

Table 12.6.	Gibbs' Reflective Cycle
6 Steps	**Reflective Questions**
Description	What happened? How would you describe the situation in detail (who, what, when, where, why)? What did you do? What did others do?
Feelings	What were the thoughts and feelings before, during, and after the situation took place? What did you feel after the situation? What do you think about the situation now? What do you think other people feel about the situation now?
Evaluation	What was good or bad about situation? What went well? What did not go well? What did you and other people do to contribute to the situation?
Analysis	How does one perceive what happened? What could have been done differently? How could this have been a more positive experience for everyone involved?
Conclusion	What did you and others learn from this situation? If you were faced with the same situation again, what would you do differently?
Action Plan	How would one act if a similar situation arose in the future? What actions must be taken to deal more effectively with this type of situation in the future?

Adapted from Mindset (2020). *Gibbs reflection cycle.* https://www.mindtools.com/pages/article/reflective-cycle.htm

feelings?), *evaluation* (what was good or bad about the situation?), *analysis* (how does one perceive what happened?), *conclusion* (what could have been done differently?), and the *action plan* (how would one act if a similar situation arose in the future?). This analytical framework is useful for breaking down complex events into concrete components to gain a better understanding of what transpired.

Kolb's Experiential Learning Theory

Kolb's Experiential Learning Cycle (Table 12.7) outlines a four-step process: *experience, reflection, conceptualization,* and *experimentation* (Kolb, 1984). During the first step, the individual identifies the concrete experience using their senses and feelings. Next, the individual assimilates the event by comparing it with previous similar events. Then, the individual conceptualizes the event by forming generalizations to learn from the experience. And finally, the individual applies what they have learned in future situations.

Table 12.7. Kolb's Experiential Learning Cycle

Steps	Actions
Experience	Individual identifies the concrete new experience or situation encountered using their senses and feelings
Reflection	Individual assimilates the event by comparing it with previous similar events, noting inconsistencies between experience and understanding
Conceptualization	Individual conceptualizes the event by forming generalizations to learn from the experience—does it give rise to a new idea or modification of an existing abstract concept?
Experimentation	Individual applies what they have learned to future situations to see what happens

Adapted from Mcleod, S. A. (2017). *Kolb – Learning styles.* https://www.simplypsychology.org/learning-kolb.html

Finding a Mentor

Mentorship can serve as the foundation for professional and leadership development (Campbell et al., 2017; Huston, 2018). A mentor is an individual who serves as an advisor, teacher, and counselor to a mentee (Starr, 2014). The word originates from Homer's *Odyssey*. Mentor is a trusted advisor of Odysseus, king of Ithaca. While Odysseus is off to war, Athena, the goddess of wisdom, takes the shape of Mentor to oversee and protect Odysseus' son Telemachus through his coming of age journeys (Homer, n.d). In modern times, a mentoring relationship is one where the mentor shares their experience, knowledge, and insight to facilitate the development of a mentee (Starr, 2014).

Mentoring is a useful tool to identify, attract, retain, and develop new nurse leaders (Hodgson & Scanlan, 2013). Leggat, Balding, and Schiftan (2014) found a formal mentoring program can assist nurse practitioner students develop their clinical leadership skills, facilitating their transition to advanced practice roles. Among university faculty, the presence of a mentor is highly predictive of a mentee's success in producing publications, obtaining grants, advancing more quickly in their career, and assuming a leadership role (Johnson, 2016; Nowell et al., 2017).

So, how does one secure a mentor? First, let us examine the motivations of a mentor to understand how they can be found and engaged. Maxwell (2008) identifies three steps for a prospective mentor to consider while preparing for a mentoring relationship. The first is "adopting a mentor mindset." In this step, the prospective mentor is encouraged to make "people development" their top priority. Maxwell argues this is a fundamental trait of a leader—the desire to lift others. During this step, the mentor must first develop a relationship with possible mentees to understand their strengths, weaknesses, aspirations, and how best to facilitate their development.

The second step is choosing a mentee that is ready for the mentoring relationship. In this step, the prospective mentor looks for new leaders who can "make things happen," even in the most difficult circumstances. Mentors understand the mentee must be driven to be successful to gain the most out of the mentoring relationship. Finally, a mentor seeks a mentee who possesses a positive attitude. Leadership is fraught with setbacks and disappointments. Effective mentors will lift their mentees in dark times and moments of self-doubt. However, a mentee must be committed to their professional development during positive and negative experiences.

The final step includes "letting the mentee fly." Mentors find this stage to be the most rewarding. It involves a sort of separation of the mentor and mentee. This does not necessarily mean the mentor and mentee will never see each other again (although this may be the case). Rather, it means, at this stage, the mentor has done all they can for the mentee's development while ensuring the mentee develops their followers and other leaders. This is the crux of mentoring—knowing one relationship will affect dozens more (Maxwell, 2008).

A hallmark of a successful leader is one who can identify and recruit mentors who will change their life (Bennis, 2004). To find a mentor, one must exude a sort of contagious desire to learn and grow. This includes a "can do" attitude. That is, the prospective mentee is willing to take risks and seize opportunities. Finally, the mentee should prepare for a time when the mentor's guidance is no longer needed. Mentoring can be a lifelong relationship but can also be time limited.

Nurse mentors can be found in and outside the mentee's institution. Inside an organization, a mentee can seek out an experienced respected practitioner and simply express a desire to be mentored. External mentors can be found online or at professional nursing events/conferences. The internal mentor can facilitate a novice leader's transition to their new role, while the external mentor provides an outsider's perspective on the mentee's experience.

Being asked to mentor someone is a humbling experience. Nurses who are in the latter stages of their careers are often looking for ways to give back and the ability to help develop the next generation of nurses; this is an opportunity many would gladly take.

Another method to find a mentor and develop one's leadership skills is to become active in professional nursing organizations. These organizations provide mentorship opportunities and resources for developing leaders. The American Association of Colleges of Nursing (AACN), Sigma Theta Tau International (STTI), and the American Organization for Nursing Leadership (AONL), formerly American Organization of Nurse Executives (AONE), among others, offer mentored leadership development programs that can help identify mentors, grow one's professional network, and facilitate one's leadership development (Smith & Johnson, 2018). In fact, active participation in a professional organization is one way to find a mentor.

Questions to Ask Yourself

1. What are my resources to find a mentor?
2. How could I benefit from a mentoring relationship?
3. What are my responsibilities in the mentoring process?
4. What traits/talents would I admire the most in a mentor?
5. What steps am I willing to take if the mentor's style of leadership is not a good fit for me?

In Their Own Words

Marcella M. Rutherford, PhD, MBA, MSN
Dean, Ron and Kathy Assaf School of Nursing
Nova Southeastern University

The key points in understanding my role are … Nursing academia is called on to adapt to today's changing environment. Healthcare is rapidly changing, and to educate tomorrow's nurses, academia is challenged to adapt course content to remain relevant. In the next decade, it is predicted that 30% of nurses in academic roles will retire. This shortage of faculty in nursing will impact the ability to educate new nurses. In addition, nursing academia will need faculty with specific competencies to teach the variety of topics included in the curriculum. All colleges are also challenged to find academic nurse faculty who wish to lead in administrative academic roles. As the Dean, it is important to keep abreast of all faculty and curriculum needs while at the same time continue to engage faculty and students in scholarship (new knowledge development) and facilitate on-going efforts in service to the college, university, and community. The dean must work with administrators to develop leadership abilities in overseeing the college's financials (budgets), fundraising, marketing, and human resource/legal needs. For nursing, the number of students enrolled impacts the need for stakeholder relationships in order to maintain clinical placements. Learning styles and a fast-paced world create changes in educational delivery style and venues. Nursing education is a very competitive business. Nursing's workforce demands of the aging population and replacing retiring nurses generates needs for the community. Accreditation standards

(Continued)

continue also to change, and data are required to support the standards and quality of each program in order to meet both regional and professional requirements. In the role of Dean, of a large, multiprogram, and campus college, it becomes essential to remain forward-thinking and innovative to continuously seek partnerships and develop a strong faculty team to maintain the success of the college. The goal remains consistent—to educate great nurses who will lead the profession.

What keeps me coming back every day is … I entered academia to fill a gap that I noted in nursing education. Nurses were expert clinicians but lacked the knowledge in finance and economics. I saw this gap as a limitation in the profession's ability to advance and be included in administrative and board roles. I felt these skills would facilitate nurses' ability to document and articulate their value to stakeholders and their community of patients. To support the needed investment into the profession, education in these areas of leadership appeared limited and in need of emphasis and inclusion in all levels of education, including the bachelor's degree. With the evolution of healthcare reform, this has become even more essential. Nursing has the experiences in healthcare to lead and shape not only healthcare but also their destiny as essential and unique professionals. In the role of faculty, I can advocate for content that will enhance the education of the nurses I teach. As Dean, I am able to use a variety of leadership skills and see the outcomes of the college's efforts—our graduates.

My greatest challenge is … To maintain effective, accurate, and open communication between and among the various faculty members in the nursing college, the nursing students in the various campuses and programs, and with the faculty and deans across the various colleges in the university. Words and actions matter. As a dean, you become the ambassador for the university and college, and these events are essential for showcasing and growing the face of the college. As in any leadership position, you are called on as the leader when issues/needs/problems arise. These situations are the most challenging and impact students and faculty lives. Developing team members who, as a team, facilitate good communication and can assist in the leadership of a college remains a challenge.

I wish someone had told me … The time and creativity that is needed to maintain the health of a college and how essential the dean's role is in advocating and gaining consensus so improvement occurs. The curriculum, for example, in each program must grow in its relevancy and align with changes occurring in healthcare and nursing. The curriculum is shaped and controlled by the faculty who teach the course, and courses are most often taught by faculty on

(Continued)

various campuses. Agreement of the collective faculty is needed for changes to the curriculum. The Dean at times is called on to facilitate, energize, encourage, and help make sure that progress continues. The greater the number of students and faculty, the more complex the effort toward advocating on the various issues.

I need to be a lifelong learner because ... The world of healthcare is always changing. In addition, the learning styles and desires of the students are always evolving. The faculty have the pleasure of being in the classroom with their students at all levels—BSN, MSN, and Doctoral—and through this interaction, both the students and the faculty learn and grow. To remain relevant and effective with nursing students, the faculty must continue to evolve and learn. As the dean, I must continue to find time to be in the classroom.

Another point to understand is ... With 4.1 million nurses, we are challenged to coalesce around one nursing voice. Nursing's greatest asset is the ability to shape change and enhance career growth. Nurses, no matter what degree level or specialty, need to remain supportive and protective of the power of nursing and remain vigilant that the variety of nursing roles and credentials do not divide or weaken nursing's voice. The power of nursing's numbers or voting power will be able to move and shape the profession by impacting policy and reimbursement legislation. This connection to the nursing profession starts in prelicensure education, and is important to dialogue at each advancement and change.

Finding Balance

Stress is the product of the body's "fight or flight" mechanism (Eblin, 2014). It occurs when one perceives their available resources are insufficient to manage physical, physiological, or emotional challenges (Eblin, 2014). In the nursing professional setting, it can be triggered by interpersonal conflict, inadequate staffing, and emotional exhaustion. The first step in dealing with stress is to identify the times the individual feels stressed. Make a list of the stressors encountered during the day. Next, identify the thoughts and emotions associated with those stressors.

Stress and emotions are inexorably linked (Matta, 2012). Thus, understanding the nature of stressors will promote an understanding of one's emotional response to stress. Emotional balance is the ability to maintain stability in the face of unpleasant states including negative thoughts and emotions. For leaders, emotional balance and stress reduction can be achieved by practicing mindfulness and effectively managing one's time.

Mindfulness

Mindfulness is the act of bringing nonjudgmental awareness to the present moment; it is a function of awareness and intention (Eblin, 2014). Mindfulness can promote emotional balance by controlling negative thoughts through recognition and regulation (Eblin, 2014). The benefits of mindfulness include reducing "mind chatter" and stress, improving memory and focus, and enhancing self-insight (Grenville-Cleave, 2012). In mindfulness, one recognizes and accepts their thoughts and emotions without labeling them "good" or "bad." They simply acknowledge their existence and allow them to drift away (Eblin, 2014).

Mindfulness brings one to the present moment and mitigates the negative effects of unpleasant thoughts. It is important to remember one cannot do this wrong. Distracting thoughts will appear; simply accept them and continue focusing on breathing and body sensations. Mindfulness practice promotes relaxation, reduces the feelings of pain and suffering, and can improve one's quality of life (Eblin, 2014). Box 12.3 presents an example of a mindfulness exercise.

Mindfulness-Based Stress Reduction (MBSR) is an evidence-based, 8-week program which promotes self-regulation and an acceptance of the present

---

BOX 12.3

▶ MINDFULNESS EXERCISE

A basic mindfulness exercise consists of the following. First, find your breath and slow it down. Study it. Follow the air as it passes through your nose, fills your lungs, and exits your body. Place your hand on your abdomen to find the natural rhythm of your breathing. Scan your body and notice how each anatomical section feels. Start from your head and move down to your toes. Do this until you have connected with each part of your body. Take one final deep breath. Do this whenever you are able throughout the day. It should take no longer than 5 min.

moment (Rush &, Sharma, 2017). MBSR encourages individuals to bring attention to the here and now (Gilmartin et al., 2017). Sensations are acknowledged but not judged as "good or "bad." Among nurses, MBSR is associated with increased self-care, improved feelings of empowerment, increased feelings of personal accomplishment, and an increased mindful presence (Mahon et al., 2017; Turkal et al., 2018). The time and resources required for a traditional MBSR program are time and cost prohibitive for many nurses. Thus, modified MBSR programs have been developed for nurses and other healthcare professionals ranging from 5 to 20 minutes a day to 30-minute sessions over a 4-week period (Gilmartin et al., 2017).

Mindfulness practices that APNs can use include yoga. Yoga improves musculoskeletal flexibility and balance and promotes inner peace (Eblin, 2014). Regular yoga practices can also promote stress reduction. In addition to meditation and yoga, other methods to cultivate emotional balance include consumption of healthy meals, reduction of processed and fast foods, consistent and regular exercise activities, and remaining socially connected with others (Matta, 2012).

It is a leader's role to provide opportunities for team members to practice mindfulness in their practice. Leaders are required to recognize the needs of staff, identify the correct training modality, and support staff through this novel process (Brennan, 2017). It is essential that leaders model mindfulness and share his or her experiences with team members.

Questions to Ask Yourself

1. How do I manage stress?
2. How effective am I managing stress?
3. How is stress affecting me physically and emotionally?
4. What steps am I taking to find a work-life balance?
5. Am I willing to make mindfulness a priority?
6. When can I practice a 10-min mindfulness exercise?

Time Management

Time management is the mindful and intentional control of time spent on activities. It can be a major stressor in a leadership position. Workload and responsibilities increase as one is accountable for administrative duties along with staff development and management. Leaders must first recognize that time is the most precious finite resource. One cannot create more time; however, one can effectively manage their time. Thus, a leader can consider *multiplying* their time by spending time today on things that will produce more time tomorrow (Vaden, 2015). This requires a new mindset where a leader focuses not on tasks but results.

Vaden (2015) argues there are several strategies that can help leaders multiply their time. Two of which include saying "no" and effective delegation. Saying "no" to additional tasks can be difficult. As a new leader, one does not want to be viewed as avoiding responsibilities. Every time a leader says "yes" to something, they are saying "no" to something else. So, rather than viewing "no" as avoidance, the leader should view it as making time for those things that will create more time in the future. Saying "yes" to reading this book can facilitate a smoother transition to a leadership role by providing practical strategies to more effectively manage oneself, relationships with others, and duties associated with a new role.

When taking inventory of tasks associated with a leadership position, it is important to ask if this is something that others can accomplish. Delegating is entrusting a task or responsibility to another. It can be difficult; leaders may have a hard time "letting go" of certain responsibilities. But, considering that time is finite and responsibilities are not, a leader should consider delegating appropriate tasks (Vaden, 2015). Questions to consider when delegating include (1) Can this task be delegated? (2) Will this task be done on time? and (3) Will it be done correctly? Follow-up is key to delegation. When delegating a task, a leader must be clear on deliverables and due dates to ensure proper completion.

Questions to Ask Yourself

1. What is my comfort level with delegation (this works better with time management)?
2. Why do I avoid delegation?
3. What success have I had with delegation?
4. Am I willing to build on that to consider other tasks that can be delegated?

Summary

In this chapter, Benner's "Novice to Expert" theory was conceptualized to the leadership development of APNs. Benner's framework can be helpful in identifying the stages associated with transitioning into a leadership role. This chapter also addressed the importance of self-awareness in leadership development. A leader must have a heightened sense of self-awareness to understand themselves, how others perceive them, and the motivators of their team. The ability to relate and demonstrate authentic empathy with one's followers promotes a sense of community and strengthens a leader's ability to influence others. Self-aware leaders recognize strengths and areas of opportunity within themselves and among those they lead. StrengthsFinder and the KTS are useful tools to begin discovering one's talents and preferences when interacting with others.

The ability to effectively communicate is a function of self-awareness and an essential competency of a leader. Leaders must be skilled communicators to articulate expectations, initiatives, and vision. Effective communication facilitates team building and cohesion. Promoting a culture of respect and collegiality can directly influence patient and organizational outcomes.

Conflict is a natural component of human communication. It occurs when two or more individuals have different opinions about a subject or course of action. Although there are different preferences with dealing with conflict, a leader must be skilled at managing conflict with and between others.

Reflection can be an effective strategy to promote self-awareness and facilitate team cohesion. Reflective practice is the intellectual and effective activities used to explore previous experiences to gain a new understanding and appreciation of those events. It can be used by an individual to analyze thoughts and feelings about previous experiences or by teams to identify more effective methods of problem-solving.

Mentorship is an essential component of leadership development. Mentors can facilitate self-reflection and introduce new leaders to resources that can promote role transition. There is no lack of nurse leaders who want to mentor; however, the onus is on the mentee to seek mentors who can change their personal and professional life. Professional nursing organizations offer programs that utilize mentorship as the foundation for professional and leadership development.

Leadership is stressful. It can be emotionally taxing, and stress reduction strategies such as mindfulness and yoga can help leaders maintain stability in the face of unpleasant states including negative thoughts and emotions. New leaders learn that time is the most precious resource and the feelings of not having enough of it can cause significant distress. Time management strategies can focus leaders on "now" vs. "later" tasks and encourage them to delegate tasks that can be successfully completed by others.

Chapter Highlights

- Benner's "Novice to Expert" theory can be applied to leadership development.
- Leadership development begins with gaining a better understanding of self.
- Effective communication is an essential competency of a leader.
- Leaders must effectively manage conflict with and between others.
- Building a cohesive team is central to accomplishing departmental and organizational goals.
- Mentorship is a fundamental competent of leadership development.
- Reflection can promote a greater understanding of self and others.
- Finding emotional balance can mitigate the negative effects of stress.
- Effective time management can reduce feelings of stress associated with increased workload.

Web Resources

Conflict Resolution in Healthcare: https://www.bing.com/videos/search?q=conflict+resolution+in+healthcare&&view=detail&mid=B78DBB9481892847B9F2B78DBB9481892847B9F2&&FORM=VDRVRV
Emotional Intelligence Test:
https://www.psychologytoday.com/us/tests/personality/emotional-intelligence-test
Six Relaxation Techniques: https://www.health.harvard.edu/mind-and-mood/six-relaxation-techniques-to-reduce-stress
The Quick Emotional Intelligence Self-Assessment: https://benefits.cat.com/content/dam/benefits/eap/EQ-Self-Assessment.pdf

---

Leadership Certifications

1. American Organization of Nurse Executives (AONE) (http://www.aone.org/):
   a. Nurse Manger and Leader Certification (CNML)
   b. Executive Nursing Practice Certification (CENP)
2. American Association of Colleges of Nursing (AACN) (http://www.aacnnursing.org/):
   a. Clinical Nurse Leader Certification (CNL)

References

Awdish, L. A., & Berry, L. L. (2017). The importance of making time to really listen to your patients. *Harvard Business Review*. https://www.physicianleaders.org/news/the-importance-of-making-time-to-really-listen-to-your-patients

Benner, P. (1982). From novice to expert. *The American Journal of Nursing, 82*(3), 402–407.

Benner, P. (1984). *From novice to expert: Excellence and power in clinical nursing practice*. Addison Wesley.

Benner, P., Tanner, C., & Chesla, C. (2009). *Expertise in nursing practice: Caring, clinical judgment, and ethics* (2nd ed). Springer Publishing Company.

Bennis, W. (2004). The seven ages of the leader. *Harvard Business Review, 82*, 46–53.

Bergstedt, K., & Wei, H. (2020). Leadership strategies to promote frontline nursing staff engagement. *Nursing Management, 51*(2), 48–53.

Bower, K. M. (2015). Coaching with Myers Briggs Type Indicator: A valuable tool for client self-awareness. *The Journal of Practice Consulting, 5*(2), 11–19.

Bradberry, T. & Greaves, J. (2009). *Emotional intelligence 2.0*. Talent Smart.

Brennan, J. B. (2017). Towards resilience and wellbeing in nurses. *British Journal of Nursing, 26*(1), 43–47.

Burton, C. W., McLemore, M. R., Perry, L., Carrick, J., & Shattell, M. (2016). Social media awareness and implications in nursing leadership: A pilot professional meeting campaign. *Policy, Politics, & Nursing Practice, 17*(4), 187–197.

Campbell, J. C., McBride, A. B., Etcher, L., & Deming, K. (2017). Robert Wood Johnson Foundation Nurse Faculty Scholars program leadership training. *Nursing Outlook, 65*, 290–302.

Consulting Psychologists Press. (2017). *Thomas-Kilmann conflict mode instrument: Profile and interpretive report*. https://www.researchgate.net/publication/265565339_Thomas-Kilmann_conflict_MODE_instrument

Consulting Psychologists Press. (2018). *A positive framework for life-long people development*. https://www.cpp.com/en-US/Products-and-Services/Myers-Briggs

Dempsey, C., & Reilly, B. A. (2016). Nurse engagement: What are the contributing factors for success. *The Online Journal of Issues in Nursing, 21*, 2. https://ojin.nursingworld.org/MainMenuCategories/ANAMarketplace/ANAPeriodicals/OJIN/TableofContents/Vol-21-2016/No1-Jan-2016/Nurse-Engagement-Contributing-Factors-for-Success.html

Dracup, K., & Bryan-Brown, C. (2004). From novice to expert to mentor: Shaping the future. *American Journal of Critical Care, 13*(6), 448–450.

Dreyfus, S., & Dreyfus, H. (1980). *A five-stage model of the mental activities involved in directed skill acquisition*. Supported by the U.S. Air Force, Office of Scientific Research (AFSC) under contract F49620-C-0063 with the University of California, Berkeley. (Unpublished study).

Eblin, S. (2014). *Overworked and overwhelmed: The mindfulness alternative.* John Wiley & Sons, Inc.

Gallup. (2020a). *The 34 Clifton strengths themes explain your talent DNA.* https://www.gallup.com/cliftonstrengths/en/253715/34-cliftonstrengths-themes.aspx

Gallup. (2020b). *The history of Cliftonstrengths.* https://www.gallup.com/cliftonstrengths/en/253754/history-cliftonstrengths.aspx#:~:text=In%202015%2C%20Gallup%20changed%20the,based%20development%20guide%20ever%20created

Gibbs, G. (1988). *Learning by doing: A guide to teaching and learning methods.* Further Education Unit.

Gillespie, C. (2019). *Difference between active listening and passive listening.* https://www.theclassroom.com/strengths-weaknesses-auditory-learner-11372616.html

Gilmartin, H., Goyal, A., Hamati, M. C., Mann, J., Saint, S., & Chopra, V. (2017). Brief mindfulness practices for healthcare providers – A systematic literature review. *The American Journal of Medicine, 130*(10), 1219.e1–1219.e12.

Grenny, J., Patterson, K., Maxfield, D., McMillian, R., & Switzler, A. (2013). *Influencer: The new science of leading change* (2nd ed.). McGraw Hill.

Grenville-Cleave, B. (2012). *Positive psychology.* MFJ Publishing.

Hodgson, A. K., & Scanlan, J. M. (2013). A concept analysis of mentoring in nursing leadership. *Open Journal of Nursing, 3*, 389–394.

Homer. (n.d). *The odyssey* (S. Butler, Trans.). Race Point Publishing.

Huston, C. J. (2018). *The road to leadership.* Sigma Theta Tau International.

Jacobs, S. (2016). Reflective learning, reflective practice. *Nursing, 4*(5), 62–64.

Johansen, M. L. (2012). Keeping the peace: Conflict management strategies for nurse managers, *Nursing Management, 43*(2), 50–54.

Johnson, W. B. (2016). *On being a mentor* (2nd ed.). Routledge Publishing.

Keirsey, D., & Bates, M. (1984). *Please understand me: Character and temperament types.* Prometheus Nemesis.

Kilmann Diagnostics. (2018). *An overview of the Thomas-Kilmann Mode Instrument (TKI).* http://www.kilmanndiagnostics.com/overview-thomas-kilmann-conflict-mode-instrument-tki

Knipfer, K., Shaughnessy, B., Hentschel, T., & Schmid, E. (2016). Unlocking women's leadership potential: A curricular example for developing female leaders in academia. *Journal of Education Management, 41*(2), 272–302.

Kolb, D. A. (1984). *Experiential learning: Experience as the source of learning and development.* Prentice Hall.

Kourkouta, L., & Papathanasiou, I. V. (2014). Communication in nursing practice. *Materia Socio-Medica, 26*(1), 65–67.

Kutney-Lee, A., Germack, H., Hatfield, L., Kelly, S., Maguire, P., Dierkes, A., Del Guidice, D. M., & Aiken, L. H. (2016). Nurse engagement in shared governance and patient and nurse outcomes. *Journal of Nursing Administration, 46*(11), 605–612.

Leggat, S. G., Balding, C., & Schiffian, D. (2014). Developing clinical leaders: The impact of an action learning mentoring programme for advanced practice nurses. *Journal of Clinical Nursing, 24*(11), 1576–1584.

Mahon, M. A., Mee, L., Brett, D., Dowling, M. (2017). Nurses' perceived stress and compassion following a mindfulness meditation and self-compassion training. *Journal of Research in Nursing, 22*(8), 572–583.

Mansel, B., & Einion, A. (2019). It's the relationship you develop with them: Emotional intelligence in nurse leadership. A qualitive study. *British Journal of Nursing, 28*(21), 1400–1408.

Matta, C. (2012). *The stress response.* New Harbinger Publications, Inc.

Maxwell, J. C. (2008). *Mentoring 101: What every leader needs to know.* Nelson Books.

Mazzoccoli, A., & Wolf, G. (2016). Mentoring through the leadership journey: From novice to expert. *Nurse Leader, 14*(4), 253–256.

Mcleod, S. A. (2017). *Kolb – Learning styles*. https://www.simplypsychology.org/learning-kolb.html

Miller, C. J., Kim, B., Silverman, A., & Bauer, M. S. (2018). A systematic review of team-building interventions in non-acute healthcare settings. *BMC Health Services Research, 18*(11), 1–21.

Mindset. (2020). *Gibbs reflection cycle*. https://www.mindtools.com/pages/article/reflective-cycle.htm

Nowell, L., Norris, J. L., Mrklas, K., & White, D. E. (2017). Mixed methods systematic review exploring mentorship outcomes in nursing academia. *Journal of Advanced Nursing, 73*(3), 527–544.

Patterson, K., Grenny, J., McMillian, R., & Switzler, A. (2012). *Crucial conversations: Tools for talking when stakes are high* (2nd ed.). McGraw-Hill.

Pietrucha, F. J. (2014). *Super communicator*. Bristol Park Books.

Rath, T. (2007). *StrengthsFinder 2.0* (2nd ed.). Gallup Press.

Rigoni, B., & Asplund, J. (2016). Developing employees' strengths boots sales, profits, and engagement. *Harvard Business Review*. https://hbr.org/2016/09/developing-employees-strengths-boosts-sales-profit-and-engagement

Rush, S. E., & Sharma, M. (2017). Mindfulness-based stress reduction as a stress management intervention for cancer care: A systematic review. *Journal of Evidence-Based Complementary & Alternative Medicine, 22*(2), 347–359.

Schon, D. A. (1983). *The reflective practitioner: How professionals think in action*. Basic Books Inc.

Sherman, R. O. (2020). Learn to manage yourself. *American Journal of Nursing, 120*(2), 68–71.

Sherrod, D., Holland, C., & Chappel-Aiken, L. (2019). Leadership: Where we've been, where we are, and where we're going. *Nursing Management, 50*(9), 1–3.

Shirey, M. R. (2007). Competencies and tips for effective leadership: From novice to expert. *Journal of Nursing Administration, 37*(4), 167–170.

Smith, M. S., & Johnson, C. S. (2018). Preparing nurse leaders in nursing professional development. *Journal for Nurses in Professional Development, 34*(3), 158–161.

Starr, J. (2014). *The mentoring manual*. Pearson Education Limited.

Thusini, S., & Mingay, J. (2019). Models of leadership and their implications for nursing practice. *British Journal of Nursing, 28*(6), 356–360.

Turkal, M., Richardson, L. G., Cline, T., & Guimond, M. E. (2018). The effect of a mindfulness-based stress reduction intervention on the perceived stress and burnout of RN students completing a doctor of nursing practice degree. *Journal of Nursing Education and Practice, 8*(10), 58–67.

Vaden, R. (2015). *Procrastinate on purpose: 5 permissions to multiply your time*. Penguin Random House LLC.

Valiga, T. M. (2019). Leaders, managers, and followers: Working in harmony. *Nursing, 49*(1), 45–48.

Vertino, K. A. (2014). Effective interpersonal communication: A practical guide to improve your life. *The Online Journal of Issues in Nursing*. https://ojin.nursingworld.org/MainMenuCategories/ANAMarketplace/ANAPeriodicals/OJIN/TableofContents/Vol-19-2014/No3-Sept-2014/Effective-Interpersonal-Communication.html

Walsh, S., & Mann, S. (2015). Doing reflective practice: A data-led way forward. *English Language Teaching Journal, 69*(4), 351–362.

Ylitormanen, T., Kvist, T., & Turunen, H. (2015). A web-based survey of Finnish Nurses' perceptions of conflict management in nurse-nurse collaboration. *International Journal of Caring Sciences, 2*(8), 263–273.

13

Advanced Practice Nurses as Leaders of Change

Carol Huston

LEARNING OBJECTIVES

After completing this chapter, you will be able to:

1. Describe forces contributing to dynamic change in contemporary healthcare organizations.

2. Identify strategies for unfreezing, movement, and refreezing planned changes.

3. Alter driving and restraining forces to promote specific changes.

4. Describe strategies change agents can undertake to increase the likelihood of a planned change being successful.

5. Identify recent successful change efforts undertaken by advanced practice nurse leaders.

6. Recognize opportunities for advanced practice nurses to plan for and be involved in future change efforts to further professional and/or consumer healthcare goals.

KEY TERMS

Advanced practice registered nurse: A registered nurse with a master's or doctoral degree, typically assuming one of the four specific roles: nurse practitioner (NP), clinical nurse specialist (CNS), certified nurse midwife (CNM), or certified nurse anesthetist (CRNA).

Change: To make something different; to alter the state of something.

Change agent: A leader skilled in the theory and implementation of planned change to deal appropriately with conflicted human emotions and to connect and balance all aspects of the organization that will be affected by that change (Marquis & Huston, 2020).

Change by drift: Unplanned change.

Change champion: An individual who encourages and supports change.

Driving forces: The forces that encourage change.

Freezing/refreezing: The reestablishment of stability once changes have been made.

Movement: Action taken to encourage change.

Restraining forces: Forces that discourage change.

Unfreezing: Creating a case for, or increasing, the readiness for change.

Change: A Pervasive Force in Contemporary Healthcare

Change is pervasive in contemporary healthcare organizations with most undergoing continual transformation related to organizational restructuring, quality improvement, and employee retention. Factors driving healthcare change include fragmentation, access problems, unsustainable costs, suboptimal outcomes, and disparities along with changing social and disease-type demographics (Salmon & Echevarria, 2017). Other factors include rising healthcare costs, declining reimbursement, new quality imperatives, workforce shortages, emerging technologies, the dynamic nature of knowledge, and a growing elderly population (Marquis & Huston, 2020).

Fundamental tenets about how value is defined have changed the healthcare landscape. Management scholar Michael Porter notes that value should always be defined around the customer (Leaf, 2018). Since value depends on results, not inputs, value in healthcare should be measured by the outcomes achieved, not the volume of services delivered or the process of care used. Leaf (2018) suggests that while science and technology will be the tools that carry us forward, it is this shift from volume to value (customer-centered value) that will continue to spur meaningful changes in healthcare. In addition, since value is defined as outcomes relative to costs, it encompasses efficiency. Cost reduction without regard to the outcomes achieved is dangerous and self-defeating (Leaf, 2018).

Questions to Ask Yourself

1. How cognizant am I of forces driving change in contemporary healthcare organizations?
2. How open am I to embracing change?
3. Do I view change as the means of improving processes and outcomes?

Lewin's Change Theory

Many theorists have suggested strategies for the effective implementation of change. For example, for effective change to occur, a thorough and accurate assessment is needed of the extent of and interest in change, the nature and depth of motivation, and the environment in which the change will occur (Marquis & Huston, 2020). Because human beings have little control over many changes in their lives, the individuals planning change must remember that people need a balance between stability and change in the workplace (Marquis & Huston, 2020).

Most of the current research on change builds on the classic change theories developed by Kurt Lewin in the mid-20th century. Lewin (1951) theorized that people maintain a state of status quo or equilibrium by the simultaneous occurrence of both **driving forces** (facilitators) and **restraining forces** (barriers) operating within any field. Driving forces advance a system toward change; restraining forces impede change. Lewin's model suggested that people like feeling safe, comfortable, and in control of their environment. For change to occur then, the balance of driving and restraining forces must be altered. The driving forces must be increased or the restraining forces decreased.

Questions to Ask Yourself

1. What changes would I like to make in my personal or professional life?
2. What are the driving and restraining forces for these changes?
3. What strategies might I use to change the status quo?

Lewin (1951) also identified three phases that must occur before a planned change becomes part of the system: unfreezing, movement, and refreezing (Figure 13.1). Unfreezing occurs when someone convinces members of the group to change or when guilt, anxiety, or concern can be elicited. Thus, people become discontent and aware of a need to change. Oftentimes, people are afraid of change, so the leader must assure that discontent/discomfort is high enough to encourage individuals to even consider change.

The second phase of planned change is movement. In movement, appropriate strategies are identified, planned, and implemented, ensuring that driving forces exceed restraining forces. Recognizing, addressing, and overcoming resistance may be a lengthy process, and whenever possible, change should be implemented gradually. Any change of human behavior, or the perceptions, attitudes, and values underlying that behavior, takes time. Indeed, addressing and responding appropriately to stress being experienced by those undergoing change is a high-level leadership skill (Marquis & Huston, 2020).

The last phase is refreezing. During the refreezing phase, the change becomes integrated into the status quo. If refreezing is incomplete, the change will be ineffective, and prechange behaviors will be resumed. For refreezing to occur, those planning for change must be supportive and reinforce the individual

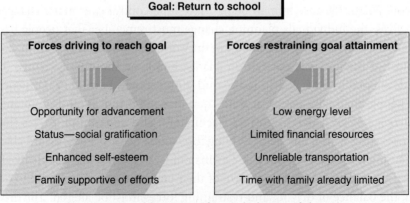

Figure 13.1. Adaptation of Lewin's theory of change.

adaptive efforts of those affected by the change. In addition, because change needs at least 3 to 6 months before it will be accepted as part of the system, those leading the change must remain involved until the change is completed (Marquis & Huston, 2020).

The Change Agent: A Critical Part of Successful Change

What often differentiates a successful change effort from an unsuccessful one is the ability of the change agent—a leader skilled in the theory and implementation of planned change—to deal appropriately with conflicted human emotions and to connect and balance all aspects of the organization that will be affected by that change (Marquis & Huston, 2020). Indeed, Larson (2015), in her interview of 50+ leaders, notes that effectively dealing with rapid change while leading ever more complex organizations was identified as both a top challenge and a critical leadership competency.

Questions to Ask Yourself

1. How much self-confidence do I have in my ability to be a successful change agent?
2. What risk-taking propensity do I typically display in initiating change?

Strategies for Successful Change

The change agent can do many things to increase the likelihood of successful planned change. Demonstrating traits such as flexibility, confidence, tenacity, and the ability to articulate vision through insights and versatile thinking establishes the change agent as a leader and give him or her credibility to carry out a change. Melnyk et al. (2017, p. 34) agree, noting "there is nothing more important to achieving success than a potent dream/vision and an ability to inspire that vision in the team." The change efforts of many leaders fail because they focus too much on process and not enough on an exciting vision, although it does need to be recognized that vision without execution will also deter success (Box 13.1).

BOX 13.1

▶ STRATEGIES FOR SUCCESS AS A CHANGE AGENT

1. Display traits such as flexibility, confidence, tenacity, and the ability to articulate vision through insights and versatile thinking.

2. Implement change only for good reasons.

3. Be cognizant of the specific driving and restraining forces within a particular environment for change.

4. Implement change gradually, not sporadically or suddenly.

5. Assure that the tools or resources necessary to implement that change are available.

6. Whenever possible, involve all those who may be affected by a change in planning for that change.

7. Expect resistance to change; it is a natural consequence of instability or a disruption of the status quo.

8. Encourage stakeholders to speak openly about their concerns and frustrations during change so that objections can be overcome.

9. Provide a feeling of control whenever possible to stakeholders during change.

10. Identify early in the planned change which stakeholders are likely to promote (change champions) or resist the change. Collaborate with the change champions on how best to address the concerns of those individuals more resistant to change.

11. Reinforce and reward desired behavior to encourage the emergence of more change champions.

12. Be a role model to stakeholders about viewing change positively and being flexible during its implementation.

Based on Marquis, B., & Huston, C. J. (2017). *Leadership roles and management functions in nursing* (9th ed.). Wolters Kluwer and Tams, C. (2018). *Why we need to rethink organizational change management*. Forbes.

In addition, change should be implemented only for good reasons. Change is never easy, and regardless of the type of change, all major change brings feelings of achievement and pride as well as loss and stress. Change for change's sake subjects stakeholders to unnecessary stress and manipulation (Marquis & Huston, 2020).

In Their Own Words

Shakira Henderson, PhD, DNP, MS, MPH, RNC-NIC, IBCLC
Senior Administrator for Research and Grants, Vidant Medical Center
Greenville, NC

How Was the Need for Change Established?

Alignment with the organization's mission, vision, operational imperatives (e.g., quality, safety), and strategic plan is key to establishing the need for change. There are times that all of the aforementioned do not always align all at once. However, the ability for the nurse leader to outline the case for change with at least one, can garner support to move the initiative forward. While this is very cliché to mention, any change that improves the financial margin is often welcomed change. In contemporary times, change that improves team member or patient experience does not always need to have a concrete return of investment as the returns are seen in satisfaction, low turnover, and organizational reputation. Another undeniable way to determine need for change is if there is a regulatory component. The latter makes this step of the change process the easiest.

No one anticipated the multitude of changes that our healthcare system would need to embark on during the protracted pandemic of COVID-19. I was tapped to lead the health system with PPE management. PPE was becoming in high demand, shortages were emerging, and in some cases, PPE was even nonexistent. The horror stories of healthcare workers not having enough or appropriate PPE when the number of hospitalized patients hit an all-time high, was the impetus for change in our current PPE management style.

(Continued)

What Was the Process to Decide "the Change"?

Most organizations have a system of management that allows decisions on who, what, when, and why change initiatives will occur in the fiscal year or over time. This involves the preparation of a formal document on the change. Some organizations use business plans. Others employ frameworks such an SBAR. Nurse leaders need to familiarize themselves with the preferred format of their organizations. Despite the formal structure for governance, the nurse leader must be prepared to navigate the informal steps and often highly political aspects of ensuring your change becomes a top priority. New leaders tend to underestimate the amount of time and effort that needs to be put into the "meetings before THE MEETING". In fact, your change initiative can be almost 100% supported if you are able to meet individually with all key decision makers prior and address any of their concerns, fears, comments, or questions.

The first thing I did as the PPE lead was to establish a system-wide Taskforce with interprofessional representation to drive, facilitate, and approve changes. Key stakeholders that were mandated to be part of the Taskforce included (1) our infection control nurse, (2) infection control MD, (3) quality nurse and MD executives, (4) operations nurse executives, (5) entity-specific operations executives, (6) legal and risk management, (7) communication, experience, and marketing leadership, and (8) supply chain management leadership. The Taskforce also included representation from nursing education, emergency nursing staff, and entity central services. The meetings were open so other key stakeholders could join or be invited as needed. To guide the changes needed in the PPE management, the Taskforce developed a PPE model that included a focus on (1) inventory, (2) conservation techniques, (3) preservation techniques, (4) use of innovation, and (5) collection of donations. All decisions also had to be data-driven and science-driven.

How Were the Nursing Staff Prepared for the Change?

Communication and roll-out plans are nonnegotiables in the preparation of nursing staff for change. Nurse champions should be chosen as far out in the process as possible to allow for input from frontline team members in both the communication and roll-out plans. These champions give updates to peers on a weekly-monthly basis to ensure team members are aware of the upcoming change. Feedback from frontline team members can also be obtained in these sessions, and this gives the entire staff ownership in the change.

One of the most controversial changes that we made as a PPE Taskforce was the decision to collect used facemasks, especially N95s, for decontamination and reuse, if we ever ran out of PPE. The decision was both data-driven, supplies were running low at the time, and science-driven, the FDA had approved

(Continued)

a decontamination process. It also fit the conservation and innovation arms of our PPE model. The collection of used PPE required that nursing staff stop wearing make-up and cut their beards, because masks with make-up or facial hair could not be safely reused after the decontamination process. To prepare the nursing staff for this change, we worked with our experience, communication, and marketing team to develop a campaign. The campaign was called the HEREOS MOVEMENT. It also had a slogan—Go Make-Up Free and Facial Hair Free for ENC (Eastern North Carolina). Our Chief Nurse and several nurses in the institution were featured in a video taking off their make-up or shaving their breads. We also held webinars for leaders and staff on the decontamination process. Once the collection bins were deployed, pictures and instructions accompanied each collection site so staff could easy ask to the "WHAT" and "WHY" of the change. Daily electronic alerts on collection status and PPE status were sent to all nursing staff as well.

What Can One Expect in the Early Period of Change?

In healthcare, change is an unfortunate constant in a system that requires consistency to meet outcomes. It is indeed the paradox of healthcare. Therefore, early periods of change tend to be chaotic even when you have well-developed communication and roll-out plans. One might say it is the "expected chaos" of change. There will be mistakes. There will be processes that do not work. There will be team members who are negative and seemingly intentionally sabotage the change. It is not always bad. There will be moments of excitement when you see planned logistics go smoothly. There will also be moments when staff fully embrace the change because they understand the need and see the positive impact.

Despite all our efforts, there were some bumps in the journey of our Make-Up Free and Facial Hair Free Campaign in the beginning. There were pockets of nurses who understandably did not like the idea of reuse of decontaminated PPE. As such, we found trash in some of the collection bins when we first launched the initiative. It is important to note, that if trash is intermingled with collected PPE, the entire bin cannot be sent for decontamination. We lost hundreds of masks in the first few weeks. Because this was occurring in only small pockets of the hospital, we decided as a Taskforce to do targeted education on the decontamination process in those areas. We explained to the nurses that we were not currently using decontaminated PPE and, in fact, it was our hope that we would never get to that point. But we wanted to make sure that if PPE supplies became nonexistent, we had PPE to keep all our nursing and other members of the care team safe. The targeted education made a major difference, we saw our viable collection rates soar. So, as you can see, there will always be bumps in the journey, but targeted interventions often pay big.

(Continued)

Were There Strategies to Keep the Staff Moving Forward?
Nursing team members need multiple channels of communication to keep the change initiative moving forward. Different team members understand the why and the what at different stages of the change. Strategies to keep the change moving forward include but are not limited to (1) team member feedback portals, suggestion boxes, unit boards, intranet blogs, and focus groups; (2) quick resolution on planned process changes; (3) daily, weekly, monthly status updates on the progress of the change to completion; (4) individual and team recognition for engagement and outcomes in the change process; and lastly (5) a debriefing session at the completion of the change initiative to ensure lessons learned are archived for future use.

The continuous stressors of the pandemic took a toll on all staff, especially nursing. As such it was important to us as a PPE Taskforce to keep our staff informed and motivated. We developed a comprehensive PPE Guidance document so that all staff would have quick access and reference to everything PPE. We also established a PPE Question email so that staff could get their immediate questions answered. To liven up the subject of PPE, we created a funny PPE mascot that delivered a PPE Fact of the Week and Monthly PPE Trivia Question.

Change agents also should be cognizant of the specific driving and restraining forces within a particular environment for change. Lewin's model suggested that people like feeling safe, comfortable, and in control of their environment. For change to occur then, the balance of driving and restraining forces must be altered (Marquis & Huston, 2020). Bradberry (2017) suggests it may be helpful to remember that the first step in leading change is always the hardest. Once you take that step, anxiety and fear often dissipate in the name of action. "People who dive headfirst into taking that brutal first step aren't any stronger than the rest of us; they've simply learned that it yields great results… and that procrastination only prolongs their suffering" (para. 7).

Change should be implemented gradually and not sporadically or suddenly. That is the very definition of planned change, in contrast to change by drift. Because change is such a complex process, it requires a great deal of planning and intricate timing. It may also take some time to assure that the tools or resources necessary to implement that change are available.

The change agent must also, whenever possible, involve all those whom may be affected by a change in planning for that change (Marquis & Huston, 2020). Stakeholders need to know and understand how a proposed change will impact them and what expectations the change agent has of them. All must have the opportunity to define their interest in the change, their expectation of its outcome, and their ideas on strategies for achieving change. There is no such thing as too much communication (Tams, 2018). When information and decision-making are shared, stakeholders feel that they have played a valuable role in the change (Marquis & Huston, 2020). Communication of the vision by the change agent then is a critical factor in success of the planned change.

Even with the involvement of stakeholders in planning for the change, the change agent should, however, expect **resistance**. Resistance to change is often just resistance to uncertainty, and to overcome resistors, the change agent must ensure that communication plays an integral role in the process (Thomas, 2018). The change agent must remember that resistance is not personal; it is a natural consequence of instability or a disruption of the status quo. Openness to creativity or change cannot thrive in an environment where divergent thinking is punished (Tams, 2018). Recognizing, addressing, and overcoming resistance is often a difficult and lengthy process since any change of human behavior, or the perceptions, attitudes, and values underlying that behavior, takes time (Marquis & Huston, 2020).

In addition, stakeholders should be encouraged to speak openly about their concerns and frustrations during change so that objections can be overcome. Attempting to intimidate resistors or to force compliance with a change guarantees the change will fail. Stakeholders need to perceive some feeling of control, if possible, during change. "Sometimes, when our proposals or ideas appear to fall on deaf ears, rather than stop and explore a disagreement or other perspectives, we push harder to make our viewpoint known. Ironically, the passion and exuberance with which we express our point of view creates more resistance than contribution and collaboration from others. Our push creates pushback from others, which may turn into a competition to determine who is right and who is wrong. Emotions will likely take over, leading to a downward spiral that will not end well" (Stoker, 2018, para. 6).

Questions to Ask Yourself

1. Is it a fundamental tenet of human behavior to resist change?
2. Do I tend to be more of an early adopter or a resistor when facing change?

It may be helpful for the change agent to identify early in the planned change which stakeholders are likely to promote (change champions) or resist the change. The change agent can then collaborate with the change champions on how best to address the concerns of those individuals more resistant to change. Change agents should also reinforce change whenever possible. Reward and celebrate those who demonstrate desired behaviors (Tams, 2018), as the likely result will be more change champions.

Finally, change agents should be role models to stakeholders about viewing change positively and being flexible during its implementation. Change and innovation are not easy, but the alternative is stagnation and obsolescence. Change agents as leaders must be catalysts for professional change as well as organizational change. "Many people attracted to nursing now find that their values and traditional expectations no longer fit as they once did. It is the change agent's role to help stakeholders confront the opportunities and challenges of the realities of emerging nursing practice; to create enthusiasm and passion for renewing the profession; to embrace the change of locus of control, which now belongs to the healthcare consumer; and to engage a new social context for nursing practice" (Marquis & Huston, 2020, p. 201).

Nurses as Leaders of Change

The Institute of Medicine (IOM, 2011) report, *The Future of Nursing: Leading Change, Advancing Health,* called for expanded opportunities for nurses to lead and diffuse collaborative improvement efforts and to innovate in practice and education. In addition, the American Nurses Association (ANA) Scope and Standards of Practice (2015) calls for all registered nurses (RNs) to be leaders within the profession, working to influence policies and encourage innovation.

Indeed, Salmon and Echevarria (2017, para. 1) suggest it is nurses who are best positioned to "contribute to and lead the transformative changes that are occurring in healthcare by being a fully contributing member of the interprofessional team as we shift from episodic, provider-based, fee-for-service care to team-based, patient-centered care across the continuum that provides seamless, affordable, and quality care. These shifts require a new or an enhanced set of knowledge, skills, and attitudes around wellness and population care with a renewed focus on patient-centered care, care coordination, data analytics, and quality improvement." Although there is no doubt that nurses are poised to assume roles to advance health, improve care, and increase value, new ways of thinking and practicing will be required (Salmon & Echevarria, 2017).

In Their Own Words

Patricia E. Thompson, EdD, RN, FAAN
Retired CEO and Past President of Sigma Theta Tau International

The key points in understanding inspiring change are… Stakeholder buy-in and an effective communication/marketing plan. Successful change also requires knowledge of the organization, its processes and culture, as well as recognizing obstacles. A formalized plan with rationale, data, and an evaluation plan is important.

To prepare for major change, one must… Expect resistance and plan to stay for the long course. Change is not an easy or short process. It requires risk-taking, so a data-driven strategic action plan with timelines is critical.

My greatest challenge in implementing change is… Consistently monitoring the people involved in the change process, decreasing stress as it occurs, and providing support and reassurance as needed. I learned early in my career to focus my energy to embrace rather than resist change.

Regarding change, I wish someone had told me… To not be afraid of change but to be a leader and embrace it as a way to move forward and make improvements.

To effectively manage change, one must remember… To not move too quickly and provide support for the people involved. It is important to consistently monitor the plan, the process, and the people. Modifying the plan as needed based on evaluation data is essential.

Another point to understand is… Change is the new normal and will always be occurring. Therefore, develop your change skills set and embrace the process.

Exemplars of Recent Advanced Practice Nurse–Led Change

Hamric et al. (2014) suggest that initiating change and diffusing and sustaining innovation are critical elements of advanced practice nursing (APN) leadership competency. Indeed, there are many recent exemplars of APNs serving successfully as advanced practice change champions. Only a few are detailed here.

Fall Prevention Collaborative

Gray-Micheli et al. (2017) describe an APN-led educational healthcare practice change intervention focused on fall prevention that was carried out in 38 hospitals in New Jersey. The project involved team training, coaching, and mentoring in falls prevention and the development of a unit-based falls prevention project. After garnering buy-in from key state administrative official stakeholders, the principal investigator, an APN, and falls prevention expert spoke to key stakeholders from the division of patient safety and quality oversight and met with the physician safety officer for acute care facilities to discuss orchestrating the delivery of the educational intervention and recruitment strategies to target key healthcare providers from the hospitals (unfreezing).

Factual content on fall demography and findings from evidence-based fall prevention interventions were then presented to 38 hospital and organizational systems, with some systems comprising two or three regional hospitals (movement). Outcomes showed that fall rates decreased ($p < .01$) following the intervention by 1.7 falls per 1,000 patient days (95% confidence limits of 0.7–2.7). In addition, there was a sustained interest by the hospitals to conduct unit-based falls prevention QI initiatives (refreezing). The researchers concluded that the active involvement of APNs was fundamental to the success of the intervention.

Providing Care to Underserved, Vulnerable Populations

Laure Marino, Doctor of Nursing Practice (DNP), a board-certified family and geriatric nurse practitioner, who had maintained a practice in Charleston since 1997, opened the first nurse-led, reverse-integrated care—meaning primary care services are placed in a behavioral health setting—practice in West Virginia (Campaign for Action, 2018c).

Gloria McNeal, PhD, MSN, ACNS-BC, grew up in a poor neighborhood in Philadelphia (Campaign for Action, 2018a). "McNeal saw firsthand that where you live, learn, work, and play determine not just your life course, but your very health. This fundamental understanding motivated her to first become a nurse, and then to do her part to change the trajectory for people from neighborhoods like hers" (Campaign for Action, 2018a para. 4). To accomplish this, McNeal brought mobile health vans to Philadelphia as well as Newark, NJ. While the van approach was effective, trust and access barriers remained.

Eventually, McNeal moved to Los Angeles and began her work in the poor Watts district. Enlisting the help of community institutions and potential partners such as local churches, community centers, and the Salvation Army (unfreezing), she set up a nurse-managed clinic at those locations on different days. Later she incorporated telehealth, bringing even greater ease and efficiency to provider-patient interaction (movement). Ultimately, McNeal was able to demonstrate that her delivery-of-care model results in her patients leading healthier lives and that cost savings come from the partnership of community organizations, a diverse healthcare team, and the use of telehealth. The end result was a model that is both scalable and replicable (refreezing) (Campaign for Action, 2018a).

Finally, there is the story of Danielle Howa Pendergrass, DNP, APRN, WHNP-BC, who grew up in an area of rural Utah without a women's healthcare provider. She changed that by opening Eastern Utah Women's Health, an independent practice that serves more than 20,000 women from teens to seniors, both insured and uninsured. In addition, in 2013, following more than a decade of advocacy efforts on behalf of NPs in Utah, Howa-Pendergrass, as part of her DNP project, helped to eliminate a clause in the Utah State Medicaid Program that prevented NPs from being paid directly by Medicaid (The University of Utah, 2014). "As an agent of change, Howa-Pendergrass networked with colleagues, joined forces with coalitions and built relationships with policy makers" (unfreezing) (Schrier, 2014, para. 3). The result was a unanimous vote by the Medical Care Advisory Committee to allow all certified NPs the ability to directly bill and be reimbursed by Medicaid (movement). The result was that patients now have access to NPs with specialties in adult and acute care, geriatrics, neonatal, psychiatric/mental health, and women's health, and NPs are paid directly by Medicaid (refreezing).

Smoking Cessation

Charlotte Parent, RN, MHCM, director of health for New Orleans, was asked to be a part of a change effort to explore a smoking ban in that city in 2012, but when the idea of improving indoor air quality in New Orleans was first introduced, city residents resisted, so the administration and Health Department dropped the idea (Campaign for Action, 2018b). Three years later, Parent again took up the cause and unfreezing began. To address pushback from businesses and members of the community, Parent and the New Orleans Health Department offered information, support, and education about the importance of the ordinance. The result was a cultural shift in the community. "More people began standing up to say, yes, we need to do this" (Campaign for Action, 2018b para. 8).

As a result, in 2015, New Orleans joined the, approximately, 700 smoke-free cities nationwide (movement). Six months after the ordinance took effect, the city's air quality drastically improved, and 8 out of 10 voters voiced support for the ordinance. Additionally, calls from Orleans Parish to the Louisiana Tobacco Quitline increased by 20% (refreezing). Parent notes "Nurses have the ability to educate, to empathize, and to navigate people toward what they need to make a change. That is a strength and key characteristic of nursing" (Campaign for Action, 2018b para. 15).

Linda Sarna, PhD, RN, FAAN, and Stella Aguinaga Bialous, DrPH, RN, FAA, have also been change agents in smoking cessation. In 2003, Sarna and Bialous received funding from the Robert Wood Johnson Foundation to create *Tobacco Free Nurses*, the first national program to help nurses stop smoking and help their patients do the same (Campaign for action, 2017b). Sarna and Bialous note that nurses generally want to quit smoking, but they still have some of the same misconceptions regarding nicotine addiction as the general public. Education as well as logistical and emotional support were the key to unfreezing.

To initiate movement, Bialous and Sarna worked with the American Academy of Nursing and the American Association of Colleges of Nursing to develop a Smoke- and Tobacco-Free Schools of Nursing Tool Kit that emphasizes the importance of self-care and includes links to smoking cessation resources (Campaign for action, 2017b). Refreezing, however, is still in progress. Many nurses continue to smoke, and the percentage of smokers among licensed practical nurses (LPNs) significantly exceeds the national average. Still, since this program launched in 2003, there has been a 36% decline in the prevalence of smoking among registered nurses as well as a proliferation of tools known to help smokers quit (Campaign for action, 2017b).

The Creation of Caregiver Tool Kits

A DNP project completed by Ashley Fuller in 2017 explored the psychological distress, depression, anxiety, social isolation, poor quality of life, and ineffective coping experienced by many individuals providing care for the chronically ill (Nursing U Mass Amherst, 2018). Following an integrative review of the literature (unfreezing), a caregiver tool kit was created (movement). This *Powerful Tools for Caregivers* (PTC) was designed to increase awareness to help caregivers cope with and communicate more effectively in the caregiving role. It also helped increase knowledge among providers and family caregivers and focused on the use of community resources, support over the caregiving trajectory, and effective communication between caregivers and providers. Awareness of the PTC program among providers and caregivers positively correlated with a decrease in this burden and improved health status and functioning, which led to enhanced coping, problem-solving, and communication (refreezing).

Questions to Ask Yourself

1. What change agents have been positive role models for me?
2. What behaviors in particular would I want to emulate if acting as a change agent?

Preventing Lead Poisoning

Mel Callan, a family nurse practitioner (FNP) from Rochester, New York, brought attention to the problem of lead poisoning in cities by writing a guest column for the *Democrat & Chronicle* in January 2016 in the wake of the Flint, MI, lead poisoning scandal (unfreezing) (Family Nurse Practitioner Heroes, 2014–2018). Rochester had passed a safe water ordinance in 2005, and over the next 10 years, the City's Office of Inspection and Compliance Services performed 129,000 inspections (movement), with a resultant 85% reduction in reported lead poisoning of children younger than 6 years in the county. In a call for awareness and action, Callan has advocated for the ongoing testing of all pre-1978 homes, as well as for all children who may have been exposed (refreezing).

The Quality and Safety Education for Nurses Initiative

To address the problem of rampant medical errors and the lack of a safety culture in most healthcare organizations, Linda Cronenwett, PhD, FAAN, and Dean of the University of North Carolina at Chapel Hill School of Nursing, spearheaded the establishment of The Quality and Safety Education for Nurses (QSEN) project in 2005. The project had three phases between 2005 and 2012 (QSEN, 2020). All three phases shared the same goal: preparing future nurses with the knowledge, skills, and attitudes (KSAs) necessary to continuously improve the quality and safety of the healthcare systems in which they work (unfreezing). With the addition of more nurse leaders to the QSEN team over the past 13 years, the project has been able to identify six competencies, integrate the competencies into pilot schools, and host successful national forums and regional faculty development institutes to teach faculty leaders about quality and safety education for use at both the undergraduate and graduate levels (movement).

What began then as a grassroots movement funded by the Robert Wood Johnson Foundation has grown into a national initiative, evident in accreditation standards in both academia and practice (Altmiller & Dolansky, 2017). The organization maintains an active website with more than 120 teaching strategies, along with annotated bibliographies, learning modules, videos, and links to related websites such as a free massive open online course about quality improvement (refreezing). In addition, the 14 Task Forces and 8 QSEN Institute Regional Centers work collaboratively to create a wider network of nurses and other healthcare professionals to contribute to quality and safety educational resources and scholarship. All these efforts inspire healthcare professionals to identify quality and safety now as core values to guide their work (refreezing) (Altmiller & Dolansky, 2017).

Future Opportunities for Advance Practice Nurse–Led Change

Clearly, APN-led changes are already impacting the healthcare landscape. Yet, opportunities still exist for APNs to be change champions in addressing ongoing scope-of-practice barriers, insufficient interprofessional collaboration, inadequate access to care for consumers, and limited reimbursement from insurance payers for APN-provided care. In addition, APNs should be front and center in taking on new roles that fill gaps in the healthcare market, particularly those that center around the coordination of care.

Removing Scope-of-Practice Barriers

Despite the IOM's (2011) assertion that nurses should be leading change and advancing health by caring for populations within complex healthcare systems, many barriers still exist that prevent APNs from practicing to the full extent of their training and education. Overlaps in professional scopes of practice, organizational policy and structure, and the inability to grant privileges to nurses based upon their education and skills continue to pose barriers for nurses in healthcare systems to fully advocate for their patients (Lucatorto et al., 2016).

For example, Moss et al. (2016) note that although nursing practice begins with a professional statement of practice and code of ethics to support decision-making, these core professional nursing tenets are then subjected to interpretation by each state, territory, and district. The result is differing scopes of practice for RNs, based solely on geographic location, with state-defined scopes of practice for RNs often being further restricted at the organizational level through enactment of policy and procedure (Moss et al., 2016).

Hain and Fleck (2014) agree that state licensure can be a barrier to NPs practicing to the fullest extent of their education and training. Licensure and practice laws for NPs vary per state, despite a main goal of full-practice authority. For example, Johnson and Garvin (2017) note that in at least 45 states, APNs can prescribe medications, but only 16 states have granted APNs authority to practice independently without physician collaboration or supervision. In states where this independent practice is not allowed, APNs must practice under the auspices of a doctor or a medical institution.

This was the case for Immaculata Inyang, an FNP who saw a need in 2013 to provide low-cost care to vulnerable populations in underserved areas. Using her own money, she started the Potter's House Family clinic, one of the 200 nurse-owned practices and clinics in Texas (Jacosbson, 2013; Potter's House Family Clinic, 2018). Despite having a statewide shortage of primary care doctors, Inyang met resistance as well as barriers to independent practice. In Texas, NPs can open an office in medically underserved areas but no farther than 75 miles from their physician supervisors. And those doctors must be present in the nurse's office at least 1 day out of 10 and review at least 10% of the cases.

At about the same time, Rose Okoro, a nurse practitioner who specialized in family medicine, opened the Daystar Family Clinic in Katy, Texas (Ura, 2014). Seven months later, she had only enough patients for part-time work. It was not a lack of demand. It was because state regulations did not allow her to be reimbursed by insurance companies unless the physician who supervised her had a contract with those companies. Texas lawmakers loosened some supervision requirements during the 2013 legislative session following a compromise with physician groups, which argued that nurse practitioners do not have the training or experience to be entirely independent, but nurse practitioners are still battling for increased autonomy in the state Medicaid program as of 2018.

Catherine Alicia Georges, EdD, RN, FAAN, President-elect of AARP, concludes that although more states are recognizing the value of authorizing APNs to provide the full scope of services, they are educated and certified to provide, "there's no way we're going to get full practice authority in all the states unless we really push to build coalitions" (Campaign for action, 2017a para. 4). "We've got to constantly affirm who we are, what we're about, and keep getting this message loud and clear to people who have not been our partners in the past. Nurses need to get to the folks who have been the naysayers, and we need to make sure that we use the science and the data that we have to move our agenda forward" (Campaign for action, 2017a para. 4). Eliminating variances in state licensure and scope-of-practice and removing barriers to independent practice are necessary elements of providing high-quality primary care (Hain & Fleck, 2014).

Increasing the Recognition of the Value of APNs

Another barrier to APNs achieving full scope of practice is insufficient interprofessional collaboration among healthcare providers from multiple disciplines (Moss et al., 2016). Some physician professional organizations, including the American Medical Association (AMA), believe that because physicians have longer and more rigorous training, NPs are incapable of providing quality, safe care at the same level (Hain & Fleck, 2014). This may contribute to the confusion among many physicians regarding the role of NPs. In addition, some physicians and other healthcare professionals do not fully understand NP scope of practice.

Other groups or organizations do not fully recognize full scope of practice for all types of APNs. In December 2016, the Department of Veterans Affairs granted only three of the four APRN roles (nurse practitioners, certified nurse midwives, and clinical nurse specialists) the ability to practice to the full extent of their education and training. The new policy excluded certified registered nurse anesthetists (Johnson & Garvin, 2017).

Assuring Continued Access to Care for Consumers

Jennie Chin Hansen, RN, MS, FAAN, former CEO of American Geriatrics Society, notes that recent congressional efforts have put the healthcare coverage of millions of people at risk (Campaign for action, 2017a). She asks "How can we continue to enable better health when people may not have the same access to care? I hope that nurses will take a leadership role and find creative ways to help people realize their best health, even if there are policy changes that create instability" (para. 8). Hansen encourages nurses to use the Institute for Healthcare Improvement's Triple Aim—better health, better care, and lower cost—as an organizing framework and concludes that nurses will have a vital role to play in safeguarding people's health even as the healthcare landscape changes in 2018 (Campaign for action, 2017a).

Mary Wakefield, PhD, RN, FAAN, acting U.S. Deputy Secretary of Health and Human Services in the Obama administration concurs, noting that an estimated 17.8 million people have coverage now through the health insurance marketplaces or through the Medicaid expansion created by the Affordable Care Act. "To see that coverage erode is highly problematic for those individuals and families that are directly impacted. Furthermore, removing the individual mandate will ultimately drive up the cost of insurance for everyone. Continued access to health insurance coverage also has an impact on the healthcare system itself. The most vulnerable components of the delivery system, such as small, rural hospitals, have fairly fragile financial bottom lines and depend heavily on people coming through the doors with insurance coverage" (Campaign for action, 2017a para. 11).

Antonia Villarruel, PhD, RN, FAAN, Dean, University of Pennsylvania School of Nursing, believes that the uneasiness in healthcare about the Affordable Care Act and tax reform will provide opportunities for nurses to lead as the emphasis will continue to be on value-based healthcare as well as costs (Stokowski, 2018). Furthermore, "increased recognition and attention to the many factors that influence health (at home, school, community, and neighborhoods) will result in a continued emphasis on creating healthy environments for all people" (Stokowski, 2018, p. 4).

Seeking Full Reimbursement for APNs From Insurance Payers

Hain and Fleck (2014) suggest that payer polices also continue to have a significant impact on the ability of NPs to practice to the full extent of their licensure and training. This is because payer policies are often linked to restrictive state practice regulations and licensure. In addition, commercial health plan payment policies vary and may not recognize NPs as primary care providers. In addition, these payers may be resistant to credentialing or directly paying NPs for services they provide.

Peter Buerhaus, PhD, RN, FAAN, director, Center for Interdisciplinary Health Workforce Studies at Montana State University College of Nursing, suggests the use of "incident to" billing by the Centers for Medicare and Medicaid Services (CMS) compounds the problem (Campaign for action, 2017a). These rules allow physicians to use their provider numbers to bill for services that were provided by an NP "incident to" the physician's diagnosis. Because physicians are reimbursed at a higher rate than NPs, there is an incentive to bill "incident to."

Buerhaus notes that the frequency of "incident to" billing is unknown because CMS does not require that it be identified as such in its claims data. This makes it difficult for researchers, policymakers, and government entities to understand the contributions of NPs providing both primary and specialty care. "If we can't figure out who actually provided which service, then the goals of MACRA (the Medicare Access and CHIP Reauthorization Act of 2015) to reward clinicians for value-based care are undermined" (Campaign for action, 2017a para. 13).

Questions to Ask Yourself

1. How much energy do I have to be involved in change efforts directed by APNs?
2. What might be my first steps to getting involved in change efforts impacting my profession?

Exploring New Roles for APNs

Other new opportunities for change focus on new emerging roles for APNs, since entrepreneurs often innovate by seeking market gaps unseen by other health disciplines (Johnson & Garvin, 2017). Many of these emerging opportunities center around the coordination of care. For example, Austin (2016) notes that APNs can play a larger role in facilitating care that crosses the divide between in- and outpatient care. Some healthcare organizations are looking at implementing models in which APNs follow patients through the continuum of care, from outpatient clinic to inpatient stay and through discharge back to clinic for follow-up.

Similarly, Antonia Villarruel notes that "nurses must be ready to provide care in unlikely places, such as drugstores and retail outlets, because we see care shifting away from the hospital and into a more home-based and community-based care model. In addition, attention to transitions in care, such as hospital to home, home to hospital, and home to hospice, provide a great opportunity to safely lead teams of caregivers to ensure safe transitions" (Stokowski, 2018, para. 3).

Villarruel adds "nurses need to be able to traverse the landscape—from home, school, community, primary care, acute care, hospice, et cetera—to support patients and families. The use of technology will not replace nurses; rather, it will open up new opportunities to communicate and support patients and families in a variety of settings" (Stokowski, 2018, para. 4).

Other emerging roles for APNs are developing globally due to the worldwide need for expert nursing care at an advanced level of practice (Kleinpell et al., 2014). Implementation challenges, however, include poor role clarification, proliferation of APRN titles, differing educational requirements and degrees, scope-of-practice conflicts, fragmentation/variability in standards, and quality of educational programs (Kleinpell et al., 2014).

Questions to Ask Yourself

1. Do I currently have the skill sets needed to be an effective change agent?
2. What is my risk-taking propensity in being a leader for change?

Summary

Baker and Williams (2016) suggest that because change is so difficult, nurses must create a guiding vision, take incremental steps toward that vision, and not lose heart when faced with obstacles. They must also "embrace revolutionary ideas that are implemented in an evolutionary manner. Nurses must not forget that they are part of a community of care providers and may need to help others embrace this vision and their role in actualizing it. Through that process, nurses can eliminate limits and barriers to their current practice and deliver on the promise of their potential" (Baker and Williams, 2016, para. 11).

Salmon and Echevarria (2017, para. 2) agree, noting that "to be a major player in shaping change, nurses must understand the factors driving the change, the mandates for practice change, and the competencies (knowledge, skills, and attitudes) that will be needed for personal and systemwide success. This new health paradigm requires the nurse to be a full partner in relentless efforts to achieve the triple aim of an improved patient experience of care (including quality and satisfaction), improved outcomes or health of populations, and a reduction in the per capita cost of healthcare."

Beaumont Health (2018, para. 1) suggests that "every nurse is a leader, no matter the position or work setting and that nurses need to articulate their value as professionals and demonstrate their leadership skills as they negotiate patient care, support and coach one another and implement changes in practice. Transforming the healthcare environment is a complex issue and nurses with strong leadership skills are the professionals who make a difference."

Beaumont Health (2018) goes on to suggest that the pace of change in healthcare is constantly increasing, which creates both challenges and opportunities for nurses and other healthcare professionals. The opportunity is that nurses can have a greater voice in articulating their value to their peers, to the nursing profession, and to healthcare organizations across the continuum of care. Advanced practice nurses must heed the call.

Chapter Highlights

- Change is pervasive in contemporary healthcare organizations.
- Lewin (1951) theorized that people maintain a state of status quo or equilibrium by the simultaneous occurrence of both driving forces (facilitators) and restraining forces (barriers) operating within any field.
- Lewin (1951) also identified three phases that must occur before a planned change becomes part of the system: unfreezing, movement, and refreezing.

- What often differentiates a successful change effort from an unsuccessful one is the ability of the change agent to deal appropriately with conflicted human emotions and to connect and balance all aspects of the organization that will be affected by that change.
- Change should be implemented only for good reasons.
- Because change is such a complex process, it requires a great deal of planning and intricate timing.
- The change agent, whenever possible, must involve all those who may be affected by a change in planning for that change.
- Resistance is a naturally occurring, expected response to change or a disruption of the status quo.
- Initiating change and diffusing and sustaining innovation are critical elements of APN leadership competency.
- There are many opportunities for APNs to lead and diffuse collaborative improvement efforts and to innovate in practice and education.

Web Resources

The Future of Nursing: Leading Change, Advancing Health: http://nationalacademies.org/hmd/reports/2010/the-future-of-nursing-leading-change-advancing-health.aspx
Change Leader's Network: http://changeleadersnetwork.com/free-resources

---

References

Altmiller, G., & Dolansky, M. A. (2017). QSEN: Looking forward. *Nurse Educator, 42*(5s), S1–S2.
American Nurses Association. (2015). *Nursing: Scope and standards of practice* (3rd ed.).
Austin, D. (2016). *New roles for nurse practitioners bring opportunities and challenges.* Science of Caring; University of California San Francisco. https://scienceofcaring.ucsf.edu/patient-care/new-roles-nurse-practitioners-bring-opportunities-and-challenges
Baker, K., & Williams, T. E. (2016). Overview and summary: Elimination of barriers to RN scope of practice. Opportunities and challenges. *The Online Journal of Issues in Nursing, 21*(3), 1. https://ojin.nursingworld.org/MainMenuCategories/ANAMarketplace/ANAPeriodicals/OJIN/TableofContents/Vol-21-2016/No3-Sept-2016/OS-Elimination-of-Barriers-to-RN-Scope-of-Practice.html
Beaumont Health. (2018). *Taking the lead 2018 leading change – The value of nurses in healthcare transformation.* https://www.regonline.com/builder/site/Default.aspx?EventID=2045275
Bradberry, T. (2017). *10 harsh lessons that will make you more successful.* The Huffington Post. http://www.huffingtonpost.com/dr-travis-bradberry/10-harsh-lessons-that-wil_b_14422346.html

Campaign for Action. (2017a). *Five nurse leaders share policy wishes for 2018.* https://campaign-foraction.org/five-nurse-leaders-share-policy-wishes-2018/

Campaign for Action. (2017b). *The great American smokeout is for nurses too* https://campaign-foraction.org/the-great-american-smokeout-is-for-nurses-too/

Campaign for Action. (2018a). *From one coast to another, nurse brings health to neighborhoods in need.* https://campaignforaction.org/one-coast-another-nurse-brings-health-neighborhoods-need/

Campaign for Action. (2018b). *Nurse helped coax the big easy to go smoke-free.* https://campaign-foraction.org/nurse-helped-coax-big-easy-go-smoke-free/

Campaign for Action. (2018c). *She opened the first nurse-led care practice in West Virginia.* https://campaignforaction.org/she-opened-the-first-nurse-led-care-practice-in-west-virginia/

Gray-Micheli, D., Mazzia, L., & Crane, G. (2017). Advanced practice nurse-led statewide collaborative to reduce falls in hospitals. *Journal of Nursing Care Quality, 32*(2), 120–125.

Hain, D., & Fleck, L. (2014). Barriers to nurse practitioner practice that impact healthcare redesign. *The Online Journal of Issues in Nursing, 19*(2), 2. http://ojin.nursingworld.org/MainMenuCategories/ANAMarketplace/ANAPeriodicals/OJIN/TableofContents/Vol-19-2014/No2-May-2014/Barriers-to-NP-Practice.html

Hamric, A. B., Hanson, C. M., Tracy, M. F., & O'Grady, E. T. (2014). *Advanced practice nursing: An integrative approach* (5th ed.). Elsevier/Saunders.

Institute of Medicine. (2011). *Future of nursing: Leading change, advancing health.* National Academies Press.

Jacobson, S. (2013). *Nurse-owned practices, clinics trying to get a foothold in Texas.* Dallas News. https://www.dallasnews.com/news/news/2013/03/20/nurse-owned-practices-clinics-trying-to-get-a-foothold-in-texas

Johnson, J. E., & Garvin, W. S. (2017). Advanced practice nurses: Developing a business plan for an independent ambulatory clinical practice. *Nursing Economic, 35*(3), 126–141.

Kleinpell, R., Scanlon, A., Hibbert, D., Ganz, F., East, L., Fraser, D., Kam Yuet Wong, F., & Beauchesne, M. (2014). Addressing issues impacting advanced nursing practice worldwide. *The Online Journal of Issues in Nursing, 19*(2), 5. http://ojin.nursingworld.org/MainMenuCategories/ANAMarketplace/ANAPeriodicals/OJIN/TableofContents/Vol-19-2014/No2-May-2014/Advanced-Nursing-Practice-Worldwide.html

Larson, J. A. (2015). *Strategy as planned change.* Jean Ann Larson & Associates. http://www.jeanannlarson.org/2015/08/05/strategy-as-planned-change/

Leaf, C. (2018). *2 forces that will drive the health industry.* Fortune/Time Inc. http://fortune.com/2018/01/03/health-care-industry-2018/

Lewin, K. (1951). *Field theory in social science: Selected theoretical papers (ed. D. Cartwright).* Harper & Row.

Lucatorto, M. A., Thomas, T. W., & Siek, T. (2016). Registered nurses as caregivers: Influencing the system as patient advocates. *The Online Journal of Issues in Nursing, 21*(3), 2. http://ojin.nursingworld.org/MainMenuCategories/ANAMarketplace/ANAPeriodicals/OJIN/TableofContents/Vol-21-2016/No3-Sept-2016/Registered-Nurses-as-Caregivers-Influencing-the-System-as-Patient-Advocates.html

Marquis, B., & Huston, C. J. (2020). *Leadership roles and management functions in nursing* (10th ed.). Wolters Kluwer.

Melnyk, B., Malloch, K., & Gallagher-Ford, L. (2017). Developing effective leaders to meet 21st century health care challenges. In Huston, C. (Ed.), *Professional issues in nursing: Challenges and opportunities* (Chap. 3). Wolters Kluwer.

Moss, E., Seifert, C. P., & O'Sullivan, A. (2016). Registered nurses as interprofessional collaborative partners: Creating value-based outcomes. *The Online Journal of Issues in Nursing, 21*(3), 4. http://ojin.nursingworld.org/MainMenuCategories/ANAMarketplace/ANAPeriodicals/OJIN/TableofContents/Vol-21-2016/No3-Sept-2016/Registered-Nurses-as-Interprofessional-Collaborative-Partners.html

Nursing U Mass Amherst. (2018). *Doctor of nursing practice (DNP) projects.* An educational intervention to alleviate the effects of burden of chronic illness care: Presentation of a caregiver toolkit to increase awareness among primary care providers and family caregivers. Scholar Works. https://scholarworks.umass.edu/nursing_dnp_capstone/95/

Potter's House Family Clinic. (2018). *Homepage.* Manta. https://www.manta.com/c/mxj3hqn/potter-s-house-family-clinic

QSEN Institute. (2020). *Project overview: The evolution of the quality and safety education for nurses (QSEN) initiative.* https://qsen.org/about-qsen/project-overview/#:~:text=Nurses%20(QSEN)%20Initiative-,The%20Quality%20and%20Safety%20Education%20for,QSEN)%20project%20began%20in%202005.&text=The%20competencies%20included%20five%20from,improvement%20and%20informatics%2C%20and%20safety

Salmon, M., & Echevarria, M. (2017). Healthcare transformation and changing roles for nursing. *Orthopedic Nursing, 36*(1), 12–25. https://www.ncbi.nlm.nih.gov/pmc/articles/PMC5266427/

Schrier, K. (2014). *Facing change to change the face of women's health.* University of Utah; Nursing News. https://nursing.utah.edu/blog/2014/changing_face_of_womens_health.php

Stoker, J. R. (2018). *Are you getting in your own way? Get more of what you want and less of what you don't.* Smart Brief. http://smartbrief.com/original/2018/02/are-you-getting-your-own-way-get-more-what-you-want-and-less-what-you?utm_source=brief&utm_source=AAL+-Clients+and+Alumni&utm_campaign=ca3286b0c6-Noteworthy_February_2018_AAL_Subscribers&utm_medium=email&utm_term=0_71cff7fbd0-ca3286b0c6-432678093

Stokowski, L. A. (2018). *What will this year bring for nurses?* Medscape. https://www.medscape.com/viewarticle/891393#vp_2

Tams, C. (2018). *Why we need to rethink organizational change management.* Forbes. https://www.forbes.com/sites/carstentams/2018/01/26/why-we-need-to-rethink-organizational-change-management/#6e65e098e93c

The University of Utah. (2014). *Facing change to face the change of women's health.* https://nursing.utah.edu/blog/2014/changing_face_of_womens_health.php

Thomas, G. (2018). *Use these 4 strategies to manage resistance to change.* Leadership First. https://www.leadershipfirst.expert/single-post/2018/03/07/Use-These-4-Strategies-to-Manage-Resistance-to-Change

Ura, A. (2014). *Nurse practitioners say that greater autonomy would cure challenges.* The Texas Tribune. https://www.texastribune.org/2014/05/18/nurse-practitioners-struggle-integrate-medicaid/

PART FIVE

Scholarship for Advanced Roles

14

Nurse Scholars

Karen Morin

LEARNING OBJECTIVES

After completing this chapter, you will be able to:

1. Identify the attributes of a scholar.

2. Differentiate between Boyer's four types of scholarship.

3. Compare different approaches with disseminating information.

4. Describe key principles to which to adhere during presentations.

5. Define critical components to include when developing an abstract.

KEY TERMS

Abstract: A brief description of a manuscript, podium presentation, or poster.

Author: A person who makes a significant contribution to a manuscript, podium presentation, or poster.

Concurrent session: A podium presentation given at the same time as other podium presentations.

Disseminate: Share information widely through a variety of means, particularly publication and presentation.

Duplicate publishing: Occurs when the same paper, or one with considerable overlap, is published when a paper with the same information has already been published.

Ghost authorship: Occurs when a person meets the criteria for authorship but is not acknowledged as an author.

Honorary author: Authorship that is assigned to persons whom do not meet the criteria for authorship.

Impact factor: A mathematical calculation that indicates the frequency with which the average article is cited in a year. Impact factor can indicate the rank of a journal by calculating the times its articles are cited.

Peer-reviewed: A person's work that has been reviewed for quality and rigor by peers.

Plagiarism: The use of another's work without proper attribution.

Plenary session: A session at which several hundred to thousands of conference attendees are present.

Podium presentation: An oral presentation at a conference of a person's work. This may be a research paper or topic of interest in which the speaker has expertise. Podium presentations are generally competitive and require submission of an abstract for judging to be selected to present.

Poster presentation: A static visual representation of a person's work.

Scholar: An individual who has advanced education, attends school, or is a learned person.

Scholarship: The communication of knowledge gained through the many forms of inquiry (research, synthesis, translation, application).

Scholarship of application: Requires scholars to apply knowledge to solve relevant problems.

Scholarship of discovery: Represents original research efforts that generate new knowledge.

Scholarship of integration: Occurs when knowledge is synthesized within a broader context to provide a comprehensive understanding of an issue.

Scholarship of teaching: Focuses on teaching practices that enhance learning.

Self-plagiarism: The use of one's own prior published work verbatim in a new publication without proper attribution.

Introduction

"You should consider making an impact on the scholarly conversation of your field, from the very beginning of your career."

(Huff, 1999, p. 9)

A scholar is an individual who has "done advanced study in a special field, attends a school, or is a learned person" (Merriam-Webster Online Dictionary, 2020). Not only do scholars have additional knowledge, but they also possess critical attributes (Conrad & Pape, 2014). Scholars think critically and solve problems. Scholars interact collaboratively and collegially with professional colleagues within and outside their discipline. Importantly, they display integrity, honesty, creativity, and passion when undertaking scholarly activities. Advanced practice nurses (APNs) qualify as scholars because the acquisition of additional knowledge and expertise in a clinical or functional area is essential to their role.

Whether procuring a master's or doctoral degree, APN graduates are expected to have skills reflective of a scholar. For example, the American Association of Colleges of Nursing's (AACN) *Essentials of Master's Education* (American Association of Colleges of Nursing, 2011) includes an essential element (Essential IV) addressing the translation and integration of scholarship into practice. Element IV highlights that being able to acquire knowledge and disseminate it to a variety of audiences is a critical skill. This skill also is emphasized in AACN's *Essentials of Doctoral Education for Advanced Nursing Practice* (DNP) (2006). Explicit expectations include preparing DNPs to "Disseminate findings from evidence-based practice and research to improve healthcare outcomes" (p. 12). Being a scholar and contributing to the professional scholarly conversation are important and integral parts of the role of an APN that reflects "a commitment to the advancement of the profession" (Conrad & Pape, 2014, p. 87). Sometimes, APNs may not believe they have information to share and could never become a scholar or not consider himself or herself a scholar. However, APNs have important knowledge to share with their professional colleagues and the lay community. Information presented in this chapter is designed to help APNs develop their confidence and their role as a scholar.

Boyer's Model of Scholarship

No discussion of scholarship is complete without clarifying what constitutes scholarship. AACN, in their position statement on scholarship, defines it as "the generation, synthesis, translation, application, and dissemination of knowledge that aims to improve health and transform healthcare" (2018, p. 2). Moreover, "scholarship is the communication of knowledge generated through multiple forms of inquiry that inform clinical practice, nursing education, policy, and healthcare delivery" (p. 2). These definitions are consistent with the model of scholarship put forth by Boyer (1990).

Boyer (1990) wrote one of the most influential works on the topic. He argued that the traditional definition of scholarship, that is, the conduct and reporting of research, did not capture all the work conducted in academic institutions. Rather, other forms of scholarship are equally valuable and contribute to increasing knowledge. He presented four unique but overlapping kinds of scholarship—discovery, integration, application, and teaching—that have been embraced by many academic institutions and professional organizations, including AACN.

APNs are most familiar with scholarship of discovery, which represents original research efforts with an emphasis on generating new knowledge. Examples include obtaining external funding for a research project, presenting research findings at a conference, and sharing findings with lay communities (AACN Position Statement, 2018).

In Their Own Words

Kim Litwack, PhD, RN, FAAN, APNP

The key points in understanding how I became a recognized speaker are…
There are several reasons I am asked to speak. However, the most important reasons are my expertise and the relevance of that expertise to the needs of the organization. The breadth of my expertise widens the potential venues at which I may be asked to speak. Take, for example, the opioid crisis. It is front and center in practice, scholarship, and policy venues. My knowledge of

(Continued)

pain assessment and management, including knowledge of opioids, may be helpful in a practice venue, but the ability to apply my expertise incorporating scholarship and evidence-based initiatives on opioid use and safety and the impact of my expertise on healthcare policy about opioids will widen the speaking opportunities I may have. Thus, not only may I be asked to speak to local healthcare providers, I may be asked to speak before a policy-making body.

Asking me to speak is not based on my education but is based on my credentials, in consideration of the intended audience. If your goal is to speak in front of national leaders, policy makers, and other scholars, degrees do matter. Certifications, if appropriate and available, matter. Your experience in the field/topic matters. Can you "walk the walk" in addition to "talk the talk"?

Asking you to speak is also based on your ability to communicate. Can you communicate well to your audience? You can develop your communication skills with practice, in small groups, in the classroom setting, and in meetings. I am a very good educator, comfortable in front of small and large groups.

You can increase your visibility as a potential speaker by… Establishing yourself as a scholar means disseminating your work with others. This includes publications, presentations, via the media, social media, and even volunteering. Publishing in journals with high impact and high readership will increase the likelihood that others come to know you and your field of expertise. Others seeking that knowledge or looking for speakers will see your name come up, consistently and repeatedly, when doing literature searches on the topic requiring a speaker. Visibility in nonrefereed lay publications with wide readership may also prove helpful if you are seen as an expert on a subject. As an example, my experience in pain management may connect me with a public audience for presentation, as well as being able to represent the consumer side of a subject at a professional meeting.

You can increase your visibility via **ACTIVE** membership in national professional organizations, where others with similar interests come to know your expertise in a given area. Many of these organizations have "special interest groups" or "expert panels" where individuals with a specific interest or expertise meet and work together to advance knowledge and policy and/or to collaborate on research. As examples, the American Academy of Nursing currently (in 2018) has 24 expert panels. Sigma Theta Tau (in 2018) maintains "Communities of Interest" in 15 different focal areas.

Another way to increase your visibility is to make yourself known to others via speakers' bureaus or expert lists often maintained by your university or places of employment. When an issue surfaces nationally, you may have the opportunity to comment on local, state, or national issues on a local TV or radio station.

(Continued)

If you have a creative streak, you may be able to increase your visibility via social media, to include the development of a blog, web site, or podcasts, as examples, to become known to others. Visibility increase the potential you will be asked to speak.

You need to determine your priorities... It will be important to determine your priorities in seeking out speaking opportunities. If, as an example, you are on a tenure track line, local or poster presentations may not have value in a tenure decision and may take time away from your ability to do your research. Presentations done at a national or even international meeting of eminence in your discipline may have tremendous value. Submitting a poster presentation may begin your visibility at a national meeting but remember that this may be at your own expense. Once you become an invited speaker, the inviting group will often cover your expenses. There are individuals who have established their expertise in continuing education or practice venues. These may prove lucrative to you, but again, consider the impact of these commitments to you as you develop as a scholar. That said, presenting at a national, well-attended clinician-dominated conference will help increase your visibility.

Why I keep accepting speaking requests... I accept speaking requests for many different reasons. When I was on the tenure track, one of the criteria for promotion and tenure was establishing myself on the local, state, national, and ultimately international level. One way to do this was to present myself and my work. I have also accepted speaking requests to advance the profession. When I first entered nursing in the field of perianesthesia care, there were no textbooks, no educational workshops, and no certification for perianesthesia nurses. I authored one of the first textbooks on the specialty and multiple articles on the specialty and, as a result, was ultimately asked to speak at 42 of the 50 state perianesthesia organizations. I looked at it as a way to advance the specialty.

I wish someone had told me... Not every email inviting you to speak is worth saying yes to. I actually knew this and never fell victim, but think it is important for new scholars. I use that word intentionally, to emails "based on your expertise in (fill in your expertise), we invite you to present at the..." conference in (fill in the international city). Daily, I find myself invited to Spain, Las Vegas, Dubai (to name a few from this past week) to present at conferences and to organizations that do not value my expertise at all, but value having a speaker, any speaker from a University, who can add to the international nature of their conference, where they (read the small print) expect you to pay all of your own travel expenses and registration to the conference.

Scholarship of integration requires "making connections across disciplines, placing the specialties in larger context, illuminating data in a revealing way" (Boyer, 1990, p. 18). It requires scholars to synthesize either their own research efforts or those of others within a broader context and emphasizes the critical need to contribute to a comprehensive understanding of an issue. Examples of integration are offering a professional development workshop or writing a systematic review.

Scholarship of application, sometimes called the scholarship of engagement (Dewar et al., 2018), requires scholars to apply knowledge to solve relevant problems. Graduates of master's and doctoral programs are well positioned to undertake this type of scholarship, as outcomes of these educational programs require graduates to demonstrate their ability to make changes in practice based on evidence. Importantly, as APNs often interact with professional organizations and perform community service, these activities also are recognized as being scholarly (Conrad & Pape, 2014). Examples include quality improvement projects and serving as a consultant on a specific topic or problem.

Scholarship of teaching focuses on teaching practices that enhance learning. As such, it is important for faculty to continue to learn so they are "not only transmitting knowledge but *transforming* and *extending* it as well" (Boyer, 1990, p. 24). An example of this type of scholarship is an innovative teaching strategy. *The Journal of Nursing Education* publishes scholarship of teaching in its "Educational Innovations" section. Additional information about Boyer's model is presented in Table 14.1.

Dissemination

A critical activity of scholarship is disseminating information reflective of an APN's expertise. There are many different forms by which APNs can share or disseminate their work. An APN can choose to offer a podium presentation or poster at a regional, national, or international conference. Perhaps writing an article for a peer-reviewed journal is a more attractive method of disseminating one's work and sharing one's expertise. Irrespective of the method of dissemination, a typical first step in dissemination is developing an abstract.

Table 14.1. Boyer's Model of Scholarship Applied to Advanced Practice Nursing

APN Scholarship Components	Explanation	Examples
Scholarship of Discovery	Generation of new knowledge through scientific inquiry in the form of quantitative or qualitative research to understand phenomena, examine relationships, or test interventions with populations of interest. Aim is to generate new knowledge, refine or expand existing knowledge that is translatable into practice. Can address social determinants of health to understand effects of healthcare and interventions on patient-centered outcomes.	Publishes or presents peer-reviewed publications or presentations of research, theory, or philosophical essays; secures competitive extramural funding for research; leads research teams at local, state, national levels; develops innovative scientific approaches that inform practice and advance healthcare methods; consults as an academic research partners in clinical setting; recognized as a scholar in an identified area at state, regional, national, or international levels; creates new theoretical frameworks and/or theory to guide, test, and disseminate the work of new phenomena.
Scholarship of Application/Practice	Application of evidence to nursing practice by implementation and translation science. Addresses the gap between theory and practice. Requires application of innovative methods to improve and transform healthcare delivery and patient outcomes. Implementation of evidence-based practices allows for testing to look for improvements to improve care and outcomes.	Establishes and disseminates best practices. Publishes to influence practice. Publishes and presents to audiences to influence practice. Serves as a clinical practice specialist in partnerships that advance research, clinical improvements, policy development, and/or implementation. Engages with stakeholders to conduct research that transforms practice. Establishes and evaluates quality improvement initiatives.

Scholarship of Teaching	Focuses on understanding, describing, and explaining teaching-learning strategies and evaluating their impact on student/patient learning. Applying theoretical concepts to guide teaching practices, curriculum development, and foster learning. Uses, evaluates, and disseminates innovative approaches to improve patient/student education.	Develops and implements evidence-based educational strategies. Develops new teaching methods and strategies to prepare students for a transformed healthcare system. Incorporates and evaluates the use of instructional technology in education of students and patients.
Scholarship of Integration	Integration of scholarship across the missions of research, practice, health policy, and teaching.	Uses data to inform population health strategies. Conducts demonstration projects and evaluates health system innovations and population health capabilities; implements quality and safety interventions across care setting and into community; supports transdisciplinary research teams with a focus on improving science and population health interventions; promotes formation of research programs in partnership with academicians, health, systems, and other professional schools.

Adapted from American Association of Colleges of Nursing. (2016). *Defining scholarship for academic nursing.* https://www.aacnnursing.org/News-Information/Position-Statements-White-Papers/Defining-Scholarship-Nursing.

Developing an Abstract

As a scholar, an APN may be required to write an abstract when submitting a manuscript for publication or in response to a professional organization's "Call for Abstracts" for conference speakers (see Box 14.1 for examples). An important skill the APN should develop is the ability to craft a well-written, clear, and succinct abstract that conveys what was done, investigated, or is being shared with an audience. In this section, what constitutes an abstract, including its importance, the types of abstracts, and what to include are discussed. In addition, helpful tips for writing an abstract are included in Box 14.2.

BOX 14.1

▶ EXAMPLES OF CALLS FOR ABSTRACTS

  Deadline: July 15, 2020

Sigma invites abstracts for Creating Healthy Work Environments. Join us 19 to 21 February 2021 in Austin, Texas, USA, at the event designed to help leaders in both academic and clinical settings develop, implement, and maintain strategies that will improve their organization's work environment.

Recommended presentation topics include the following:

- Enhancing Professional Well-Being

- Implementing the AACN Healthy Work Environment Standards

- Optimizing Patient Outcomes

- Promoting Interprofessional Collaborations

- Strengthening Healthy Work Environments

- Moral and Ethical Strategies and Solutions

- Supporting the Mental Health of Nurses

- Advocating for the Workforce and Environment

Deadline: Extended to January 6, 2021
46th Biennial Convention

Abstracts of translational research, evidence-based clinical projects, and leadership initiatives are invited. Abstracts must demonstrate a direct link to the convention theme above. NOTE: Selected guidelines are presented in this example. Abstract topics can address clinical practice, research, leadership, evidence-based and translational, or education topics.

Submission Guidelines. A complete oral or poster presentation submission includes the following:

Abstract Text Step:

The abstract should be a minimum of 300 words (not more than 500 words). We suggest that abstracts be developed in a word processing program before accessing the online submission form. Use the spell check and word count features of your word processor to check the text of the abstract before submitting it. There is no need to shorten lines so that they fit inside the box; the text will wrap automatically to fit. Please remove all references to the title and author information on the abstract before completing the submission. Authors should review the information submitted very carefully for spelling, punctuation, and grammatical errors. It will not be possible to change any information in the abstract once it is uploaded and posted to the Sigma Repository.

Bibliographic References Step:

Recommended references should include more than five scholarly references (e.g., science journal articles, books). References should be recent and/or appropriate for the abstract (references should be no older than 5 years, unless they are a seminal work).

From Sigma, 2020. *Sigma Call for Abstracts*. https://www.sigmanursing.org/connect-engage/meetings-events/calls-for-abstracts

BOX 14.2

▶ ABSTRACT WRITING TIPS

1. Including labels when crafting an unstructured abstract can help assure that relevant information is not ignored. These labels can be removed before submitting the abstract.

2. Organize your thoughts and follow a systematic approach when writing an abstract.

3. Plan enough time to rewrite and revise the abstract and to have a colleague review your work before submission.

4. Consider highlighting the date on the "Call," as conferences typically adhere to submission deadlines without exception.

5. Read abstract guidelines carefully whether the abstract is part of a manuscript or conference presentation submission.

6. Follow the guidelines explicitly.

The National Information Standards Organization (NISO) (2015) defines an abstract as a "brief, objective representation of the contents of a primary document or an oral presentation" (p. 1). Note the critical terms in this definition: brief, objective, document, and podium presentation; they are relevant to all types and structures of an abstract. According to the American Psychological Association (APA) (2020), an abstract "needs to be dense with information" (p. 26) and reflect the following characteristics: accuracy, conciseness, readability and coherence, and nonevaluative. Addressing these characteristics is important, as the abstract is the first opportunity a reader—whether in the role of a journal editor or a journal or conference reviewer—has to evaluate what the author is proposing.

The abstract can be the most important (APA, 2020) and visible (Heseltine, 2012) paragraph an APN writes. Journal editors use the abstract associated with a manuscript to decide whether to send a manuscript out for review. Manuscript reviewers use the abstract to determine whether to accept an invitation to review it. Conference planners use the abstract to determine the scientific integrity of a study or the relevance of a topic for their audience. A well-written abstract presenting accurate information facilitates reviewers' assessment of whether required key information is present. A well-written abstract enhances the possibility of a manuscript being accepted in a journal or of a presentation being accepted at a conference.

Types of Abstracts

Abstracts can vary in type, such as structured or unstructured (Leggett, 2018; Mott, 2014). A structured abstract has specific headings (see Boxes 14.3 and 14.4) that facilitate reviewer understanding and enhance consistency with information is presented. When crafting an unstructured abstract, a narrative paragraph approach is used. This type of an abstract does not include labels or headings; rather, it is comprised of continuous text in several paragraphs (Khasseh & Biranvand, 2013) (see Box 14.5). Including labels when crafting an unstructured abstract can help ensure that relevant information is not ignored. These labels can be removed prior to submitting the abstract.

BOX 14.3

▶ EXAMPLE OF A STRUCTURED RESEARCH ABSTRACT

Maternal Child Health Nurse Leader Academy: Comparison of North American and South African Outcomes

Purpose: To compare Leadership Mentor/Fellow knowledge, skills and leadership practices and patient outcomes of a leadership development program involving two cohorts in the Maternal-Child Health Nurse Leadership Academy (MCH NLA): The 2014 to 2015 North American (NA) cohort and the 2014 to 2015 South African (SA) cohort. Both cohorts were participants in a program to strengthen the leadership base of maternal-child bedside nurses in the United States and South Africa.

Rationale: Nurse Leaders have recognized the critical need for leadership development in nursing since the early 2000s. Consequently, healthcare institutions, professional nursing organizations, and academic institutions have offered leadership development programs that vary in structure, length, and outcome. Although these programs provide insight into leadership development, information about international leadership development programs is limited. The MCH NLA, sponsored by Sigma Theta Tau International, the Honor Society of Nursing, in partnership with Johnson & Johnson Corporate Contributions, and developed and facilitated by experts in maternal-child health, leadership, and organizational development, is an exception to this gap. The program, based on an established leadership model, engages participants in an 18-month mentored leadership experience within the context of an interdisciplinary team project. Leadership Mentor/Fellow dyads are paired with a faculty member during the leadership journey. Review of results from earlier North American cohorts indicates significant growth in leadership over time. Given differences in context and healthcare cultures, Leadership Mentor/Fellow and patient outcomes may be different in different areas of the world.

Methods: Retrospective cohort comparative study using secondary analysis. Data were collected at four points: baseline, following workshop 1, following workshop 2, and at convention.

Results: Twelve Leadership Mentor/Fellow dyads comprised the SA cohort; 14 dyads comprised the NA cohort. Leadership Mentors and Fellows in both cohorts increased in leadership outcomes; the most significant increase was between baseline and workshop 1. No significant differences were obtained between cohorts. Patterns of growth were similar. Review of project reports revealed they had the potential to impact more than 1,000 women, children, and healthcare providers.

Conclusions: A leadership program based on a global leadership model facilitates leadership development and has an impact on patient outcomes and is very implementable.

Word count: 351 (Could have 500 words)

Morin, K. H., Klopper, H. C., & Der Walt, C. V. (2016). *MCH Leadership Development: A Retrospective, Comparative Cohort Study*. Sigma Theta Tau International 26th Research Congress. Cape Town, SA, July 20, 2016.

BOX 14.4

▶ EXAMPLE OF A STRUCTURED PROFESSIONAL ISSUE ABSTRACT

Retiring? Some Things to Consider

Background: Within the next 10 years (by 2024), approximately 700,000 nurses will retire. Nurses approaching retirement age need to be proactive in planning for retirement. Adjustment to retirement is enhanced when individuals consider their possibilities several years before retirement occurs. Organizations benefit from being proactive in terms of leadership succession and wisdom sharing.

Framework for the Talk: Retirement is discussed within the context of a transitions framework (Bridges, 2004) and the most recent retirement literature. Bridges views transition in terms of endings, a neutral zone, and new beginnings. Interestingly, much of the work that occurs during the endings phase is internally driven and requires individuals to reflect on several factors, including how to disengage from the familiar that reflects an ending of a past life. Part of the transition process calls for being comfortable with some ambiguity, as new life possibilities present over time.

(Continued)

Implications for Practice: Reflection is not an activity in which nurses participate on a regular basis. Participants can use this information as a starting point for discussions about retirement with their significant others and their employer, explore financial retirement options, and examine work options that may be available. For example, a nurse could explore "phased retirement" possibilities. Doing so would help the nurse experience free time while still being able to provide expertise at the workplace.

Word count: 252 (Could have 300 words)

Morin, K. (2017). *Retiring? Some things to consider.* Specialty Session, 2017 AWHONN Conference, New Orleans, LA, June 27, 2017.

BOX 14.5

▶ EXAMPLE OF AN UNSTRUCTURED RESEARCH ABSTRACT

A Survey of Delaware Acute Care Facilities' Use of Research

The importance of using research findings to guide nursing practice has been well recognized by the profession. Yet, incorporating research findings into practice remains difficult. The purpose of this study was to examine research utilization practices in the acute care agencies in the state of Delaware. Specifically, this study sought to ascertain (1) the process of developing, implementing, and revising (or updating) research-based protocols; (2) examples of research-based protocols currently being used in the acute care specialties of critical care, emergency, general medicine, general surgery, obstetrical, and psychiatric nursing; (3) how reflective the submitted research-based protocols were in terms of accuracy and consistency with current research findings. Currently, a database on the existence of research-based protocols does not exist in the state of Delaware. This study will provide insight into the current use of research utilization strategies in acute care agencies within the state, and across a variety of clinical specialties. Furthermore, the information obtained from this study will be used to formulate a plan to assist agencies to develop and expand their research utilization activities. Nurse leaders in 13 acute care agencies were contacted to identify those resources nurses (ARNs) who were most familiar with the agency's protocols, their development, and revision. ARNs from each of the six specialties were asked to participate in an interview and to submit examples of research-based protocols. Sixty ARNs were interviewed. The interview guide, adapted from Haber et al. (1994) and consisting of 22 questions categorized in four sections, was reviewed by a panel of 6 nurse researchers. A content validity index of 1.00 was achieved. All interview data were compiled and analyzed to identify similarities and differences in development, implementation, and revision processes of research-based protocols used by all agencies. Many agencies reported having research-based protocols, although inspection of the protocols often did not support this. Most of the ARNs were unclear about the research process and what constitutes research-based protocols. Few protocols had documented references. The most frequent references cited were textbooks. A gap between perceptions and reality was identified.

Note: Margins for this abstract were: 2½ inches from the top; 1 14/16 from the left. Abstract was not reviewed if not in this format.

Word count: 344 (could have 500 words)

Morin, K., Plowfield, L., Bucher, L., Hayes, E., Mahoney, P., & Armiger, L. (1997). *A survey of Delaware acute care facilities' use of research.* 9th Annual Scientific Session of the ENRS, Philadelphia, April, 1997.

Headings

Headings or labels for a structured abstract vary by type. An abstract describing the report of research will have different headings than an abstract describing an innovative clinical program. Examples of headings for different types of abstracts are provided in Table 14.2. Irrespective of the type of abstract, it is important to organize your thoughts and follow a systematic approach when writing an abstract.

Title

Cook and Bordage (2016) admonish authors to devote significant time to crafting the title, although it is often the last thing an author creates. The title plays a critical role, as it is what a reader sees first. They recommend asking colleagues for input by identifying a variety of key words. The goal is to have an "informative and indicative title" (p. 1101) that invites the reader to learn more.

Table 14.2. Typical Structured Headings for a Variety of Abstracts

Type of Abstract	Typical Structured Headings
Research	Background (relevance, aims, purpose)
	Methods (design, setting, participants, instruments)
	Results (findings)
	Conclusions (implications/recommendations for future study)
Review papers	Depends on the type of review undertaken (narrative, systematic, scoping). In general, the following are included.
	Introduction (could include theoretical framework)
	Methods (search strategies, key words, etc.)
	Findings (results)
	Discussion (synthesis, summary)
	Implications
QI papers	Refer to Squire Guidelines http://www.squire-statement.org/index.cfm?fuseaction=page.viewpage&pageid=471 for a complete listing of headings. Note headings are required for a journal or conference abstract.
Innovative clinical papers	Statement of clinical problem leading to the program
	Program development (steps involved in its development)
	Summary of the literature
	Program description (detailed description of the program)
	Outcomes (what happened)

Based on Leggett, T. (2018). Getting to the heart of the matter: How to write an abstract *Radiation Therapist, 27*(1), 76–78; Oermann, M. H., & Hays, J. C. (2016). *Writing for publication in nursing* (3rd ed.). Springer Publishing Company; and Wood, G. J., & Morrison, R. S. (2011). Writing abstracts and developing posters for national meetings. *Journal of Palliative Medicine, 14*, 353–359. https://doi.org/10.1089/jpm.2010.0171.

Before You Write

If submitting for a conference presentation, pay attention to the submission date included in the "Call for Abstracts." Consider highlighting the date on the "Call," as conferences typically adhere to submission deadlines without exception. This strategy ensures the cut-off date is not missed along with the chance to share your work.

Calls for abstracts for conferences may have a theme or a special focus and may accept completed as well as works in progress (Foster et al., 2019; Kara, 2015; Mott, 2014). Read abstract guidelines carefully irrespective of whether the abstract is part of a manuscript or conference presentation submission (McCurry, 2018). Given the competitive nature of the selection process, not adhering to guidelines may result in a rejection (Kara, 2015; Mott, 2014).

Typically, a call for abstracts includes information about the number of words permitted and the font size. Most journals limit the number of words to between 250 and 350 (Leggett, 2018). Conference abstracts may range from 150 to 500 words (Mott, 2014). Adhere to the word limitations. There are organizations and reviewers who will reject abstracts outright when the abstract exceeds the word limitations. Using Times New Roman, a serif font, or Arial, a sans serif font, is recommended for readability. Follow guidelines explicitly.

Writing the Abstract

Writing an abstract takes time. Plan enough time to rewrite the abstract several times and to have a colleague review your work before submission. If what is being submitted is part of a group effort, build in time for your partners to review and comment. Do not forget to build in enough time to account for potential technical issues that may arise when employing an online submission platform (Wood & Morrison, 2011).

As you develop the first draft of the abstract, keep these questions in mind: "Why did you start? What did you do? What answer did you get? What does it mean?" (Heseltine, 2012, p. 204). These questions are broad enough to be helpful irrespective of whether the abstract describes the report of research or some other form of scholarship.

Break the information into sections, and clearly identify each section of the abstract. Even if a narrative abstract is being crafted, such an approach helps highlight whether a crucial part of the abstract is being inadvertently omitted. Abbreviations are used sparingly and spelled out with first use. Given the emphasis on word count, consider whether an abbreviation is necessary. Reference citations and tables are rarely included in an abstract.

Mott cautions, "Remember that words do make a difference" (2014, p. 383). Scholars follow grammar rules, avoid abbreviations and local jargon, employ simple, clear sentences, and use an active voice, thus enhancing readability of an abstract.

As with other forms of scholarship, a good practice is to give the guidelines and completed abstract to a colleague to determine whether abstract guidelines have been addressed appropriately and that ideas are clearly and succinctly conveyed. His or her objective critique of your work contributes to a better product.

Lastly, create an electronic or paper folder in which to place relevant manuscript or conference information. Some conference submission systems will request additional information such as learning objectives, a content outline, references, and a brief description of the presentation. Knowing where to find them once the abstract is accepted contributes to a more positive experience.

Abstracts generally will not be accepted when they either provide too much or too little information, do not highlight the importance or relevance of the work, do not follow abstract guidelines, or do not pay attention to grammar, spelling, or typographical issues (Foster et al., 2019; Happell, 2008). APNs can keep these pitfalls in mind as they develop abstracts to enhance their success.

Writing an abstract takes time and requires considerable revision. The challenge is to include information critical to a project in a concise, clear, and consistent manner. Being familiar with information in this section can enhance successful outcomes. APNs certainly have the skills and ability to share their knowledge in this format.

In Their Own Words

Carol Klingbeil, NDP, RN, CPNP-PC

The key points in understanding my roles are… My roles include being a full-time Clinical Assistant Professor of Nursing at the University of Wisconsin in Milwaukee as well as practicing part-time as a Pediatric Nurse Practitioner at Children's Hospital of Wisconsin in the Urgent Care. Throughout my career I have committed to not only the education of nurses but also to continuing to

(Continued)

practice nursing in a variety of clinical roles to synergistically grow and contribute to nursing in a variety of important ways. Early on in my career I realized that the combination of both education and practice roles could facilitate a rich and personally rewarding career. That belief is exemplified and anchored theoretically in the Boyer (1990) Model of Scholarship that focuses on four areas critical to academic work. These include the scholarship of discovery (research), the scholarship of teaching, the scholarship of application, and the scholarship of integration. When addressing clinical practice aspects of scholarship, the scholarship of application refers to clinical practice and integration focuses on working in an interprofessional manner with multiple disciplines. Clinical practice allows me to practice what I teach and experience the reality, challenges, and joys of providing high-quality care to children and families over the course of my career. After 37 years of practice, many things have changed yet so much remains the same when it comes to communication and practicing family-centered and developmentally appropriate care. Continuing to be clinically and educationally relevant and reality oriented becomes much more possible when immersed in a clinical practice on a weekly basis. Patient stories and clinical scenarios enhance the quality of teaching and support student engagement in the classroom or during online discussions. Teaching students in all levels of education programs (prenursing, undergraduate and graduate levels) requires not only knowledge of the course content and excellent teaching skills but also an ability to facilitate student content application in the course and the clinical practice arena.

What keeps me coming back every day is… I believe nursing is pivotal to high-quality, safe, and accessible healthcare for all and that it is a critical profession contributing to quality of life across the lifespan for people across the world. Sharing this belief with students and practicing professionals not only contributes to the growth of the profession through higher education but also development of highly collaborative, satisfying, and healthy work environments. Providing high-quality care to children and families comes from working with a high-functioning interprofessional team in an organization that values a culture of safety and clinical excellence. Leadership in nursing education and at the bedside brings tremendous personal and professional satisfaction as well as confidence that what you are doing in your career makes a difference for others, for one's self, and for the society in general. It is easy to go to work every day when you enjoy your work and believe you are making an important contribution and impacting the lives of others. Hearing from students, colleagues, leaders, and supervisors that my contributions are meaningful, valuable, and appreciated also keeps me engaged in teaching the next generation of nurses

(Continued)

and caring for children and families. Reciprocating that feedback to others is also a critical aspect of supporting and valuing others' contributions to the work environment, patient care, and student success.

My greatest challenge is… To practice in a clinical environment, there are many requirements for a minimal number of hours practiced, education, credentialing and professional meetings that go beyond the academic requirements for teaching nursing. The academic environment also requires professional development, mandatory meetings, committee work, student advising responsibilities, and university advancement requirements. Academia also has additional scholarship requirements for publication and leadership that are on-going and provide evidence of contributing to the science of nursing and the advancement of the profession. Finding balance in one's personal life and professional life is always a priority and can easily become challenging when two roles are demanding and full of commitments that require focus, energy, and planning.

I wish someone had told me… I wish someone had told me the value of self-reflection and developing reflective practice early in my career. Deeper learning comes through regular reflection of one's practice as both an educator and a clinician. I wish I had been told and understood that enjoying the process more than the outcome would add tremendous growth and depth to my practice and my career as it evolved. I wish someone had told me that in some jobs you will work with some of the most interesting and gifted educators and clinicians and to take the time to access their wisdom whenever you can. I wish someone had told me to be sure to laugh and cry and have fun every day at work and at home to get the most satisfaction out of your work and home life. While this wisdom has developed over time through hours of practice as an educator and clinician, I wish I had started self-reflection and appreciating and regularly accessing other's wisdom earlier in my career.

I need to be a lifelong learner because… Lifelong learning is central to nursing and any healthcare-oriented career. Change is accelerated and ever present in the clinical practice arena. Teaching students who will function in a nursing role in the future in a variety of roles requires agility, retooling one's skill sets, and humility that one will never remember or know everything that is needed daily. Understanding that knowing how to problem solve and use resources to answer important clinical or research questions and knowing your limitations especially in the clinical practice setting is essential for safe practice. Working in a clinical practice as well as academia fosters lifelong learning which is perhaps one of the strongest driving forces for me professionally as a nurse educator and clinician.

(Continued)

> **Another point to understand is…** Nursing professionals are challenged by the intensity and scope of the role whether it is in an in-patient, out-patient, or community setting. As resources dwindle, policy changes, and financial models impact care delivery, healthcare professionals are more stressed and more at risk for illness and burn-out than ever. Educators must prepare students to face the realities and challenges of providing safe, efficient, and quality health-care while understanding the need for professional boundaries and self-care to remain healthy. A rewarding professional life and as well as a quality personal and home life is essential over the lifetime of a career. Role modeling and articulating ways to balance one's career responsibilities and personal goals are essential in preparing students to stay in the nursing profession when challenges seem overwhelming and a career no longer feels satisfying. We must seek better ways to prepare students for the nursing profession over a lifetime to grow and maintain a viable work force.
>
> Boyer, E. (1990). *Scholarship reconsidered: Priorities of the professorate. The Carnegie Foundation for the Advancement of Teaching*. Jossey-Bass.

Presentations

Many people fear speaking in public (Levoy, 2010). Dwyer and Davidson (2012), in a sample of 815 students drawn from a large Midwestern university, found that 61.7% of men and 65.9% of women ranked fear of speaking before a group before financial problems and death. Knowing others' experience anxiety when presenting can be reassuring as you are not alone with these experiences. Knowing there are resources and strategies available to decrease presenter anxiety makes the experience less intimidating.

Questions to Ask Yourself?

1. How do you feel about speaking in public?
2. Does your current employment position require public speaking? Will your future position require it?
3. Do you currently give presentations but do not seek out the opportunities? Do you actively seek opportunities to speak?
4. Do you wish to establish a national reputation?

A critical first step is determining the type of presentation: an oral podium presentation or a poster presentation. Tierney (1996) challenges presenters to keep four principles in mind relative to presentations:

- Be responsible to the audience.
- Make conscious decisions about what you are presenting and not rely on your intuition alone.
- Make decisions before, during, and after you speak.
- Become aware of your strengths and weaknesses as a presenter and practice using techniques that will enhance your talk (p. 6).

These four principles are relevant whether you develop an abstract, craft a podium or a poster presentation, or write a paper.

Podium

A recent Google search using the phrase "Call for nursing abstracts 2021" yielded more than 7,000,000 results. Thus, APNs have many opportunities to present a podium presentation at a conference. Podium presentations range from a plenary session delivered to several hundred to thousands of conference attendees, a concurrent session to fewer attendees, or a workshop prior to conference. APNs who wish to practice podium presentation in a setting less daunting than a national or international conference might consider presenting at Grand Rounds in your organization, to colleagues on the unit, to nursing students, or to a lay audience. Important public-speaking practices should be following irrespective of the venue and the size of the audience.

Responsibility to the Audience

A critical practice is developing expertise about the topic; you must know the material you are presenting (Foster et al., 2019; Longo & Tierney, 2012). Experts recommend 10 hours of preparation time for 1 hour of presentation (Baker, 2017). Consequently, allowing sufficient time to prepare a presentation can help decrease anxiety while respecting your responsibility to the audience.

Take time to learn about your audience before the event (Cottingham, 2019; Levoy, 2010). Ask the conference planners for information about the possible number of people attending your presentation and the level of education of attendees. For example, are they students or experts in your field? Having this information helps you structure your presentation.

Speakers often develop a handout for attendees. Slutsky and Baum (2017) suggest distributing a handout following your presentation so the audience remains focused on you and what you are saying. Rather than simply providing a copy of the PowerPoint (PPT) slides, consider creating a one-page handout in which you provide the most salient points of your presentation (Slutsky & Baum, 2018).

Equally important is knowing your style of verbal and nonverbal communication (Happell, 2009). You must convey not only a clear message but also use clear speech. Practice how to pronounce difficult words to avoid mispronouncing them during your presentation. Crick (2017) advises using specific rather than nebulous terms. For example, the word "huge" can be interpreted in many different ways, while the word "1000" cannot. If appropriate, use analogies to reinforce the point being made. Consider varying the pace and tone of your delivery, as speakers who present at a rapid-fire pace or speak too slowly may lose the audience (Crick, 2017; Levoy, 2010). The audience is more engaged when you vary delivery.

Body language, a form of nonverbal communication, is important when presenting (Medina & Avant, 2015). Watch your posture and avoid leaning on the podium. Pay attention to how you use your hands, as excessive hand movement can distract the audience. Exude confidence as a speaker.

Conscious Decisions About What to Present

A beneficial practice when deciding on the content is to remember you want to tell the audience what you will be discussing, discuss it, and then remind them of what you discussed. Consequently, it is critical to have a clear message (Tierney, 1996). Take time to craft the message and develop an outline to ensure you convey the key points. Experts suggest the presentation be broken into three parts: opening, middle, and closing (Longo & Tierney, 2012; Slutsky & Baum, 2017).

Opening

Because evidence indicates "the first and last 30 seconds of any speech have the most impact" (Slutsky & Baum, 2017, p. 89), spend considerable time crafting the opening and ending of your presentation. This is your opportunity to get the audience's attention and to establish your role as an expert. Several authors advise not using the phrase "I am going to talk about" or "I'm delighted to be here" as an opening statement (Slutsky & Baum, 2018;

Tierney, 1996). Rather, tell the audience what they will learn during your presentation by reviewing presentation objectives. Another approach is to ask participants what they hope to gain from attending your presentation. Consider whether you want to reinforce the relevance of the presentation, review the presentation objectives, or tell a joke or a humorous story. These are effective strategies that engage the audience quickly. Presenters experiment with various formats to determine which are most comfortable for them. In addition, the type of presentation and the audience influence how you begin the presentation. Reasons for attending a report of research may be very different than for attending a clinical session.

Middle

The body of your presentation contains the bulk of the content you are presenting. Be deliberate about the amount of information you provide, as too much can overwhelm an audience. DeCoske and White (2010) encourage presenters to "leave your listeners wanting more and show them where to find it, instead of leaving them with information overload and a headache" (p. 1226).

The amount of time devoted to the delivery of a podium presentation can range from 20 minutes (typical when reporting research) to 60 to 90 minutes (typical for a conference concurrent session). Given the "adult attention span is approximately 10 to 15 minutes" (Medina & Avant, 2015, p. 1092) and a typical session has between three and six objectives, a presenter should devote about 10 to 15 minutes per presentation objective. As you prepare the content relevant for each objective, consider using numbers to highlight the key points. Numbering key points helps the audience "effectively chunk the content and know what to expect" (Medina & Avant, 2015, p. 1092).

Adults need to hear things more than once to retain information, so do not hesitate to use repetition (Phillips, 2019). Repetition also can evoke an emotional response—think of the emotional impact Martin Luther King's "I Have a Dream" speech had. Consider what you want to accomplish by using repetition and then build opportunities to repeat information into the talk.

Once critical content is determined, you need to decide the type of visual aids to use. Most audiences anticipate a presenter will use audiovisual aids. While PowerPoint (PPT) slides, props, flip charts, and videos are possibilities, the most common visual aids are PPT slides. When preparing slides, keep in mind that less is more. Use fewer words per slide, employ less glitz, and use a consistent background and font. Lastly, allot enough time to enlist the help of a colleague to proofread the slides. Key points to consider when developing PPT slides are presented in Table 14.3.

Table 14.3. PowerPoint Development Tips	
Color	Use contrasting colors; e.g., black, dark blue, white, and yellow; provide good contrast
	Refer to a color wheel
	Do not use color for decoration
	Do not use a different color for each point
	Avoid red and green, which cannot be seen by persons who may be experiencing color-blindness
Font style	Serif: Times Roman, Bookman, Century, Garamond, Lucinda, and Palatino
	Sans serif (recommended): Arial, Century Gothic, Helvetica, Lucinda Sans, Tahoma, and Verdana
	Script: Brush script, Freestyle script
Font size	Title: 36–44 point
	Main body: 28–32 point
	First-level subpoint: 24–28 point
	Second-level subpoint: 24–26 point
Slide layout	Use bullet points to convey key points
	Sentences only when quoting
	Use a consistent style
	Observe 6 × 6 guideline (six words, six lines)
	Title each slide
	Replace text with graphs when possible

(continued)

Table 14.3. PowerPoint Development Tips (continued)	
Other	Use high-quality pictures
	Limit use of clip art, sounds, and slide transitions
Number of slides	A general rule is no more than one slide/minute; for a 20 min presentation, no more than 20 slides should be prepared.

Based on Baker, J. D. (2015). Professional versus predatory publishing: Cautions for perioperative nurse authors. *Journal of Perioperative Nursing in Australia, 29*(4), 48–49; Longo, A., & Tierney, C. (2012). Presentation skills for the nurse educator. *Journal for Nurses in Staff Development, 28*, 16–23. https://doi.org/10.1097/NND.0b013e318240a699; and Medina, M. S., & Avant, N. D. (2015). Delivering an effective presentation. *American Journal of Health-System Pharmacy, 72*, 1091–1094. https://doi.org/10.2146/ajhp150047.

During the presentation, it is critical that you do not read the slides verbatim. Your audience can read the slides; your role is to elaborate what is on the slide with additional information. Observe how the audience is responding to your presentation (Levoy, 2010; SpeakerHub, 2017). If you note disinterested behaviors (yawning, restlessness, playing with electronics), you need to be ready to shift the presentation to reengage the audience. One way to do this is incorporating questions that require an audience response into your presentation.

Closing

At the end of the presentation, summarize your key points (Medina & Avant, 2015). The last couple of slides can serve this purpose. Remember to build in time for audience questions. Thank the audience once questions have been answered or time runs out. As you consider how to end the presentation, take time to evaluate whether there are sections of the presentation that can be removed if time is an issue (Longo & Tierney, 2012).

Know Your Strengths and Weaknesses

Consider the following questions: Do you need to write the speech out completely? Should you use note cards? What about using an outline? How comfortable are you interacting with the audience? Are you versed in techniques to engage the audience? Can you build in a think-pair-share activity? Answers to these questions can help you prepare more effective presentations.

While you may feel more comfortable writing out the complete presentation, reading it may not sound natural and be stiff (Branch, 2017). Reading your talk limits eye contact with the audience. One way to address these criticisms is to use an outline to jog your memory. Note cards are another option. They are less obtrusive and more flexible, as additional cards can be added as needed. Note cards with important information relevant to more than one topic can be used interchangeably, decreasing preparation time.

Practice Using Techniques to Enhance Presentation

The goal in practicing is to familiarize yourself with the content, not to memorize it. Given the importance of establishing a connection with the audience early and maintaining it during the presentation, practicing the presentation prepares you to address content in your slides without referring to them (Slutsky & Baum, 2017). Otherwise, the connection you have established with the audience is lost when you look repeatedly at the slides.

Continue rehearsing until you feel comfortable recovering from mistakes you may make. Practicing decreases the number of times you use fillers and pet phrases, such as "um," "ah," and "you know" that can distract the audience. Importantly, practicing your presentation ensures you will not exceed your allotted time (Slutsky & Baum, 2017).

Consider how to respond to challenging audiences. Audience members sometimes conduct sidebar conversations, monopolize the conversation, or challenge speakers (Longo & Tierney, 2012). Speakers deal with such issues in a variety of ways. You might stand next to the audience members who are conversing, shift the focus to other members of the audience to limit monopolizing, or invite comment from the challenger.

Public speaking need not be intimidating. Strategies in this section are designed to lessen presenter anxiety and nervousness. Ultimately, a good speaker stands up to be seen, speaks up to be heard, and sits down to be appreciated (Figure 14.1). The information in this section prepares the APN to do just that. Lastly, take the feedback and convert your podium presentation into a publication. You have a great start: you have the knowledge, you have an outline, now all you need to do is elaborate on your thoughts. The section on publishing can help you (Box 14.6).

BOX 14.6

▶ SELECT WRITING RESOURCES

General Texts

Heinrich, K. T. (2008). *A nurse's guide to presenting and publishing. Dare to share.* Jones and Bartlett.

Huth, E. J. (1999). *Writing and publishing in medicine* (3rd ed.). Williams & Wilkins.

Oermann, M. H., & Hays, J. C. (2016). *Writing for publication in nursing* (3rd ed.). Springer Publishing Company.

Slaver, C. (2011). *Anatomy of writing for publication for nurses.* Sigma Theta Tau International.

Grammar Texts

Brohaugh, W. (2007). *Writeright. Say exactly what you mean with precision and power.* Sourcebooks, Inc.

Graff, G., & Birkenstein, C. (2014). *They say. I say. The moves that matter in academic writing.* W. W. Norton & Company.

Swales, J. M., & Feak, C. B. (2012). *Academic writing for graduate students. Essential tasks and skills* (3rd ed.). The University of Michigan Press.

Truss, L. (2003). *Eats, shoots and leaves. The zero-tolerance approach to punctuation.* Gotham Books.

Poster

Perhaps a podium presentation is not your desired scholarly activity, but you still have important information to share. A poster presentation is a suitable alternative, as it typically takes place in a more informal manner. It gives the presenter the opportunity to interact with individual conference participants one-on-one. Poster presentations also provide the opportunity to present work in progress, that is, work for which findings may not yet be determined. Obtaining conference

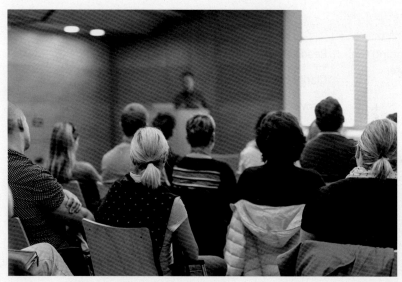

Figure 14.1. Audience showing gratitude toward speaker. (Source: Shutterstock/ESB Professional.)

participant input about a research or quality improvement project can enhance the end product and increase the contribution your scholarly work makes.

A **poster** is a static visual representation of your work that is more than words. The challenge is to design a poster that is visually appealing and conveys creativity while not violating common and evidence-based practices. Posters can be presented using a cork standing board of varying dimensions: 3 feet by 6 feet or 4 feet by 8 feet is common. However, there are times when tabletop posters are used. These dimensions will be different from those of the cork standing boards; thus, it is essential to read the directions before developing the poster.

Although most posters are offered in a stand-alone format, conferences may now provide select poster presenters an opportunity to present a short oral summary (Zerwic et al., 2010). These narrated posters typically occur as a separate session where several people present.

For any type of poster presentation, there are critical poster elements. Siedlecki (2017), in her study of 180 clinical nurses, advanced practice registered nurses (APRNs), nurse educators, and nurse managers, found that relevance and visual appeal were essential. Other elements include font/headings, color, graphics, and layout. Poster presentation tips are provided in Table 14.4.

Table 14.4.	Poster Presentation Tips
Planning the poster	Read the directions
	Clarify what is to be presented
	Know the audience
	Plan sufficient time
Developing the poster	Avoid busy backgrounds
	Apply common visual practices (font size, white space)
	Use colors cautiously, not more than four
	Use sections and headings to divide the content
	Ensure symmetry of content—a three-column format is typical
	Ensure font size readable from 3 to 5 feet
	Omit abstract and references
	Center title at the top of the poster
	Make certain title conveys the project clearly
	Tables and visuals can replace text effectively
Presenting the poster	Have handouts available
	Have contact information readily available to distribute
	Be present when required and available if needed

Based on Sherman, R. O. (2010). How to create an effective poster presentation. *The American Nurse, 5*(9). https://www.americannursetoday.com/how-to-create-an-effective-poster-presentation/; Siedlecki, S. (2017). How to create a poster that attracts an audience. *American Journal of Nursing, 117*(3), 48–54; and Zerwic, J. J., Grandfield, K., Kavanaugh, K., Berger, B., Graham, L., & Mershon, M. (2010). Tips for better visual elements in posters and podium presentations. *Education for Health, 23*(2), 1–6.

Font/Headings

Type and size of fonts play a critical role in whether a conference attendee will read your poster. A sans serif font is recommended for the titles (Bingham & O'Neal, 2013; Sherman, 2010), while a serif font is best for text (see Table 14.2 for examples of fonts). A font size of "20 to 40 point for text and 36 to 50 for headings" (Connelly, 2018, p. 65) is recommended. Font sizes vary by level of heading: larger fonts are used for the title of the abstract, smaller for section headings. Viewers should be able to read the content from between 3 and 10 feet away (Bingham & O'Neal, 2013; Connelly, 2018; Siedlecki, 2017).

What is included in a heading varies by type of project being presented and can be influenced by conference guidelines. As with other forms of scholarship, reading guidelines is an important first step. A major heading is the title. Best practice is to keep the title brief (fewer than 10 words) (Connelly, 2018). The title should be compelling and avoid professional jargon. "The title should be readable from 15 to 20 feet away, with letters 2- to 3-inches high" (Sherman, 2010, n.p.).

Color

Color plays a critical role enhancing visual appeal, highlighting differences, and contributing to esthetic appeal. The rules that are followed when creating PPT slides apply when developing a poster. Zerwic and associates (2010) suggest limiting colors to four including white, red, black, green, and/or blue; Scout (2015) advises no more than three colors. Other colors, such as yellow and pink, do not show up well. An alternative is to use variations or shades of one or two colors. A lighter background with darker text is easier to read (Buckley, 2014; Sherman, 2010).

Graphics

Graphics play an important role in poster development, as a picture, figure, table, or diagram can convey information more succinctly than words. If using pictures or photos, make certain they are well-defined and not blurry. A good rule is to limit the number of images to no more than four (Bingham & O'Neal, 2013).

Layout

Balance is key when developing the poster (Connelly, 2018; Siedlecki, 2017). Typically, three columns are used: left, middle, and right. Information is presented starting top left, proceeds down the left column, and then to the middle. The same process is used for the remaining columns.

A good idea is to sketch where the content will be placed before developing the poster. Sketching helps identify the headings needed, where to place visual aids, and what connectors (arrows, numbering) to use to help the viewer follow the linkages between the information on the poster (Connelly, 2018). Judicious use of white or empty space enhances readability (Sherman, 2010; Whitespace Marketing, 2018).

Too much information on a poster overwhelms the viewer. Do not use complete sentences; bulleted information is better and more visually attractive. Lastly, avoid large sections of text; use quotations with many lines of text sparingly.

Producing the Poster

Many prepare posters using one slide in PPT. Although an excellent resource, it is not always easy to see errors or misalignment of content while developing it. One way to check for errors is to project the slide "on a screen to get a better idea of what it will like from 5 feet" (Connelly, 2018, p. 65). Your employer or organization may have templates to use.

The Poster Session

Poster presenters usually spend some dedicated time at their poster. Frequently, these times are during coffee or meal breaks in the program. Prepare a short 1- to 2-minute summary of the poster to share with the viewer (Connelly, 2018). Interact with viewers but avoid bothering them. Making eye contact with viewers helps you gauge their level of interest and interaction. Have a copy of the poster with your contact information and the abstract available to share with conference participants. Lastly, take time to visit other posters to see how others present information.

Presenting a poster is a suitable alternative to a podium presentation. The information in this section, Table 14.4, and Box 14.7 provides a good foundation for your work. Lastly, do not let the energy generated by presenting disappear. Take your hard work and convert it into a publication, the topic of the next section.

BOX 14.7

▶ PODIUM PRESENTATION TIPS

Before the Conference

- Practice.

- Proof.

Day of Conference

- Bring a backup paper copy of the presentation and a USB (notes, slides).

- Arrive early (at least 10–15 minutes before your presentation).

- If possible, practice your presentation with the IT personnel.

- Inspect the room and check audiovisual equipment.

- Interact with audience members before you speak (makes presenting less intimating).

Before Speaking

- Perform relaxation techniques, such as shoulder rolls and deep breathing.

During the Presentation

- Observe audience response.

- Vary the pace and tone of your delivery.

- Repeat the audience question before responding.

Remember

- You are the expert.

Based upon Medina, M. S., & Avant, N. D. (2015). Delivering an effective presentation. *American Journal of Health-System Pharmacy*, 72, 1091–1094. https://doi.org/10.2146/ajhp150047 and Slutsky, J., & Baum, N. H. (2017). Public speaking for the podiatric physician – part I. *Podiatry Management*, 36(8), 87–90.

Publications

While podium and poster presentations are excellent venues in which to share expertise, converting these presentations to publications ensures information reaches the widest audience. Some experts encourage scholars to convert their work to publications within a few months of the presentation. There are good reasons for making the effort. The information is fresh and foremost in your

BOX 14.8

▶ TYPES OF MANUSCRIPTS

- Opinion piece
- Letters to the editor
- Short reports
- Discussion papers
- Research reports
- Clinical practice articles
- Quality improvement projects
- Clinical reviews/state of the science
- Book chapters
- Nursing narrative

Based upon Oermann, M. H., & Hays, J. C. (2016). *Writing for publication in nursing* (3rd ed.). Springer Publishing Company and Slaver, C. (2011). *Anatomy of writing for publication for nurses*. Sigma Theta Tau International.

mind, so preparing a publication is easier sooner than later. The information is important—it would not have been accepted for presentation otherwise. The outline is already developed, making writing an easier undertaking. Finally, your productivity and self-confidence improve when you make a valuable contribution to disciplinary knowledge (Levett-Jones & Stone, 2012). However, before beginning the journey, consider four factors: the enthusiasm you have for the topic, its relevance to the discipline (refer to the quote at the beginning of the chapter), the contribution your work will make, and how the contribution influences your career (Huff, 1999). Each of these plays a role in the speed with which you accomplish the task, so take time to reflect on them. The resources in Boxes 14.6 and 14.8 can help with your writing efforts.

Reasons for Writing

Individuals publish for various reasons. Scholars often publish to meet requirements for promotion and tenure or clinical ladders. Perhaps there is an innovative clinical endeavor worth sharing that improved patient outcomes (Oermann & Hays, 2016; Slaver, 2011). Researchers publish to report findings and to get feedback on their work. Other reasons for writing include provoking dialogue on a relevant disciplinary or professional topic, refining one's abilities and knowledge, and garnering self-gratification (Oermann & Hays, 2016). There is something special about seeing your own work in print, particularly when this form of dissemination may not be your strength.

Barriers to Writing

If the benefits of writing are many, why, then, do individuals not write for publication? Frequently heard reasons are a lack of confidence (Slaver, 2011) and a fear of rejection (Oermann & Hays, 2016). Confidence is developed by building a writing skill set. However, while graduate students often write papers to meet course requirements, writing a manuscript for publication requires different skills frequently not addressed while in graduate school. This fact need not hinder you, however, as embracing and incorporating writing into your life is the best way to build confidence and help you deal with rejections you may encounter. It is a rare author who has not experienced rejection of a manuscript. Confidence helps authors deal with the disappointment inherent in receiving a rejection. Confidence provides the foundation for authors to address reviewer issues and to submit again to another journal.

Another reason is lack of time. Everyone is busy; however, successful authors commit to writing and employ numerous strategies to honor their commitment. Shirley Moore, PhD, RN, FAAN, Associate Dean for Research in the Frances Payne Bolton School of Nursing at Case Western University, recently shared how she manages her scholarship. She builds 20 to 25 minutes into her daily schedule to write. The time of day may vary but she writes something every day. Slaver (2011) suggests thinking about writing when doing other activities such as showering, biking, or commuting to work, reinforcing that crafting a paper need not occur only when seated before a computer. Enlisting help as you address completing is another strategy. Would your writing efforts perhaps be more productive by enlisting the contributions of a colleague? Many authors employ this strategy to share the work and the accountability. It is not as easy to postpone writing when someone else is depending on your work.

Getting Ideas

Nurse authors get ideas from many places: quality improvement projects, research projects, policy issues, a unique role, reviews of the literature, a unique clinical care case, and new solutions to practice problems. Think about issues you deal with daily or about which you are passionate. They are better options than writing about an esoteric topic. Once a potential topic has been identified, the next step is becoming knowledgeable about the topic by conducting a thorough review of the literature. It is possible the topic or focus may change after reviewing the literature. A change in focus is not a bad thing if the end product makes a significant contribution to the scholarly discussions on the topic.

Selecting a Journal

Choosing which journal to submit to is one of the most important activities an author can do, as submitting to the wrong journal can delay review and possible publication by months (Oermann & Hays, 2016). Moreover, making the selection prior to writing the paper can save time.

What factors does an author consider in journal selection? The topic, type, and purpose of the article, audience, quality and reach of the journal, and frequency of publication play important roles in journal selection. The topic should be relevant to journal readers and contribute new information. A letter to the journal editor can help determine whether a journal you have selected is appropriate. Another strategy is to speak with journal editors when you attend a conference. Editors enjoy interacting with prospective authors.

The type of manuscript submitted, and its intended audience, also influences journal selection. Manuscripts can range from a letter to the editor to a state of the science (Box 14.8). For example, a "Lessons Learned" paper would not be appropriate for the journal *Nursing Research* but could be considered for the *American Journal of Nursing* or *JPN: The Journal for Nurse Practitioners*. A good practice is to scan the table of contents of possible journals to get an idea of the type of manuscripts published.

Equally important in selecting a journal is whether it is peer-reviewed, that is, one in which submitted manuscripts are reviewed for quality and rigor by peers. Some journals implement peer review through a blind process in which neither author nor reviewers are known to each other, while with other journals, the author and reviewers may be known.

The distribution of the journal, frequency of publication, and acceptance and response rates also are considered (Oermann & Hays, 2016). Distribution can be important if the author's goal is to reach an international audience. Frequency is important when considering how quickly an author wants information published. If achieving tenure is the focus, then selecting a journal with a monthly publication cycle is more advantageous than selecting one published quarterly. How quickly a journal gets back to the author with a response (response rate) is important, as an author does not want to wait an excessive amount of time. Most journals aim for a response rate of about 3 months from time of submission until editor decision. A journal's goal is to expedite the process, not serve as an impediment to the process, and they work hard to get articles to publication expeditiously. Lastly, authors consider a journal's acceptance rate. If the goal is to get published quickly, selecting a journal that only accepts 10% of manuscripts submitted may not be the best choice.

Selecting a journal to which to submit is not undertaken lightly. A good practice is to craft a list of between three to five journals that would be appropriate for the manuscript being developed. Having a list facilitates the revision and resubmission processes should they be necessary. Many authors rank the journals and submit to their top-ranked journal first. Their choice of which is the top-ranked journal may be based on the journal's impact factor (Oermann & Hays, 2016).

Types of Journals

Historically, professional journals were published in a paper format and available to a limited audience either through individual or institutional membership. Recent advances have made them available electronically but with the same membership restrictions. For example, fees associated with membership in a professional organization often include access to publications produced by the organization. Similarly, libraries pay fees to publishers to make journals to their users.

The newest type of journal is the open-access quality journal. Quality open-access journals are peer-reviewed, very accessible, and provide rapid dissemination of information. They are reputable professional journals. There are, however, fees associated with these journals that are covered by the individual author, their institution, or possibly a funding agency. Consequently, while open-access journals are reputable, are transparent with their publishing practices, and accelerate the rate of dissemination, they can be quite costly for an author.

Determining Authorship

An author is a person who makes a significant contribution to a manuscript, presentation, or poster. The International Committee of Medical Journal Editors (ICMJE) (2017) provides four criteria for authorship:

1. Substantial contribution to the conception or design of the work; or the acquisition, analysis, or interpretation of data for the work;
2. Drafting the work or revising it critically for important intellectual content;
3. Final approval of the version to be published; and
4. Agreement to be accountable for all aspects of the work (p. 2).

Oermann and Hays (2016) emphasize "Authorship establishes both credit and responsibility for work in nursing, other health fields, and science in general" (p. 38). Moreover, being clear about what constitutes authorship is important as there are implications associated with authorship (ICJME, 2017). Not only can authorship influence tenure decisions, employment, professional reputation, and financial remuneration but also there have been ethical issues associated with the assignment of authorship (Holland & Watson, 2012; Kennedy et al., 2014; Oermann & Hays, 2016). Authorship may be assigned to guest or honorary authors, that is, to persons who have limited or no knowledge of the work. For example, authorship could be assigned to the head of department as recognition of his or her position. This practice does not reflect the established criteria for authorship and is considered unethical. Unethical, ghost authorship occurs when a person who meets authorship criteria is not included as an author. Kennedy et al. (2014) reported both these practices were more common in nursing rather than medical journals. As an author, be transparent in recognizing the efforts of others in your work but avoid giving undue credit. It is critical to the discipline and the profession that such practices be avoided.

Ethical Issues

Two other ethical issues are particularly relevant: duplicate publishing and plagiarism. Duplicate publishing occurs when the same paper, or one with considerable overlap, is published when a paper with the same information has already been published (King, 2009; Slaver, 2011; Villar, 2015). When this occurs, the impact of an author's work can be exaggerated (Watson et al., 2014).

Plagiarism occurs when one uses another's work without giving them credit. Self-plagiarism occurs when an author uses prior published work verbatim in new work (King, 2009). Plagiarism detection technology and excellent citation records can help authors avoid plagiarizing or self-plagiarizing (Oermann & Hays, 2016).

Process of Writing

Writing is a repetitive process, so build in time to write and rewrite many times. The goal in writing is to be clear and precise. Achieving this goal takes time and critical review. Writing occurs in phases: preparing, writing, reviewing, revising, finalizing, and submitting. As you contemplate the process, consider finding a writing mentor. This person could be a current or former faculty or a colleague who has been successful as an author. Several professional organizations have developed mentoring programs to assist with writing. Also review the writing tips in Box 14.9.

Preparing

In preparing for writing, authors must become knowledgeable about the topic. They take time to become conversant with how the topic is being discussed in all types of literature. Being conversant with the literature reaffirms that they are creating a product that provides important and original work based on an extensive command of current knowledge (Morin, 2017). Oermann and Hays (2016) suggest authors review journal guidelines and clarify the audience they wish to reach. Reviewing guidelines also provides information

---

BOX 14.9

▶ WRITING TIPS

1. Be passionate about your topic.

2. Find someone to guide you on the journey—a mentor would be most helpful.

3. Develop a system: Write a little every day or build in longer blocks of time.

(Continued)

4. Acknowledge you have something to contribute.

5. Keep the audience and your message in the forefront.

6. Develop an outline.

7. Have a beginning and an ending thought.

8. Do not wander.

9. Write and rewrite—being an author is possible.

about the journal's writing style preference (Bowling, 2013). This is the phase during which a schedule for writing is crafted, a writing place is established (office, kitchen, bedroom), and distractions are identified, limited, and/or eliminated.

Writing

Developing an outline is a critical first step in the writing phase (Bowling, 2013; Oermann & Hays, 2016). Although outlines vary by type of article being written, all include an "introduction, the body of the paper, and the conclusion" (Bowling, 2013, p. 617). An example of an outline for a clinical paper is presented in Box 14.10. An outline helps an author maintain conceptual consistency, provides the basis for manuscript headings, and enhances flow of ideas. The absence of conceptual congruency reflects fuzzy author thinking. Moreover, the absence of conceptual congruency, along with poor writing, are reviewer pet peeves (Morin, 2017).

New authors often think they need to start at the beginning and then continue to write until the manuscript is finished. Bowling (2013), however, argues, "You want to start at the end and then work your way backward" (p. 617). Some authors start in the middle or a section of the paper. The important point is to start writing so that your thoughts are documented (Oermann & Hays, 2016). The opportunity to revisit your thoughts is present in the reviewing phase. Watson (2012) recommends setting a word goal each time you write; his was 500 words at every writing session.

BOX 14.10

▶ CLINICAL PAPER OUTLINE

- Introduction

- Type of feeding
  - Breast
  - Bottle

- Nutrient supplementation
  - Iron
  - Zinc

- Introduction of solids
  - Recommended time
  - Associated issues

- Use of juices
  - Current parental practices
  - AAP recommendation

- Vegetarian mother

- Infant colic
  - Definition
  - Nutrition implications

- Clinical implications

Note: The author developed this outline after an extensive review of the literature. Headings were determined once she determined there was inconsistent or limited literature about the topics that warranted being highlighted.

Morin, K. H. (2004). Current thoughts on healthy term infant nutrition: The first 12 months. *MCN: The American Journal of Maternal Child Nursing, 29*, 312–317.

Reviewing

Plan to write and rewrite the manuscript several times with a goal of greater clarity with each revision. Become your most critical reviewer. Review your use of complex language or jargon, convoluted sentences, past tense, and passive voice (Raimes & Miller-Cochran, 2017) and correct them. For example, evaluate how you use language. Do you employ the term "utilize" rather than "use"? Remember simpler is better. Evaluate whether you attribute appropriate credit to sources and whether they are in the appropriate reference format for the journal you selected. Once you are satisfied with the manuscript, give it to a colleague to review against the author guidelines. Assure your colleagues that you are seeking truthful and helpful feedback so that your success in publishing is enhanced. Encourage them to be ruthless but kind.

Finalizing

Finalizing your writing includes addressing all concerns identified by your colleague and then crafting a title and the abstract. Huff (1999) suggests the following: Construct three possible titles, then indicate a couple of reasons for its use or nonuse, have others read the titles, and then make your decision. Bowman and Kinnan (2018) also suggest using less than 15 words, containing key words in the title, and avoiding abbreviations, question marks, and exclamation points. While the title should reflect the purpose of the manuscript, avoid using excessively long titles. Once you have attended to these details, the manuscript is ready to be submitted. Although most manuscript management systems allow you to track the progress of your manuscript, anticipate waiting about 3 months before you receive a decision from the journal. Decisions range from reject to accept, or authors may be asked to revise a manuscript based on peer-reviewer comments. Rarely does a manuscript get accepted on the initial submission. A rejection decision, although disappointing, provides an opportunity to create a better manuscript. All authors know there is a home for their manuscript; they simply need to find it.

Summary

Advanced practice nurses are well positioned to become scholars. Irrespective of the type of scholarship embraced—podium presentation, poster presentation, or publishing—there are key points to keep in mind: Read the directions more than once; allow sufficient time to prepare the work; adhere to common practices; know the audience; have a clear message; practice, practice, practice; revise, revise, revise. Information in this chapter provides a solid foundation for your scholarship journey and your contributions to the profession. Now start the journey.

Chapter Highlights

- Being a scholar is a professional expectation that can be a learned skill.
- Scholars possess integrity, honesty, creativity, and passion for their work.
- APNs are well positioned to become scholars.
- The four types of scholarship are discovery, integration, application, and teaching.
- Disseminating information has different approaches, including podium and poster presentations and publications.
- There are four key principles to respect when disseminating information.
- Dissemination requires effort and dedicated time.
- Practice and revision are key practices.
- Many resources are available to help learn the skill.
- The title is developed after the abstract, paper, or presentation is completed.

Web Resources

Poster Presentations

- The Owl at Purdue: https://owl.purdue.edu/owl/subject_specific_writing/healthcare_writing/writing_as_a_professional_nurse/list_of_nursing_resources.html
- Tips on Poster Presentations at Professional Conferences: http://www.csun.edu/plunk/documents/poster_presentation.pdf
- Guidelines for Poster Presentations: http://www.pitt.edu/~etbell/nsurg/PosterGuide.html
- Poster Presentations: http://www.people.eku.edu/ritchisong/posterpres.html
- https://www.utoledo.edu/nursing/pdfs/Designing%20Posters%20in%20PowerPoint.pdf

---

Publishing

- Nurse Editor & Author: https://nursingeditors.com/journals-directory/
- Listing of Nursing Journals: http://en.wikipedia.org/wiki/List_of_nursing_journals
- Nurse Editor &Author: https://nursingeditors.com/resources/writing-for-publication/
- University of Utah College of Nursing: https://nursing.utah.edu/journalwriting/
- Directory of Open Access Journals: http://doaj.org
- Thomas Long's blog: "Nursing Writing": https://nursingwriting.wordpress.com

References

American Association of Colleges of Nursing. (2006). *Essentials of doctoral education for advanced nursing practice.*

American Association of Colleges of Nursing. (2011). *Essentials of master's education in nursing.*

American Association of Colleges of Nursing. (2018). *Defining scholarship for academic nursing task for consensus position statement.*

American Psychological Association. (2020). *Publication manual of the American psychological association* (6th ed.).

Baker, J. D. (2017). Presentation skills: A necessity for perioperative nurses [Editorial]. *AORN Journal, 105*, 136–140. https://doi.org/10.1016/j.aorn.2016.12.016

Bingham, R., & O'Neal, D., III. (2013). Developing great abstracts and posters: How to use the tools of science communication. *Nursing for Women's Health, 17*, 131–138. https://doi.org/10.1111/1751-486x.12021

Bowling, A. M. (2013). SPN Column. Writing for publication: You can do it. *Journal of Pediatric Nursing, 28*, 616–619.

Bowman, D., & Kinnan, S. (2018, September). Creating effective titles for your scientific publications. *VideoGIE, 3*(9), 260–261.

Boyer, E. (1990). *Scholarship reconsidered: Priorities of the professorate. The Carnegie foundation for the advancement of teaching.* Jossey-Bass. ISBN:7879-4069-0.

Branch, J. (2017). *How to become a successful motivational speaker.* Lulu Press.

Buckley, J. (2014). *Type and background color in research posters.* https://blog.postersession.com/2014/03/20/type-and-background-color-in-research-posters/

Connelly, L. M. (2018). Designing effective conference posters. *MEDSURG Nursing, 27*(1), 64–65.

Conrad, P. L., & Pape, T. (2014). Roles and responsibilities of the nursing scholar. *Pediatric Nursing, 40*, 87–90.

Cook, D. A., & Bordage, G. (2016). Twelve tips on writing abstracts and titles: How to get people to use and cite your work. *Medical Teacher, 38*, 1100–1104. https://doi.org/10.1080/0142159x.2016.1181732

Cottingham, R. (2019, July 17). *Why and how you should get to know your audience before a speech.* https://www.prdaily.com/why-and-how-you-should-get-to-know-your-audience-before-a-speech/

Crick, N. (2017). *Rhetorical public speaking: Civic engagement in the digital age* (3rd ed.). Routledge.

DeCoske, M. A. & White, S. J. (2010). Public speaking revisited: Delivery, structure, and style. *American Journal of Health-System Pharmacy, 67*, 1225–1227. https://doi.org/10.2146/ajhp090508

Dewar, J., Bennett, C., & Fisher, M. A. (2018). *The scholarship of teaching and learning: A guide for scientists, engineers, and mathematicians.* Oxford University Press.

Dwyer, K. K., & Davidson, M. M. (2012). Is public speaking really more feared than death? *Communication Research Reports, 29*, 99–107. https://doi.org/10.1080/08824096.2012.667772

Foster, C., Wager, E., Marchington, J., Patel, M., Banner, S., Kennard, N. C., Panayi, A., Stacey, R., & GPCAP Working Group. (2019). Good practice for conference abstracts and presentations: GPCAP. *Research Integrity & Peer Review, 4*(11). https://researchintegrityjournal.biomedcentral.com/articles/10.1186/s41073-019-0070-x

Happell, B. (2008). Conference presentations: A guide to writing the abstract. *Nurse Researcher, 14*(4), 79–87.

Happell, B. (2009). Presenting with precision: Preparing and delivering a polished conference presentation. *Nurse Researcher, 16*(3), 45–56.

Heseltine, E. (2012). Writing an abstract: Window to the world on your work. *Australian and New Zealand Journal of Public Health, 36*, 204–205.

Holland, K., & Watson, R. (2012). *Writing for publication in nursing and healthcare. Getting it right.* Wiley – Blackwell.

Huff, A. S. (1999). *Writing for scholarly publication.* SAGE Publications.

International Committee of Medical Journal Editors. (2017). *Recommendations for the conduct, reporting, editing, and publication of scholarly work in medical journals.* http://www.icmje.org/icmje-recommendations.pdf

Kara, H. (2015, January 7). *How to write a killer conference abstract: The first step towards an engaging presentation.* The London School of Economics and Political Science (LSE). https://blogs.lse.ac.uk/impactofsocialsciences/2015/01/27/how-to-write-a-killer-conference-abstract/

Kennedy, M. S., Barnsteiner, J., & Daly, J. (2014). Honorary and ghost authorship in nursing publications. *Journal of Nursing Scholarship, 46*, 416–422. https://doi.org/10.1111/jnu.12093

Khasseh, A. A., & Biranvand, A. (2013). Structured vs. unstructured abstract: a different look at Iranian journals of library science. *International Research Journal of Applied and Basic Sciences,* 4(7), 1706–1709.

King, C. R. (2009). Issues and best practices related to ethical writing and publishing. *Journal of the Association for Vascular Access, 14*, 40–45. https://doi.org/10.2309/java.14-1-7

Leggett, T. (2018). Getting to the heart of the matter: How to write an abstract. *Radiation Therapist,* 27(1), 76–78.

Levett-Jones, T., & Stone, T. (2012). Writing for publication: Turning the conference paper into publishable work. In Holland, K. & Watson, R. (Eds.), *Writing for publication in nursing and healthcare* (pp. 145–161). Wiley-Blackwell.

Levoy, B. (2010). More tested tips for public speaking. *Podiatry Management, 7*, 187–190.

Longo, A., & Tierney, C. (2012). Presentation skills for the nurse educator. *Journal for Nurses in Staff Development, 28*, 16–23. https://doi.org/10.1097/NND.0b013e318240a699

McCurry, D. (2018, April 6). *Learning how to write an abstract for a conference is a matter of following a simple formula for success.* Here it is. https://www.exordo.com/blog/how-to-write-an-abstract-for-a-conference/

Medina, M. S., & Avant, N. D. (2015). Delivering an effective presentation. *American Journal of Health-System Pharmacy, 72*, 1091–1094. https://doi.org/10.2146/ajhp150047

Morin, K. (2017). *Retiring? Some things to consider.* Specialty Session, 2017 AWHONN Conference, New Orleans, LA, June 27, 2017.

Morin, K. H. (2017). What reviewers say: Authors listen up! [Editorial]. *Journal of Nursing Education, 56*, 63–64. https://doi.org/10.392801484834-20170123-01

Morin, K. H., Klopper, H. C., & Der Walt, C. V. (2016). *MCH Leadership Development: A Retrospective, Comparative Cohort Study.* Sigma Theta Tau International 26th Research Congress. Cape Town, SA, July 20, 2016.

Morin, K., Plowfield, L., Bucher, L., Hayes, E., Mahoney, P., & Armiger, L. (1997). *A survey of Delaware acute care facilities' use of research.* 9th Annual Scientific Session of the ENRS, Philadelphia, April, 1997.

Mott, S. (2014). The process of writing an abstract. *Journal of Pediatric Nursing, 29*(4):383–385. https://doi.org/10.1016/j.pedn.2014.04.008

National Information Standards Organization. (2015). *Guidelines for abstracts.* [ANSI/NISO Z39.14-1997 (R2015). ISSN:1041–5653.

Oermann, M. H., & Hays, J. C. (2016). *Writing for publication in nursing* (3rd ed.). Springer Publishing Company.

Phillips, B. (2019, April 10). *Nine rhetorical devices for your next speech*. https://www.throughline-group.com/2011/03/15/nine-rhetorical-devices-for-your-next-speech/

Raimes, A., & Miller-Cochran, , (2017). *Pocket keys for writers* (6th ed.). Cengage Learning.

Scholar. (2020). In *Merriam Webster Online Dictionary*. https://www.merriam-webster.com/dictionary/scholar

Scout, J. (2015). *The best colours to make your posters pop*. https://www.clubink.ca/blog/print/best-colours-make-posters-pop/

Sherman, R. O. (2010). How to create an effective poster presentation. *The American Nurse, 5*(9). https://www.americannursetoday.com/how-to-create-an-effective-poster-presentation/

Siedlecki, S. (2017). How to create a poster that attracts an audience. *American Journal of Nursing, 117*(3), 48–54.

Slaver, C. (2011). *Anatomy of writing for publication for nurses*. Sigma Theta Tau International.

Slutsky, J., & Baum, N. H. (2017). Public speaking for the podiatric physician – part I. *Podiatry Management, 36*(8), 87–90.

Slutsky, J., & Baum, N. H. (2018). Public speaking for the podiatric physician – part 2. *Podiatry Management, 37*(3), 113–118.

SpeakerHub (2017, August 21). *How to read your audience in 10 seconds*. https://medium.com/@speakerhubHQ/how-to-read-your-audience-in-10-seconds-619e9a2a2383

Tierney, E. P. (1996). *How to make effective presentations*. SAGE Publications.

Villar, R. (2015, October). What is this duplicate publication thing? *Journal of Hip Preservation Surgery, 2*(3), 203–205.

Watson, R. (2012). The basics of writing for publication and the steps to success: Getting started. In Holland, K., & Watson, R. (Eds), *Writing for publication in nursing and healthcare. Getting it right* (pp. 7–21). Wiley – Blackwell.

Watson, R., Pickler, R., Noyes, J., Perry, L., Roe, B., & Hayter, M. (2014). How many papers can be published from one study? [Editorial]. *Journal of Advanced Nursing, 71*(11), 2457–2460.

Whitespace Marketing. (2018). *Why use white space*. https://www.whitespacemarketing.com.au/why-use-white-space/

Wood, G. J., & Morrison, R. S. (2011). Writing abstracts and developing posters for national meetings. *Journal of Palliative Medicine, 14*, 353–359. https://doi.org/10.1089/jpm.2010.0171

Zerwic, J. J., Grandfield, K., Kavanaugh, K., Berger, B., Graham, L., & Mershon, M. (2010). Tips for better visual elements in posters and podium presentations. *Education for Health, 23*(2), 1–6.

15

Funding Your Project

Valerie A. Adelson

LEARNING OBJECTIVES

After completing this chapter, you will be able to:

1. Designate the sources of grant funding, including foundations, corporations, and federal awarding agencies.

2. Understand how to research prospective funding from foundations, corporations, and federal awarding agencies.

3. Communicate how to build relationships with foundations and corporations for grant funding.

4. Describe the key elements of a competitive grant proposal.

5. Explain the key elements of a project budget, including the budget justification.

6. Recognize general federal grant requirements, including the mechanics of applying for a federal award.

7. Distinguish general reporting and compliance requirements of a grant award, in particular, as a recipient of federal funding.

8. Identify the functions of a consultant and how the consultant may support the applicant organization or institution with grant funding.

KEY TERMS

501(c)(3): The Internal Revenue Code section that designates an organization as charitable and tax-exempt. Organizations seeking foundation or corporate funding secure a Section 501(c)(3) classification from the Internal Revenue Service.

Allowable costs: Budget costs approved for required work performed under grants with the federal government.

Awards: Financial assistance, including grants and other agreements, to an eligible recipient.

Budget: The proposed financial plan for a project or program that a foundation, corporation, or federal awarding agency (or pass-through entity) approves during the grant award process or in subsequent amendments to the grant award. A federal awarding agency may request the applicant to document the federal and nonfederal share of a budget or only the federal share.

Close-out: The process by which the foundation, corporation, or federal awarding agency (or pass-through entity) determines that all appropriate administrative actions and all required work of a grant or contract have been completed to officially close the grant award or contract.

Contract: A legally binding agreement by which a nonfederal entity purchases property or services needed to carry out the project or program under a federal award.

Discretionary funds: Grant funds distributed at the discretion of one or more trustees, which usually do not require prior approval by the full board of directors.

Financial report: An itemized accounting that shows how grant funds were used by the recipient organization.

Form 990/Form 990-PF: The Internal Revenue Service forms filed annually by public charities and private foundations, respectively. PF refers to "private foundation." Both forms list organization assets, receipts, expenditures, and compensation of officers. Form 990-PF includes a list of grants made during the year by private foundations.

Four-Factor Analysis: Developed by the U.S. Department of Justice and recognized by federal agencies as the fundamental first step in determining how to comply with the language assistance mandates of Title VI of the Civil Rights Act of 1964 and how to provide people with limited English proficiency (LEP) with meaningful access to federally funded programs. (1) The number or proportion of LEP persons eligible to be served or likely to be encountered by the grantee; (2) the frequency with which LEP individuals come into contact with the program; (3) the nature and importance of the program, activity, or service provided by the program to people's lives; and (4) the resources available to the grantee/recipient and costs.

Funding cycle: The time line that includes the proposal review, decision-making, and applicant notification, which may operate at established intervals (e.g., quarterly, semiannually) or annually.

Funding opportunity announcement: A publicly available document by which a federal agency declares its intentions to award discretionary grants or cooperative agreements. Funding opportunity announcements may be referred to as program announcements, notices of funding availability, or solicitations; the name of the announcement varies depending on the agency or foundation and type of program.

Goals: A broad statement about the long-term expectations of the proposed program that serves as the foundation for developing proposed program objectives.

Grants: An award of funds to an organization or individual to undertake charitable activities including research, health, education, arts, and culture, as well as alleviating poverty.

Grant agreement: The terms of the foundation or federal agency grant award. A grant agreement with a federal awarding agency does not provide for substantial involvement between the awarding agency (or pass-through entity) and the recipient in accomplishing the activities stipulated by the award.

Grant monitoring: An ongoing assessment by the foundation or federal awarding agency of the progress of grant-related activities to determine if the terms and conditions of the grant are being met and if the goals of the grant will be accomplished by the recipient organization or institution.

Grantee: The individual, organization, or institution that receives a grant award.

Grantor: The foundation, corporation, or federal awarding agency that makes a grant award.

Guidelines: The established goals, priorities, criteria, and procedures of a foundation, corporation, or federal awarding agency for applying for a grant award.

In-kind contribution: A donation of goods or services rather than cash or appreciated property.

Logic model: A visual tool that shows the logic, or rationale, behind a proposed program or process included in a grant application.

Object classes (object class categories): Federal budget categories that may include personnel salaries, fringe benefits, travel, equipment, supplies, and contractual obligations.

Objectives: The expected results and how they will be achieved. Objectives establish program priorities to measure progress and provide for accountability.

Operating support: A financial award to cover an organization's general, ongoing expenses, such as salaries, utilities, and office rental.

Pass-through entity: A nonfederal entity that provides a subaward to a subrecipient in order to carry out part of a federal program.

Preliminary proposal: Also known as a *query letter*, a brief draft of a grant proposal (or a brief letter) used to learn if sufficient interest from a foundation warrants submission of a proposal to save time for the prospective foundation donor as well as the time and resources of the prospective applicant.

Principle investigator (PI): The lead researcher and primary contact for the proposed project.

Program officer: A staff member of a foundation or corporate giving program who may recommend policy, review, and process grant applications for the board of directors and manage the foundation budget.

Restricted funds: Charitable assets that are restricted in use, such as in the types of organizations that may receive grants from the fund or the process to award grants from such funds.

Site visit: Visiting an applicant organization at its office location or area of operation and/or meeting with its staff or directors or with recipients of its services.

Technical assistance: Operational or management assistance to a nonprofit institution or organization, including, for example, fundraising assistance, budgeting and financial planning, program planning, legal advice, and marketing. Assistance may be offered directly by a foundation or corporate staff member or in the form of a grant to offset the costs of retaining an outside expert or consultant.

Unrestricted funds: Funds not specifically designated to particular uses by the donor.

Introduction

Advanced practice nurses (APNs) are employed in all types of organizations—universities, colleges, nonprofit hospitals or healthcare systems, nongovernmental organizations, and not-for-profit organizations—that qualify for funding from foundations, corporations, or the federal government. However, despite the availability of grant funding, there is strong competition between applicants. APNs need to familiarize themselves with key terms, strategies, and techniques to determine how they can best find funding for their proposed project. These projects—whether a pilot study, unit-based project, or systems-wide approach—could be worthy of funding if the APN can identify appropriate funding sources and submit a proposal that reflects funding priorities and complies with requested information. These projects can make a significant impact and bring about long-term results. This chapter provides information that prompts APNs to ask and answer several questions in understanding and applying for grant funding.

Types of Grants and Funding Sources

Total giving by U.S. foundations in 2003 was more than $30 billion. By 2013, overall giving by the nation's private and community foundations reached $54.7 billion, surpassing previous record levels after adjusting for inflation. In 2016, total contributions from several sources—including individual giving, bequests, foundations, and corporations—totaled $390.05 billion. Of the total amount, foundations represented 15% or $59.28 billion, an increase of 3.5% from the previous year; corporate giving represented 5% or $18.55 billion, an increase of 3.5% from the previous year. The modest increase in corporate giving may be attributable to slower growth in the gross domestic product (GDP) as well as minimal growth in the share of pretax profits directed to charitable giving (Annual Report on Philanthropy, 2016).

Though giving by foundations increased at a slower rate in 2016 as compared to stronger increases in recent years, foundations are eager to engage and to collaborate with organizational and institutional partners to further the foundation's impact on diverse issues (The Annual Report on Philanthropy, 2016).

The Foundation Center (2016) defines a foundation as, "…a nonprofit corporation or a charitable trust, with the purpose of making grants to unrelated organizations or institutions or to individuals for scientific, educational, cultural, religious, or other charitable purposes."

The Foundation Center (2014) notes that foundations have flexibility in determining all aspects of their grantmaking activities, including who, what, when, where, and how they will provide funding. Foundations can fund local or global projects. Some foundations provide funding for a small number of large, targeted grants to achieve organizational goals, while others emphasize providing many small, unrestricted grants as being most effective in achieving their goals. Similarly, some grant makers focus their giving on specific populations. This range of priorities and approaches illustrates the role of foundations as critical sources of support for new strategies and opportunities throughout higher education and social sectors, including colleges, universities, academic health centers, and nonprofit entities.

Though several different terms are used within the field of philanthropy to describe how a grantor or foundation operates and awards grants, foundations are established to aid social, educational, religious, or other charitable needs. Generally, a board of directors makes discretionary giving decisions, often within specific guidelines as to the charitable field of interest and/or geographic area (The Council on Foundations, 2020a, 2020b). Awards from corporations are typically more focused on branding, visibility, and corporate opportunities for social responsibility with the nonprofit sector.

In seeking funding opportunities, it is important to understand that foundations can take many different forms: **independent**, **operating**, **corporate**, and **community** (Box 15.1).

More than 90% of U.S. foundations annually distribute approximately 5% of their net investment assets for charitable purposes (The Foundation Center, 2012). Private nonoperating foundations, which constitute the majority of U.S. grantmaking foundations and include most **family**- and company-sponsored foundations, must meet the minimum 5% legal requirement. Private operating foundations, which directly operate charitable programs (rather than making grants) as their primary activity, have a different distribution requirement. Community foundations, which are classified as public charities, are not subject to any payout requirements (Box 15.2).

BOX 15.1

▶ TYPES OF FOUNDATIONS

- **Community:** A tax-exempt, nonprofit, philanthropic institution that uses funds from multiple donors to assist residents of a particular community. A community foundation consists of permanent funds established by many separate donors, including individuals, families, and businesses, from a defined geographic area.

- **Corporate:** A private foundation whose grantmaking funds are derived from a profit-making business. While the company-sponsored foundation may maintain a close relationship with the donor company, it is a separate organization subject to the same rules and regulations as other private foundations.

- **Family foundation:** A foundation whose funds are derived from members of a single family. At least one family member must continue to serve as an officer or board member of the foundation, and as the donor, they or their relatives play a significant role in governing and/or managing the foundation.

- **Independent foundation:** A private foundation usually founded by one individual, typically through a bequest. They are also termed *nonoperating* because they do not run their own programs; instead, independent foundations make grant awards to other nonprofit organizations and institutions.

- **Operating foundation:** A private foundation that uses much of their income to provide charitable services or to run charitable programs of their own. They make few, if any, grants to outside organizations or institutions.

- **Private foundation:** A nongovernmental, nonprofit organization with funds (usually derived from a single source, including, for example, an individual, family, or corporation) and programs managed by its own trustees or directors.

- **Public foundation:** Public foundations, along with community foundations, are recognized as public charities by the Internal Revenue Service. Although they may provide direct charitable services to the public, the primary focus is on grantmaking.

Based on The Council on Foundations, The Council on Foundations. (2020a) and The Council on Foundations. (2020b). *Foundation basics.*

BOX 15.2

▶ TYPES OF GRANTS AS IDENTIFIED BY THE FOUNDATION CENTER

- **Matching grants:** Grant funds paid only if the recipient is able to identify additional sources of funding and not rely solely upon the award of grant funds. The grant applicant may be asked to include in the proposed project budget a percentage or amount of financial support from sources other than the grant award. Matching grants are made with the intent that the amount donated must be matched on a one-for-one basis or according to some other prescribed formula.

- **Demonstration grants:** Grants made to establish an innovative project or program that will serve as a model, if successful, and may be replicated by other organizations or institutions.

- **Discretionary grants:** Grants made by foundation officers or foundation staff without review by the foundation board. Though discretionary grants are awarded without oversight by the foundation board, the grants must follow the foundation's mission. Discretionary federal grants are grants for which the federal awarding agency may select the recipient from among all eligible recipients and make or do not make an award based on the programmatic, technical, or scientific merit of an application. The federal awarding agency can also determine the amount of funding to be awarded to a recipient.

- **Foundation-administered program awards:** Given to programs, including research programs, which are administered by the foundation.

Typically, federal government grant applications are much more complex than a grant proposal for a foundation and involve standard forms, assurances, and certifications as well as a broad multidisciplinary approach by the applicant organization. The funding opportunity announcement, published by the federal awarding agency, will stipulate the required forms and documents for a specific funding opportunity.

In Their Own Words

Jodie C. Gary, PhD, RN
Texas A&M University
College of Nursing

What Prompted You to Apply for Your First Grant?

From 2013 to 2016, I served as the RN-BSN Program Coordinator for the College of Nursing (CON). As I started this role, two scenarios presented opportunities for positive impact. First, our new program had a largely homogenous population of nursing students with only 2.8% of our 2012 graduating nursing students self-identified as Black or Hispanic. The demographics of Texas is approaching 40% Hispanic, and our university is a land-grant institution dedicated to serving the needs of the entire state. Second, the CON was in the beginning stages of developing partnerships in South Texas, an area with a large Hispanic population. The prospect of increasing the diversity of the nursing workforce while leveraging the early stages of partnerships in South Texas was the launching point for a project.

What Grant Opportunity Presented a Match to Your Interest?

A request for applications (RFA) was posted by the Texas Higher Education Coordinating Board (THECB) Minority Health Research and Education Grant Program (MHGP) for a Recruitment and Retention grant opportunity. The RFA called for projects to enable more African Americans and Hispanics to enroll in and graduate from health-degree programs. The RFA requested a brief emailed "intent to apply" with a deadline of early January.

How Did You Approach the Intent to Apply?

I began by assembling a small team of three key faculty to begin brainstorming. The team identified the challenge of recruitment and retention of minorities into nursing as one that could be best addressed through the developing partnerships in South Texas. The focus of the project was centered on Hidalgo County in South Texas where the online course delivery of our RN-BSN program could afford an opportunity to recruit, educate, and graduate Hispanic students within the communities of South Texas and allowed the CON partnerships to develop for potential program expansion. We submitted a letter of intent and waited to learn if an application would be requested.

(Continued)

Once You Were Requested to Submit a Full Application, How Did You Proceed?
The team broke the application down into sections and crafted an outline that assisted in organization of the process and created a diagram of the program we wanted to accomplish. Our overall program objective was to recruit, retain, and foster success of minority baccalaureate nursing students. This meant increasing minority student engagement with our CON programs, fostering student success for all students, and promoting excellence in all of our CON programs. Taking our successful email outline and submitting a full project proposal meant our team needed to meet at regularly scheduled intervals in order to submit the grant on time. We had to consider ongoing assessment, analysis, and evaluation in the project proposal.

What Writing Strategy Did You Use?
The writing strategy that worked for our team was to have myself and a coinvestigator meet and work on a draft simultaneously from a projected screen. This assisted in writing the proposal in one cohesive voice as well as having multiple sets of eyes on the mechanics of the application. We used a large dry erase board to diagram the process and outline specific components during these writing times. This was instrumental to the brainstorming aspects as well as ensuring we were connecting the work components of the project in a logical way as well as being instrumental in the budget formation. This process led to the development of phases for the project where the first phase informed the second. The third team member was called for specifics related to her expertise and we also consulted our CON administrative team such as student affairs, academic affairs, and the instructional designer for key aspects related to the program in development.

Phase 1 was to advise the refinement and implementation of programmatic strategies as quantitative and qualitative data were to be evaluated for effective strategies in facilitating performance outcomes to improve minority student recruitment, retention, and success. Community explicit needs were deemed invaluable and plans were made to assess this from multiple perspectives. Then in the second phase, we planned to collect quantitative and qualitative data to evaluate the effectiveness of the strategies in facilitating outcomes of specific activities tied to the goals. In diagramming the project, it was clear that a mixed methods design would allow cyclical process improvement and ongoing refinement of strategies to increase application and enrollment of minority students.

(Continued)

Was Your Application Successful?

We were notified that our application had been tentatively accepted with conditions to be discussed with the program officer. The revising of the project narrative was completed to strengthen the focus of program development, implementation, and evaluation. The revised application was funded.

How Did the Implementation Phase Proceed?

There were more challenges to the initial start-up of the project than initially and naively anticipated. We had created an extremely ambitious timeline and that did NOT sufficiently include time for challenges. The first order of business was to adjust the overly ambitious timeline proposed. We worked with the program officer during the first reporting period, and this actually ended up becoming more positive as there was time for best practices in literature to be identified and for more thoughtful consideration in the implementation of the first phase.

Of particular challenge to initiating the project was the lack of understanding concerning the specific needs for institutional review board (IRB) approval. This caused a setback as grant funding could not be released until IRB approval was awarded, but at the same time, the team needed to purchase supplies such as laptops and software in order to design and address specifics for the IRB application as well as project design. Modified IRB approval was sought for the release of funds with the caveat that no contact with human subjects would occur until an amendment was submitted and approved. Direct communication with the university research services representative also assisted in overcoming some of the challenges. Hindsight was clear that engagement with the IRB could have been initiated for guidance at as the proposal was being written.

Communication, flexibility, and patience became key components in completing the grant as well as attributes learned for application to current and future grant awards. Despite the learning moments, the project was successfully completed.

What Was Involved in Reporting?

Due dates for the reporting requirements were placed on each team members' calendar at the beginning of the grant to ensure advanced notification. The team scheduled times 10 days ahead of the due dates to accommodate the procurement of required data and signatures as needed depending on the report. It also helped to send calendar invites to those administrative roles or compliance offices from which information was requested. As a first time principal investigator, this open communication was instrumental in the success. Going forward, I will keep communication with future program officers at the forefront of any project.

(Continued)

> **How Did You Benefit From Writing Your First Grant?**
> Beyond the scholarship, the impact of the grant was far more for my personal scholarship journey. Grant work is *not* a linear process. It requires thoughtful consideration of assessment, analysis and evaluation and more importantly aspects of communication, flexibility, and patience.
>
> *The author reports no conflicts of interest. This work was supported in part by a grant from the Texas Higher Education Coordinating Board (THECB). The opinions and conclusions expressed in this document are those of the authors and do not necessarily represent the opinions or policy of the THECB.*

The Award Process

For graduate students completing a dissertation or a clinical project, seeking and obtaining external funding for a research or training grant can be daunting. Whether originating with a foundation or federal awarding agency, the grant process has a life cycle that includes identifying funding options, submitting a grant application, award notification, project implementation, grant reporting, and closing out of the grant award, all of which have individualized variables and dynamics (Grants.gov, n.d.). There are typically three distinct stages of the grant life cycle: pre-award phase, award phase, and post-award phase (Figure 15.1).

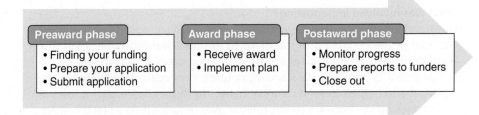

Figure 15.1. Three stages of grant cycle.

Pre-Award Phase

The pre-award phase includes foundations and federal awarding agencies announcing the availability of grant funding through a funding opportunity announcement or a request for proposal. The process of researching, writing, and submitting a grant proposal is considered as the pre-award phase of the grant funding cycle.

Some foundations may not accept unsolicited grant proposals. An organization or institution interested in applying for grant funding may need to submit a letter of inquiry to the prospective foundation partner. This **query letter** is an introduction by the applicant organization or institution and should briefly describe why the organization or institution is interested in applying for grant funding, the proposed project and its relevance to the foundation's program areas, and an estimated budget for each year of the proposed project. The letter should succinctly present the case for the worthiness of funding a proposed project or program.

The foundation program officers will consider the letter of inquiry, and if the proposed project aligns with the foundation's funding criteria, the organization may be invited to submit a formal grant proposal. Alignment between the letter and foundation's funding criteria is imperative. Regardless of how worthy or intriguing a project or program may appear to be, if the foundation's priorities do not align with your organization, the foundation will decline your request for funding. Given the competition for grant funding, an organization should not expect that the invitation to submit a formal grant proposal is a certainty that the funding request will be approved by the foundation's program officers or board of directors.

Writing the Grant Proposal

"The development of effective strategies and methods in identifying funding opportunities takes time, requires practice, and needs patience."
(U.S. Department of Health and Human Services, Office of Minority Health Resource Center, 2015).

An applicant organization or institution must have an appreciation of the nature of grant seeking and grant writing—the process is long term, fraught with frustration, and requires taking a broad, objective approach in identifying funding prospects (U.S. Department of Health and Human Services, 2015). Logic

---

BOX 15.3

▶ LOGIC MODELS

Definition: A logic model is a picture that presents the relationships between resources, activities, outputs, and outcomes/impacts for your program.

Purpose: Its purpose is to depict the relationship between your program's activities and its intended outcomes.

Components:

- Inputs: The resources needed to implement the activities

- Activities: What the program and its staff do with those resources

- Outputs: Tangible products, capacities, or deliverables that result from the activities

- Outcomes: Changes that occur in other people or conditions because of the activities and outputs

- Impacts: The long-term outcomes

Adapted from Centers for Disease Control and Prevention (CDC). (2018). *Logic models: CDC approach to evaluation.* https://www.cdc.gov/eval/logicmodels/index.htm

---

models are increasingly required as part of a grant application (see Box 15.3). No matter the passion and experience the staff of an organization or institution has, in order to gain funding support, the proposed project or program must be realistic from the perspective of the potential funder.

Finding Funding Opportunities

Foundations may restrict grant funding to a specific geographic area. For example, foundations may only award grants to nonprofit organizations serving specific states or counties. In pursuing grant funding, consider that foundations may not offer the type of grant support your organization requires such as clinical trials; the foundation may offer restricted funds or unrestricted funds. Foundations, as well as federal agencies, typically fund programs or projects rather than provide general operating support for administrative expenses.

Identifying funding prospects can be daunting. Gathering and analyzing information directly from the foundation's Form 990/Form 990-PF tends to be more current and relevant than many directories. For example, from a foundation's website, you can accumulate significant information about the foundation, including what motivates the foundation, the focus of the foundation's program areas, as well as eligibility criteria or restrictions on the use of grant funds.

The Catalog of Federal Domestic Assistance (CFDA) is a government compendium available at www.cfda.gov that lists general information about federal programs, including grants. Each program listed has a unique identifier code or CFDA number. For example, the U.S. Department of Health and Human Services programs are listed with the prefix 93.XXX (Administration for Native Americans, 2018).

A funding opportunity announcement is published by federal grantmaking agencies for potential applicants. The funding opportunity announcements are based on related legislation and their budgets. The funding opportunity announcement includes pertinent information and requirements for an applicant to assess their eligibility, competency, and interest in the funding opportunity.

Questions to Ask Yourself

1. Does your project or program have common goals with the foundation or federal agency?
2. Do your board members have a relationship with leadership or staff of a foundation?
3. Which foundations or federal agencies offer grant funding relevant to your area of research interest?

The Grant Proposal

The grant proposal is the tangible manifestation of the proposed project or program. The Foundation Center (2019) notes that elements of the grant proposal may have implications for different departments of an organization. Potential principle investigators should coordinate with additional departments (for example, communications and finance) for guidance in preparing the grant proposal and in submitting necessary documents. Table 15.1 presents the sections of a typical grant proposal.

Table 15.1. Components of a Grant Proposal

Grant Proposal	Purpose	Content	Hints for Writing
Executive summary	The executive summary is a brief overview of the organization and institution, including the history and the mission.	The executive summary also serves as an abstract of the grant proposal and provides an overview of the research question and proposed program or project for which an organization or institution is seeking funding.	Be compelling and convincing; the executive summary should capture the interest and imagination of the potential funder.
Narrative statement	The narrative describes in greater detail the purpose of the proposed project or program. Addresses the level of effort for each team member.	Includes the qualifications and experience of the key team members who will work on the proposed project and program, as well as the support and resources of the participating institution.	It is also important to articulate how team members will collaborate, especially if several facilities are participating in the grant program.
Statement of need	The statement of need should describe the specific problem or need an institution or organization seeks to address.	What evidence exists to support the stated need? Providing anecdotes specific to the project or program is important but also provide data—for example, demographic data—in order to create context and to help understand the changes the proposed project or program may bring about in the community.	The goals of the proposed project or program should align with the statement of need.

Project description	The project description should address why the organization or institution and staff are uniquely qualified to conduct the proposed research. The description should also include the outcomes that the organization or institution is trying to achieve along with the plan of approach.	The project description must identify the staff responsible for oversight of the proposed program or project (for example, the **principle investigator**), their credentials, qualifications, and experience with similar grant-funded projects. If appropriate, address the supervision of staff, including consultants, from institutions.	Provide specific goals and related strategies to be accomplished to achieve the desired outcomes.
Evaluation	The evaluation plan documents how the applicant organization or institution will evaluate the proposed grant project or program, for example, how relevant data indicators will be collected or measured to demonstrate a successful outcome.	The evaluation plan should also justify that the outcome measures are appropriate and validated for the proposed study.	Increasingly, foundations and federal agencies are requesting specific measures of project or program outcomes, including **logic models.**

(Continued)

Table 15.1. Components of a Grant Proposal   (continued)

Grant Proposal	Purpose	Content	Hints for Writing
Organizational information	Organizational information should include a biography of the applicant organization or institution as well as the qualifications of the researchers. Consider, for example, if the organization or institution received an award or other recognition for its innovative programs in the community. Does the principal investigator have demonstrated experience conducting grant-funded projects that are similar in scope and complexity?	Understand competing organizations with mission statements similar to the applicant organization or institution; an applicant must be able to explain to a foundation how the organization's services or programs are unique and differ from other organizations or institutions.	It is important to remember that an applicant is competing with many worthy organizations and institutions for grant funding. An applicant may have a sterling grant proposal. However, if the organization or institution is poorly organized or managed or has an inconsistent record of accomplishments and problematic financial statements, a foundation will likely be reluctant to agree to fund the proposed project or program and risk its own reputation; a dependable partner will be selected rather than entering into an arrangement with an unreliable organization.
Conclusion	The conclusion should reiterate how the applicant intends to address the awarding agency or foundation's program guidelines and interests.	Summarize all sections of the proposal.	No new information should be presented in this section. Instead, emphasize key points of the application.

Preparing a Responsive Grant Application

Foundations will also request that applicants demonstrate the impact of the proposed project or program through various outcome or performance measures. Foundations, as well as federal funding agencies, may require an applicant to describe dissemination activities to relevant audiences, including, for example, professional societies and how the applicant will engage in communication efforts with various lay and professional audiences.

Before writing the grant application, it is imperative that the potential principle investigator have the approval and support of the appropriate leadership or authority. Universities, colleges, and academic medical centers may have an Office of Sponsored Research (OSR). The OSR is responsible for pre-award proposal review, approval, and submission and post-award services for externally funded grants. In addition, an institution may have an Office of Corporate and Foundation Relations (CFR). The CFR coordinates with corporations, foundations, and association philanthropies on behalf of faculty and staff seeking research grant funding. Applicants may also need to have approval from an institutional review board (IRB). The role of an IRB is presented in Figure 15.2.

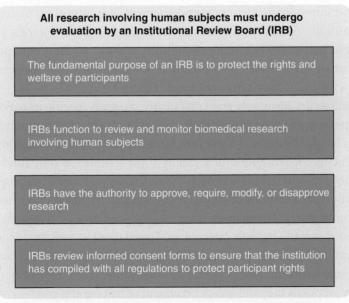

Figure 15.2. Role of institutional review board (IRB).

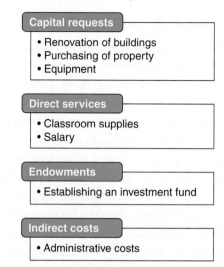

Figure 15.3. Types of funding costs with examples.

Foundations may also consider the tenure of an organization and the availability of resources to conduct the proposed project or program. Newly established organizations can establish credibility in other ways, for example, with a dedicated board of directors or evidence of strong community collaboration and partnerships through letters of endorsement. It is important to demonstrate your organization's or institution's impact through various metrics, including, for example, outreach work in the community and successful programming. It is also important when researching potential philanthropies that applicants wisely consider what foundations may not fund (Figure 15.3).

Foundations are invariably and consistently program specific in making grants and may not support general operating costs. It is important to research how grant funds may be used by the **grantee** or how funds are restricted. Approaching a funder for construction or renovation of a facility if the foundation only funds research grants is not a recommended approach. Indeed, ignoring foundation program rules and priorities may impair the ability of an organization or institution to successfully obtain future funding. Foundations favor making grant awards to organizations and institutions that abide by their preferences. Foundations as well as federal funding agencies can always identify and partner with worthy applicants that comply with the requirements of a funding opportunity. Also, foundations may restrict the number of new proposals they will accept because of other ongoing grant commitments. The applicant organization or institution should be clear and direct in its approach to facilitate separating itself positively from the competition.

Prior to applying for grant funding, either from a foundation or federal agency, ensure that your organization is registered as a 501(c)(3). Foundations and federal agencies generally do not award grants to for-profit entities. Foundations do not typically award grants to individuals and may give preference to specific organizations such as institutions within a particular geographic area. For-profits may wish to consider partnering with or collaborating with a nonprofit organization in order to apply for grant funding. However, grant applicants should be judicious when considering a collaboration with another organization or institution. It is important to identify a credible and financially viable partner.

Applicants for federal agency funding must have a Data Universal Numbering System (DUNS) number from Dun & Bradstreet. In addition to the DUNS number, applicants applying online through the federal government's Grants.gov must register with the System for Award Management (SAM). Applicant organizations must also register with Grants.gov; applicants must provide the organization's DUNS number in order to complete the Grants.gov registration. Completing the application process with Grants.gov prompts the applicant to receive an email request to designate an E-Business Point of Contact (E-Biz POC) and Authorized Organization Representatives (AORs). In order to apply for federal grants online on behalf of an organization, the individual applicant must be recognized as an AOR in Grants.gov.

Partnerships

Collaborations are the way forward. In preparing a competitive grant application, consider collaborating with other organizations that complement your organization's expertise. Collaborating with another not-for-profit or public sector organization or institution may enhance the possibility of grant funding for your organization. Foundations, as well as federal funding agencies, are increasingly encouraging partnering organizations to apply for grant funding. Consider engagement efforts with partner organizations or institutions, including negotiating with potential partners in advance of preparing and responding to a funding opportunity. Philanthropies may request the applicant describe the period of time that the collaborating organizations have worked together on relevant projects, programs, or services. Philanthropies may expect organizations to develop a record of successful partnerships and collaborations to demonstrate an organization's bonafides and strength of reputation. Lastly, describe in the grant application the specific contributions of partnering organizations and institutions as well as the roles and responsibilities of staff.

Letters of Support

Signed letters of support are statements from the leadership of other public or private sector organizations or institutions that support the proposed project or program for grant funding. Letters of support address the roles of partnering organizations and institutions with the proposed project or program. Though letters of support may not be required, one that recommends the applicant's project or program enhances the grant application or proposal.

Overview of the Budgeting Process

Writing a responsive budget and budget narrative may be more challenging than preparing the project or program narrative. All grant applicants are required to follow guidelines in submitting a budget for the proposed project and program; federal funding agencies also request a budget justification with the application. The proposed federal project or program budget is provided on SF-424A (https://www.sba.gov/sites/default/files/SF-424A.pdf) or SF-424C (https://www.nsf.gov/bfa/dias/policy/docs/sf424c.pdf), Budget Information Standard Form.

The federal budget justification includes a budget narrative and line-item budget detail. The line-item budget detail involves specific project budget calculations for object class categories. The object class categories may include personnel, fringe benefits, travel, equipment, and supplies and are listed on the federal awarding agency's Budget Information Standard Form. It is important to ensure that each line item in the proposed budget throughout the grant award period is reasonable and **allowable**.

If matching or cost-sharing is required by the foundation or federal awarding agency, applicants must provide evidence of other reliable funding sources in direct support of the proposed activities; other funding sources may include foundations, corporations, federal or state government agencies, or individuals.

Foundations as well as federal agencies that award grant funding will specify allowable direct and indirect costs. For example, SAMHSA (2017) defines direct costs as "…costs that can be identified specifically with a particular sponsored project, an instructional activity, or any other institutional activity, or that can be directly assigned to such activities relatively easily with a high degree of accuracy." Indirect costs include costs which cannot be identified specifically with a particular research project or program, including, but not limited to, taxes, administration, personnel (not directly related to the project), and security costs (SAMHSA, 2017).

Federal grant applicants will be required to provide a detailed plan to ensure oversight of federal funds as well as how the proposed grant activities and partnering organizations will follow relevant federal and programmatic regulations (Administration for Native Americans, 2018). The applicant organization or institution may need to demonstrate sustainability of the proposed project or program goals, outcomes, and objectives after the grant award has expired. For example, the applicant may be required to describe the specific strategies and efforts to financially support and continue a project beyond grant or contract funding.

Award Phase

The process for reviewing grant applications and making funding decisions differs between foundations and federal agencies. A program officer is a staff member of a foundation who reviews grant proposals and processes applications for the foundation's board of trustees. In reviewing the grant application, program officers will ask questions such as:

- Is the organization or institution well known and engaged in its community?
- Does the organization or institution provide programs or services that meet a need in the community?
- Does the organization or institution have strong leadership?
- Does the organization or institution have a strong financial and organizational infrastructure?

The program officers and foundation leadership, in reviewing requests for grant funding, will determine if the applicant organization has a compelling mission and focus that is compatible with the foundation's mission and focus. In order to ensure a fair review process by the foundation, program officers request experts external to the foundation to review proposals. When the application review process is complete, the program officer will inform the applicant organization or institution if the applicant has been successful or unsuccessful. If successful, the terms of the foundation award and binding agreements will be negotiated with the program officer.

The peer-review process is integral to the decision by federal agencies in awarding discretionary grant funding. The peer review involves a panel of experts without conflicts of interest who evaluate the applications following a rating or scoring system that has been determined by the agency. After conducting an independent review, the peer reviewers will meet either in person or via teleconference to discuss the merits of the applications and discrepancies in scores. The discussion is moderated by federal agency staff to ensure fairness and objectivity with the review process.

Once the final award decisions are made, the federal awarding agency sends a Notice of Award to the entities selected for funding. The Notice of Award serves as a legally binding issuance of the award. As the recipient of a federal grant award, organizations are subject to uphold federal statutory and regulatory requirements, including federal civil rights laws. Applicants are required to review and accept assurances and certifications, which indicate that the entity will abide by a particular requirement if awarded a federal grant (SAMHSA, 2017). These assurances are sometimes given under criminal penalty of perjury for submitting incorrect information. An applicant should consult competent legal counsel with experience in federal grant compliance to advise about legal obligations as a recipient of a federal grant.

The applicant must comply with assurances in order to receive federal funds. It is the responsibility of the recipient of the federal funds to fully understand and comply with these requirements. Ignorance of the law is not considered an excuse. Failure to comply may result in the withholding of funds, organizations, or institutions being asked to return federal grant funds received, termination of the award, or other sanctions.

One federal civil rights law that recipients of federal financial assistance must administer in their grant-funded program is Title VI of the Civil Rights Act of 1964. Many foundations have adopted the federal award requirements with a focus on equity, diversity, language and disability access, and inclusion. Because of potential foundation compliance with federal laws and career opportunities with organizations and institutions that receive federal funding or reimbursement, it is important for healthcare practitioners to understand and appreciate the legal obligations of grant recipients. The awarding organization or institution and the award recipients have distinct federal legal obligations that include federal civil rights laws.

Grants and Federal Legal Obligations

Let us consider the example of a healthcare provider organization that has been awarded a federal grant. Healthcare providers encounter clients and their families who are limited English proficient (LEP), who speak little or no English. Being able to communicate with LEP clients and providing them with effective language assistance are essential and required by federal law (United States Department of Justice, 2013). The U.S. Department of Health and Human Services has stated, "With 80% of hospitals encountering LEP individuals frequently, there is an increasing demand for effective language access services" (United States Department of Health and Human Services, 2014).

Many federal laws address language assistance and translation requirements. The federal law that requires federally funded and assisted healthcare providers to provide effective and meaningful language assistance is Title VI of the Civil Rights Act of 1964, 42 US Code sections 2000d-2000d-7. Understanding how to provide federally required language assistance, in what languages, and to which communities can be a daunting task. It is axiomatic that the "languages spoken by … LEP individuals with whom the agency has contact determine the languages accommodated by [the] agency" (United States Department of Justice, 2011). However, each federally funded agency and organization has its own requirements beyond language identification to inform providing the legally mandated "meaningful access" to federally funded "programs, activities, and services" (Title VI of the Civil Rights Act of 1964).

The Four-Factor Analysis

Organizations need a formula or rubric to help them determine the how, when, where, and to whom of federally required language assistance. The Four-Factor Analysis, developed by the U.S. Department of Justice, is recognized by federal agencies as the fundamental first step. The analysis is also a key box to check for federal regulators when conducting Title VI investigations or evaluations of an organization's language assistance compliance and compliance with federal grant obligations in the Certificate of Assurance. For example, as the U.S. Department of Health and Human Services has stated: "[Federal funding] recipients may want to consider documenting their application of the four-factor test to the services they provide" (United States Department of Health and Human Services, 2003). As an essential tool, the Four-Factor Analysis (Figure 15.4) is also mandated by federal agencies in their consent agreements.

The first factor pinpoints the Title VI language access starting point—"The population to be served by race, color, and national origin" (U.S. Department of Justice, Title VI Regulations). This factor must be applied to each non-English language group in the federally funded organization's service community.

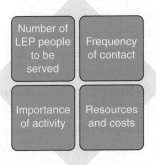

Figure 15.4. Four-Factor Analysis.

To apply the first factor correctly, organizations must determine those LEP people who actually interact with the organization and those LEP people the organizations are "likely" to encounter (U.S. Department of Justice, Title VI Regulations). The "likely to encounter" requirement can be challenging and requires organizations knowing their communities and how to provide them access to their federally funded services. This information may be gleaned "by reviewing available data from federal, state, and local government agencies, community, and faith based organizations" (United States Department of Justice, 2011).

The second factor calls for information about how often LEP people use particular federally subsidized programs and services. Analysis of this factor will involve data from the entire organization and each individual department and agency within the organization about frequency of use. Determining such frequency can be aided by staff-conducted surveys of patients, for example.

The third factor involves objectively determining how important the federally subsidized program, activity, or service is to people in the community. One way to evaluate this factor is provided by the U.S. Department of Justice: "A recipient needs to determine whether denial or delay of access to services or information could have serious or even life-threatening implications for the LEP individual." (United States Department of Justice, 2003).

The more important and crucial the service, the higher the level of language services needed to comply with Title VI. For example, public education, public transportation, healthcare, law enforcement, and access to the courts are considered to be among the most important of federally subsidized services. Consequently, they require the highest level of language access services and resources, such as in-person qualified interpreters.

The fourth factor concerns an organization's resources and the cost of language services. This factor examines the size of the federally subsidized organization and its overall budget. In essence, the larger the organization, such as an urban 1,000-bed hospital, and its budget, the more it will be expected to provide language access compared to smaller entities, such as a rural 50-bed hospital.

The fact that language services and language assistance cost money and resources is not an excuse for not providing them. Once an organization accepts federal financial assistance, the organization must comply with the law, in this case Title VI's language assistance mandates.

As the U.S. Department of Justice has explained:

> "[F]iscal pressures are not a blanket exemption from civil rights requirements, and our investigation has determined that financial constraints do not preclude [an organization] from taking several further reasonable steps to comply with its federal non-discrimination obligations, for several reasons. [L]anguage services must be considered part of the cost of doing business."

In Their Own Words

Martha Johnson
Deputy CEO/Chief Development Officer
Rosemount Center
Washington, DC

Finding a Grant-Writing Consultant
Fundraising and/or grant-writing consultants can help with federal grant applications as well as private foundation proposals. There are many people willing to help with grant writing, but it is important to find the right person for your particular needs.

How does one find a good grant-writing consultant? Attending a professional conference will help you find consultants who present workshops and trainings on fundraising and are knowledgeable in your field. Networking with

(Continued)

colleagues at organizations similar to yours is another way of finding competent consultants. Program officers at local foundations are usually willing to give guidance and share resources if you contact them for advice on consultants. Searching online for local fundraising consultants is another way of finding someone to interview. Local chapters of service organizations in your field can also be good resources for consultants. There are consultancy firms all over the country who provide fundraising advice, but you will have to do research to see which one has the best reputation—and you may be better off finding someone local, rather than working with someone who will have to travel to your site if you want to work with them in person.

Interviewing consultants will take up a significant amount of your time, but will be worth the time spent if you want to find a good match for your organization. You should expect to schedule an interview or an introductory meeting with a potential consultant free of charge. You will need to give an overview of your organization, share your goals in working with a consultant, review the scope of the project needing to be funded, and be clear about your expectations. After the initial meeting, the consultant should send you a proposal specifying the scope of work and the cost involved. A written contract is helpful to set parameters and to agree on the price of the work to be produced. You can decide whether you want the consultant to help you with one project only, or you may want help on an ongoing basis. In any case, you will need to decide what your budget is and how much you are willing to spend before starting to work with a consultant. It is always a good idea to ask an attorney to review the contract on your behalf. Many organizations work with pro bono attorneys or have an attorney on their Board of Directors who is willing to review a contract. Since most consultants are independent contractors, their hourly fee will be significant, but some consultants will provide an **in-kind contribution** as part of their billing to help support the organization. It is advisable to get a proposal from more than one consultant for comparison purposes.

When you start to work with a consultant, beware of the following:

- The consultant is depending on receiving correct information in order to write an effective grant proposal. You will need to spend time not only giving the consultant information about your organization but also information on the project you are looking to fund.
- Always proof drafts of the proposal along the way in order to guide the consultant in the right direction.
- If the consultant is getting information from others in your organization, make sure this information is accurate and not out of date.

(Continued)

- Always set false deadlines so if the consultant's work needs to be corrected or changed, you have ample time to return it to the consultant for additional edits before the actual grant deadline. Many consultants will create a time-line with scheduled tasks so the consultant gets what is needed in order to complete the work in a timely manner.
- Clarify who will be submitting the proposal or application (you or the consultant?) and make sure you have a system in place as required by the funder in order to submit the proposal/application by the deadline.

Consultants can sometimes help with other areas of your organization including facilitating strategic planning, providing board training, working on a community assessment, supporting program staff, providing fundraising advice, etc. Of course, make sure you get separate proposals from the consultant for any additional projects you ask the consultant to complete.

Monitoring

It is important to keep in mind that grants are **contracts** to undertake a specific project or program. Involve your organization's or institution's general counsel in understanding the obligations of a grant award. An award involves substantial **grant monitoring**, including significant legalities. A best practice is for recipients of grants and awards from foundations, corporations, or federal agencies to implement rigorous evaluation and monitoring systems to ensure ongoing compliance with the terms of the grant award.

Once an institution or organization has been notified of a successful request for grant funding, there is often a delay between notification and receipt of the grant funds. The delay should be considered before costs are incurred related to the proposed project or program.

Reporting

Reporting requirements, including the performance progress and **financial reports**, is included in the Notice of Award from the foundation or federal agency. An officer of the organization or institution may be asked to sign and return the Notice of Award or letter of agreement.

The awardee will coordinate with the recipient organization or institution to ensure progress with the grant-funded project or program. For example, the U.S. Department of Health and Human Services, Administration for Children and Families, Administration for Native Americans (ANA) will review "… grantee semiannual and annual reports to determine whether the grantee is meeting its goals and objectives and completing activities identified in the [Objective Work Plan] OWP. ANA also performs ongoing monitoring of grantee progress throughout the project period by Program Specialists through telephone interviews and **site visits**. The grantee will submit a non-competing continuing application to receive additional funding. Prior to funding the next budget period of a multi-year grant, ANA requires verification from the grantee that objectives and outcomes proposed in the preceding year were accomplished" (Administration for Native Americans, 2018).

Performance Progress Reports

Federal grant recipients submit performance progress and financial reports throughout the grant award period. These reports may include both expense-related data and quantitative information about the project or program impact based on performance metrics included in the grant agreement (Office of Management and Budget's [OMB, 2017] *Uniform Administrative Requirements, Cost Principles, and Audit Requirements for Federal Awards* [commonly called "Uniform Guidance"]).

Grant recipients of awards from foundations or corporations may also be required to submit periodic reports, including project data, to demonstrate that (1) the grantee is fulfilling the goals and objectives of the grant-funded project or program and (2) that the grant-funded project or program is having the intended impact on the community (United States Department of Justice, 2015). Program officers from the awarding foundation may conduct site visits of the award recipient. The federal awarding agency may also assign a grants management officer who is tasked with site visits and reviewing the award recipient's progress reports. Federal agencies may offer technical assistance to ensure that the grant recipient is complying with the terms of the award agreement.

Audits may also be conducted by foundations and the federal government. According to the Single Audit Act Amendments of 1996 (31 U.S.C. 7507 Chapter 75), a federal grant recipient may be audited to ensure compliance with government regulations and evaluate the grant recipient's financial information, including expenses paid for with federal award funds.

Close-Out

The close-out refers to the final step in the grant award process. Typically, this involves the grant award recipient submitting the necessary final financial and programmatic reports to the foundation or awarding agency. The foundation or federal awarding agency will review the reports to ensure compliance with the terms of the grant agreement and that the grant funds were spent as stipulated by the terms of the grant agreement. Grant recipients may be required to retain all records related to the grant funding for a period of at least 3 years from the date of the final expenditure report.

Questions to Ask Yourself

1. Is the applicant organization or institution eligible for grant support according to Internal Revenue Service regulations?
2. What trends in grantmaking from philanthropic organizations or the federal government may impact external funding of the applicant organization's proposed program or project?
3. Does the applicant organization or institution have the necessary policies and procedures in place to support and sustain grant funding?
4. Does the applicant organization or institution have the necessary organizational and financial infrastructure in place to support and sustain grant funding?
5. Does the applicant organization or institution have the experience to successfully manage a grant award?

Working With a Consultant

Engaging with institutional donors, as well as preparing and writing a successful request for funding, requires significant time. Before committing to securing support from a foundation, corporation, or federal agency for grant funding, applicants should determine who is best qualified to write the grant proposal—an individual who is internal to the applicant organization or institution or a consultant who will provide specific services or subject matter expertise for a fee.

Proposal writing involves timely coordination across departments, for example, human resources and finance. Professional help from a grant-writing consultant can be crucial to developing a successful grant application, especially in responding to a federal agency's funding opportunity announcement with often complex requirements. In addition to offering an organization the benefits of expertise in grant writing and grant management, an experienced consultant may optimize funding opportunities for an organization by recommending grant funding opportunities that best align the projects and programs of an organization or institution with the priorities of a foundation or corporation.

Expanding and managing partnerships with grantmaking entities or federal agencies requires a daily commitment to succeed. Funding opportunities often arise unexpectedly. There may also be multiple opportunities that an organization or institution decides to pursue simultaneously. To ensure that an organization or institution is prepared when opportunities arise, consider retaining a consultant to research new sources of support and provide regular updates about trends or issues related to foundation and federal grants.

An organization or institution interested in retaining a consultant should conduct interviews with prospective candidates and request writing samples as well as references. Before retaining a consultant, prepare a written contract that states the terms of the relationship with the organization or institution. Consider expanding the scope of services that a consultant may provide beyond writing a grant application; the scope of work will also determine the amount of the fee or retainer agreement:

- Preparing grant proposals, budgets, reports, and other ancillary materials
- Conducting ongoing research funding opportunities to support work across a range of programs and events
- Monitoring financial progress against established fundraising goals
- Identifying and cultivating relationships with a select group of new funders
- Preparing progress reports and all other correspondence following the awarding of a grant
- Assisting with post-award reporting obligations for active awards
- Preparing funding renewal applications as appropriate
- Serving as a representative and attending meetings, briefings, and conferences with corporate and foundation funders
- Collaborating with organization staff to identify opportunities for external funding
- Participating in monthly grant planning meetings with leadership

Summary

Researching and understanding the requirements for applying for grant funding from a foundation, corporation, or federal agency is critical before an organization or institution commits to planning and writing a proposal. This chapter presents detailed information in understanding the types of grants and the work required in completing a grant application. Various organizations may offer grants, including community institutions, corporations, family foundations, independent foundations, operating foundations, public foundations, and private foundations. Types of grants include matching grants, demonstration grants, discretionary grants, and foundation-administered program awards. An applicant must focus on the motivation and interests of the philanthropy or federal agency in establishing measurable goals and objectives of the proposed project or program. Grant requirements may include long-term sustainability of a proposed project or program, requiring reliable financial support from myriad funding sources. Grant requirements, including compliance and reporting, differ between foundations, corporations, and federal funding agencies.

Chapter Highlights

- Researching and understanding the requirements for applying for grant funding is critical in planning and writing a proposal.
- Different organizations may offer grants, including community institutions, corporations, family foundations, independent foundations, operating foundations, public foundations, and private foundations.
- Types of grants include matching grants, demonstration grants, discretionary grants, and foundation-administered program awards.
- An applicant must focus on the motivation and interests of the philanthropy or federal agency in establishing measurable goals and objectives of the proposed project or program.
- Grant requirements may include long-term sustainability of a proposed project or program.
- Grant requirements, including compliance and reporting, differ between foundations, corporations, and federal funding agencies.

Web Resources

- How to Write a Grant Proposal: https://www.arc.gov/funding/HowtoWriteaGrantProposal.asp
- How to Write a Winning Grant Proposal: https://www.thebalancesmb.com/how-to-write-a-grant-proposal-2501980
- Nonprofit Grant Writing Guide: https://snowballfundraising.com/nonprofit-grant-writing-guide/
- Owl at Purdue Introduction to Grant Writing: https://owl.purdue.edu/owl/subject_specific_writing/professional_technical_writing/grant_writing/index.html
- HRSA Grant Workshops: https://www.hrsa.gov/grants/manage-your-grant/training/workshops
- Government Grant Search Engine: https://www.grants.gov/

Professional Organizations

American Grant Writers Association (AGWA): http://www.agwa.us/
Grant professionals Association (GPA): https://www.grantprofessionals.org/
National Grants Management Association (NGMA): https://www.ngma.org/
Association of Fundraising Professionals: https://www.afpnet.org/

References

Centers for Disease Control and Prevention (CDC). (2018). *Logic models: CDC approach to evaluation*. https://www.cdc.gov/eval/logicmodels/index.htm

Giving USA Foundation. (2017). *The annual report on philanthropy for the year 2016*. Giving USA. http://lclsonline.org/wp-content/uploads/2017/12/GUSA-2017-Report-Download.pdf

Grants.gov. (n.d.). *Grant lifecycle timeline*. https://www.grants.gov/web/grants/learn-grants/grants-101/grant-lifecycle.html

Office of Management and Budget's (OMB). (2017). *Uniform administrative requirements, cost principles, and audit requirements for federal awards, 78federal register 78589*. https://www.federalregister.gov/documents/2017/05/17/2017-09909/uniform-administrative-requirements-cost-principles-and-audit-requirements-for-federal-awards

The Council on Foundations. (2020a). *Glossary of philanthropic terms*. https://www.cof.org/content/glossary-philanthropic-terms

The Council on Foundations. (2020b). *Foundation basics*. https://www.cof.org/content/foundation-basics

The Foundation Center. (2012). *Understanding and benchmarking foundation payout*. https://foundationcenter.issuelab.org/resources/14076/14076.pdf

The Foundation Center. (2014). *Key facts on U.S. foundations*. http://foundationcenter.org/gainknowledge/research/keyfacts2014/pdfs/Key_Facts_on_US_Foundations_2014.pdf

The Foundation Center. (2016). *Introduction to finding grants.* https://grantspace.org/training/courses/introduction-to-finding-grants/

The Foundation Center. (2019). *Philanthropy classification system.* https://taxonomy.candid.org/resources/downloads/full-pcs-taxonomy-with-definitions. http://taxonomy.foundationcenter.org/organization-type

United States Department of Health and Human Services. (2003). Federal financial assistance recipients regarding title VI prohibition against national origin discrimination affecting limited English proficient persons. *Federal Register, 68*(153), 47314.

United States Department of Health and Human Services. (2014). *Compliance review initiative: Advancing effective communication in critical access hospitals.* https://www.hhs.gov/sites/default/files/ocr/civilrights/activities/agreements/compliancereview_initiative.pdf

United States Department of Health and Human Services, Office of minority health resource center. (2015). Webinar. *Getting to know the federal government and funding opportunities.* https://www.minorityhealth.hhs.gov/assets/pdf/Getting_to_Know_the_Federal_Government_OMHRC_Webinar-Nov_5_2015-final.pdf

United States Department of Health and Human Services. (2017). *Substance abuse and mental health services administration. Glossary of terms and acronyms for SAMHSA grants.* https://www.samhsa.gov/grants/grants-glossary#C

United States Department of Health and Human Services, Administration for Children and Families, Administration for Native Americans. (2018). *Native American language preservation and maintenance.* HHS-2018-ACF-ANA-NL-1342. https://www.federalgrants.com/Native-American-Language-Preservation-and-Maintenance-63822.html

United States Department of Justice. (2003). *Guidance to federal financial assistance recipients regarding title VI prohibition against national origin discrimination affecting limited English proficient persons.* 67 Federal Register 41464. https://www.hhs.gov/civil-rights/for-individuals/special-topics/limited-english-proficiency/guidance-federal-financial-assistance-recipients-title-vi/index.html

United States Department of Justice. (2013). *Title VI Regulations. 28 C.F.R. section 42.101 et seq.* https://www.hhs.gov/civil-rights/for-individuals/special-topics/needy-families/civil-rights-requirements/index.html

United States Department of Justice. Civil Rights Division. Federal Coordination and Compliance Section. (2011). *Language access assessment and planning tool for federally conducted and federally assisted programs.* https://www.lep.gov/sites/lep/files/resources/2011_Language_Access_Assessment_and_Planning_Tool.pdf

United States Department of Justice. Office of Justice Programs. (2015). *United States Department of Justice grants financial guide.* https://www.justice.gov/ovw/file/892031/download

PART SIX

Professional Practice

16

Nurse Entrepreneurs

Annie Moore-Cox

LEARNING OBJECTIVES

After completing this chapter, you will be able to:

1. Differentiate between innovators, entrepreneurs, social entrepreneurs, and intrapreneurs.

2. Describe the characteristics of entrepreneurs in nursing.

3. Discuss ways to overcome barriers, perceived and actual, to nurse entrepreneurship.

KEY TERMS

Innovators: Those who work within systems to bring new ideas to modify or improve those systems.

Nurse innovators: Nurses who implement new techniques, from finding a new way to suction a patient to bringing innovative management techniques to their institutions.

Entrepreneurs: Individuals who tend to be confident, bold risk takers who are able to see opportunities, act decisively to create new opportunities, and bring that creation to the world overcoming any and all obstacles.

Entrepreneurship: The ability to recognize opportunity and act with out-of-the-box thinking and dogged determination to create a completely new product or service of value to the world.

Nurse entrepreneurs: Nurses who use their knowledge and skills to start their own healthcare-related business. This may include marketing of a new product or a service based on the nurse's creativity, innovation, and business savvy.

Intrapreneurs: Employees who work outside the mainstream of their workplace to develop and promote new and innovative products and services for their employer.

Nurse intrapreneurs: Nurses who develop and promote innovative ideas in a healthcare setting.

Social entrepreneurs: Change agents who develop products and services to solve a societal problem or to help those in need by combining social mission passion with the discipline and drive usually associated with industries such as technology (Dees, 2001).

Introduction

Nurses have never been bystanders in the drive to improve the health of the patients they serve. A nurse educator used to admonish her graduating students by saying, "If it isn't happening in your community, it's because you haven't done it yet." Her call to action echoes throughout nursing and is never more relevant than it is now. From Clara Barton and Florence Nightingale in the 19th century to the 21st century when two nurses from Nebraska created a tool to remove body piercings in emergency departments (Bunger, 2008), nurses have been innovators in addition to caregivers. The nurses described in this chapter and many others like them are pushing the boundaries of their roles and solving problems in healthcare in the United States and abroad. Despite their example, the healthcare system has not embraced or encouraged the unique and innovative contributions nurses have made to patient care over the past century and a half (Institute of Medicine [IOM], 2010; Vannucci & Weinstein, 2017; Wilson et al., 2012). As a result, innovation that might emerge from nurses, who make up the largest percentage of the healthcare workforce (American Association of Colleges of Nursing, 2019), is discouraged and often lost. This happens even with rapid change in the healthcare industry in the last 2 decades in the United States caused by increased numbers of older adult patients with higher health needs, an influx of insured individuals into the healthcare system, unsustainable costs, and an explosion of information technology. These factors, among others, have increased opportunities for innovation by nurses and entrepreneurs. Our evolving healthcare system cannot afford to continue losing great ideas from nurses who make up the majority of its workforce.

For some nurses, innovation means coming up with new ideas to meet the needs of patients or populations within their existing job description, for example, the nurse practitioner (NP) who starts a foot care clinic in her practice to help older adult patients with foot care challenges. For others, becoming an innovator means expanding their job description to encompass new roles, like a psychiatric NP who sees her community's lack of addiction recovery services and obtains the necessary credentials to serve them. Innovation in nursing sometimes requires a complete departure, a disruption in the status quo, that may lead to a new business altogether, such as an independent community care service or a revolutionary product. For some nurses, innovation may mean bringing the unique perspective and skill set of nursing to industry, either through a job in a for-profit company or by entering local, state, or national politics.

Because nurses touch every aspect of people's lives and because of advanced education in specialty areas and progressive state legislation expanding autonomy for advanced practice registered nurses (APRNs), there are fewer boundaries today for nurses who have entrepreneurial, intrapreneurial, and social entrepreneurial ideas for improving the lives of the people they serve. Globally, the entrepreneurial movement is growing as nurses seek to reclaim independence in practices and services around the world (International Council of Nurses [ICN], 2004). The IOM report (2010) exhorts nurses to be full partners in the redesign of the healthcare system, another sign that healthcare is ready for nurse innovators, entrepreneurs, and intrapreneurs willing to be imaginative and innovative agents of improved patient care.

This chapter explores the opportunities for nurses to assume roles outside the traditional roles in advanced practice nursing. Readers will learn to describe the differences between innovation, entrepreneurship, intrapreneurship, and social entrepreneurship; to discuss some of the history of innovation and historical barriers to innovation and entrepreneurship in nursing; to hear the stories of a new group of nurses who are pushing the boundaries of their profession; and to inspire those seeking advanced practice roles to look beyond current roles and responsibilities and imagine new and creative ways to serve patients. Innovative nurses will discover more entrepreneurial opportunities in the years to come.

History and Evolution

The role of the nurse has been governed by market and societal forces that, for much of history, have reduced the autonomy of the profession. Nursing emerged as a profession in the latter half of the 19th century with the creation of nursing schools in Britain, largely because of Florence Nightingale. Prior to its professionalization, nursing was usually provided by family members, considered part of a woman's duty, and unpaid. Even when practiced by trained and "registered" individuals, nursing remained a women's profession and was undervalued. While many graduates of nurse-training programs went into private-duty practice as independent business women (Whelan, 2012), training continued to center around "domestic order created by a good wife, the altruistic caring expressed by a good mother, and the self-discipline of a good soldier" (Reverby, 1987, p. 41). Early training stressed duty and submissiveness, character traits that were taught and learned as skills (Reverby, 1987). These characteristics are precisely the opposite of those required of the entrepreneur, whose work requires boldness, rule breaking, and unconventional thinking. It is not hard to see why nursing's history is not replete with stories of entrepreneurs. "As a result of much oppressed group behavior in nursing, opportunity is often missed" (Porter-O'Grady, 2001). Table 16.1 identifies some of nursing history's notable figures as innovators or entrepreneurs.

Nurse training did turn out well-prepared hospital employees, and that is where most nurses found themselves employed after World War II (ICN, 2004). As employees of large healthcare institutions, nurses rarely practiced on equal footing with other care providers, and their important skills as caregivers and patient advocates often were underutilized. As a result, nurses rarely were encouraged to propose and implement the improvements they envisioned for their patients and within their own work environments. In recent decades, as inefficiencies have driven up healthcare costs, the federal government has taken steps to increase quality, accessibility, and cost effectiveness. The Affordable Care Act (ACA) of 2010 expanded the role of APRNs and other mid-level providers. The ACA has improved both the availability and quality of primary care. The ACA also funded NP education, while promoting NP-staffed Federally Qualified Health Centers and Nurse-Managed Health Centers (NMHC) (Robert Wood Johnson Foundation [RWJF], 2015). However, the scope of NP practice is determined not by education and training but rather by rules that vary from state to state. Since 2010, some states have changed their practice rules to remove

Table 16.1. Notable Innovators and Entrepreneurs in Nursing History	
Innovator	**Entrepreneur/Social Entrepreneur**
Dorothea Dix (1802-1887) campaigned tirelessly for the rights of the mentally ill through testimonials about horrific conditions in asylums and prisons (Parry, 2006).	Florence Nightingale (1820-1910) used her experiences in the 1850s serving soldiers in army hospitals in the Crimea to gain support and funding to begin her own nursing schools in England. She is considered the founder of modern nursing.
Mary Adelaide Nutting (1858-1948) was among the first superintendents of the Training School for Nurses at The Johns Hopkins Hospital and made great advances training nurses there and at Columbia Teachers College.	Clara Barton (1821-1912) was compelled by her experience as an untrained nurse for Union soldiers in the Civil War to lobby, lecture, and persevere to form The American Red Cross and become its first president in 1881 (Michals, 2015).
Isabel Hampton Robb (1854-1910) founded the American Nurses Association and the National League for Nursing, launched the American Journal of Nursing, and served as superintendent of Training School for Nurses at The Johns Hopkins Hospital.	Lillian Wald (1867-1940), shocked by conditions of the poor, raised money, and organized people to create the Henry Street Settlement in New York City. She invented the term and concept of public health nursing to bring nurses into the homes of the poor. She also began a program of health insurance to cover the cost of in-home nursing visits that was ahead of its time (Buhler-Wilkerson, 1993).
Lavinia Dock (1858-1956) worked at the Henry Street Settlement House and is renowned for her efforts to persuade people to work for women's suffrage and to support the rights of workers to strike (Garofalo & Fee, 2015).	Charlotte Rhone (1874-1965), at a time when African Americans were refused admission to hospitals even in emergencies, was among the first African Americans to be registered as a nurse in North Carolina. Among her many social entrepreneurial efforts, she created a garment factory in her community to employ African Americans after a fire destroyed most homes and businesses (Pollitt, 2015).

restrictions on NP practice, although the majority of states continue to restrict practice to some extent.

Though there are many examples of nurses leading innovative efforts to improve healthcare, barriers remain to entrepreneurship (IOM, 2010) including restrictive limits on APRN practice, payment and reimbursement issues, and professional resistance from other healthcare providers. For facility or agency-based nurses, the designation of nursing as a cost center rather than as a profit center discourages innovation because it relegates nursing to the same category as bed linen and housekeeping, which are drains on resources rather than potential sources of increased revenue.

Nurse Practitioners

Especially in states that enable full practice authority, NPs today are finding more entrepreneurial opportunities (Hahn & Cook, 2018). NPs are in a unique position to identify gaps in service and to fill those gaps creatively and entrepreneurially by creating new and innovative services. However, they can do this only if they are granted practice authority that frees them to create such services. Since the 1960s, NMHCs, usually affiliated with a school of nursing, have offered an expanded array of clinical services. The number of NMHCs has grown by more than 8% since 2010, when the RWJF began tracking them through the Campaign for Action to measure the extent to which states allowed APRNs to practice to the full extent of their licenses. The ACA identified these centers as key players in meeting the growing need for services as more insured patients enter the healthcare system (Ely, 2015). Since 2011, when there were 132 NMHCs, their numbers have grown to 153, of which 63.4% are in medically underserved areas (Campaign for Action, 2018). NMHCs offer fertile soil for innovative nurses willing to create new patient services.

Certified Nurse Midwives

The first freestanding birth center called the Childbearing Center, staffed by certified nurse midwives, opened in 1975 in New York City because a group of social entrepreneurial nurses saw that low-income women lacked access to low-cost, low-intervention maternity care (Ernst & Bauer, 2012). At the time of the birth center's creation, low-intervention birth was unavailable to most women who gave birth in hospitals and underwent unwanted procedures that arguably have limited benefits to mothers and babies. Today, the American Association of Birth Centers helps midwife-owned and midwife-operated centers around the country provide safe and cost-effective care in more than 345 freestanding birth centers in the United States (American Association of Birth Centers, 2016).

Informatics Nurses

Nurse informaticists put technology to use in the healthcare setting by managing health information. As managers, interpreters, and communicators of data, they are improving the quality of patient care services (Electronic Health Reporter, 2016). Documentation now occurs automatically and transmits quickly to patient records. This helps nurses improve their decisions about patient care services and quickly adjust to changes. This ability to respond quickly and appropriately has helped reduce medical errors and medical costs, while improving the coordination of patient care. Not only has the nurse's environment become easier to navigate, patients also benefit from having their information accessible by everyone involved in their care. Nurse informaticists are charged with improving the quality of patient care through adoption of technology-enabled processes.

The advent of the electronic health record (EHR) has opened doors for innovative and entrepreneurial nurses in informatics, many of whom develop business acumen working with large vendor organizations that exposed them to entrepreneurs in other fields. Informatics nurses have found new careers as consultants, as clinical informatics staffers in hospitals, and as data analysts.

In Their Own Words

Rose E. Sherman, EdD, RN, NEA-BC, CNL, FAAN
Professor Emeritus, Florida Atlantic University
Editor in Chief, Nurse Leader
Author—*The Nurse Leader Coach: Become the Boss No One Wants to Leave*

How Did You Become Interested in Nursing Leadership?
I spent the first 25 years of my career working for the Department of Veterans Affairs at five medical centers in different parts of the country. I went to work for the VA initially as a staff nurse and later a Clinical Nurse Specialist. It was a Chief

(Continued)

Nursing Officer who saw my leadership potential and urged me to switch gears from my advanced clinical work to leadership. Her most convincing argument was the impact I could have if I moved into leadership. At the time, she saw something in me that I did not see in myself. I took her advice, moved into a leadership role, and never looked back. While I was highly effective as a CNS, the only real power I had was my professional influence. Moving into leadership gave me a role where I had not only influence but also the authority to change practice. I often tell leaders my story because I think it is essential that when nurse leaders see staff with leadership potential they have the conversation that my CNO did with me.

What Skills Will Be Important for Nurses to Develop in the Coming Years?

Leadership skills are always relevant regardless of what your role is in nursing. I believe that nurses will need to be continuous learners to adapt to environmental changes. Organizations will depend on nurses to help with strategic thinking about how to plan most effectively to meet the healthcare needs of populations they serve. Nurses who are creative and innovative will be highly valued. Healthcare is changing so rapidly that adaptability and resiliency are also critical.

How Do You Believe Technology Will Change Practice?

I think technology will profoundly change many aspects of nursing practice. Nurses currently spend a great deal of time on hunting and gathering activities, whether it be for supplies, drugs, or information. This is an area where robotics has the potential to make positive changes in the day-to-day practice of nurses, so they have more time to spend with patients. Artificial intelligence could significantly improve nurse decision-making by helping us to process the vast amounts of information that nurses are expected to know. Nurses today are in cognitive overload so having expert decision support could help reduce the stress levels we see. Nurses will need to be open to these new technologies as a way to make us more productive. Technology will not replace nurses. We are in a hands-on humanistic profession and that will not change.

What Advice Would You Give Nurses Beginning Their Career Today?

I would say that it is essential to stay open to possibilities because there will be new fantastic career roles available that do not exist today. Say yes more than you say no when you are given an opportunity to do something that scares you. When we begin our careers, we often have a very narrow view of nursing opportunities. Over time, we learn that a nursing skill set is invaluable in many roles, including some completely outside of healthcare. We know that companies like Amazon, Google, and Microsoft are now hiring nurses. Healthcare is a multi-trillion-dollar industry, and there will be many companies entering healthcare who want and need nursing expertise. Keep an open mind and look beyond the traditional roles. You may even want to be an entrepreneur and start your own business. When you meet someone who has a role that you are interested in, ask them about their pathway to that position.

What Do You Wish You Had Understood at the Beginning of Your Career?
Two things that I probably did not know at the beginning of my career was the role that timing and luck play in your career. We can have well laid out plans and be on a clear path to achieve them. However, life has a way of throwing us curve balls. It may be because of personal circumstances, or things can change with our employers. When this happens, a well thought out path may not seem as doable. As you gain more life experience, you realize that complete control of your career path is an illusion. You also begin to see that even the detours you take can turn out to be lucky breaks that in the end provide you with valuable experience. In his address to the 2005 graduating class at Stanford, the late Steve Jobs noted that *"You can't connect the dots looking forward; you can only connect them looking backward. So you have to trust that the dots will somehow connect in your future. You have to trust in something—your gut, destiny, life, karma, whatever. This approach has never let me down, and it has made all the difference in my life."* This was such wise advice.

Clinical Nurse Specialists

Clinical nurse specialists (CNSs) with an intrapreneurial streak can assume roles within their institutions as case managers and navigators and out of institutions as, for example, independent community care nurses. Just as they have with NPs, some states are easing practice limitations placed on CNSs in the United States. In 28 states, CNSs may now practice independently (National Association of Clinical Nurse Specialists, n.d.). This independence promises to open doors for innovative CNSs who want to become entrepreneurs or intrapreneurs.

Nurse Executives

Acknowledged for the unique insight they bring to an ever-changing healthcare delivery environment, nurse executives are increasingly moving beyond the Chief Nursing Officer (CNO) role and taking jobs as Chief Operating Officers and Chief Executive Officers (CEOs) of hospitals and healthcare systems (Carlson, 2011). When they receive advanced education in business and leadership, nurses can bring the voice of the patient to the decision-making table while preserving the institution's financial health.

Nurse Educators

Nurse educators often discover entrepreneurial and innovation opportunities because they work in the increasingly cost-constrained fiscal environment of most colleges and universities and find they need to come up with new and creative teaching methods. Most academic institutions experience nursing faculty shortages and have trouble securing clinical sites for student practice. While these conditions pose challenges, they also create opportunities for nurse educators who want to become entrepreneurs and intrapreneurs. Some educators develop their own websites, either free or behind a pay wall, to help fellow teachers teach or students learn. Others work as adjunct instructors, sometimes from their own homes, as online courses and programs proliferate. Nurse educators sometimes start their own companies to educate healthcare providers using their particular area of expertise or to provide teachers or students with educational products. A groundbreaking study by the NCSBN (Hayden et al., 2014) on the efficacy of teaching nursing students through simulation led to new grants and other capital investments further opening up possibilities for nurse educators. Entrepreneurs and intrapreneurs in simulation write scenarios for their own use or for sale, develop innovative simulation products, and even go to work for simulation companies.

A nurse educator's traditional academic trajectory involves advancing from faculty member to department chair to director or dean. But some are also able to move beyond the nursing school or department to become academic officers serving an entire institution. In many cases, their success came from years of performing a rigorous balancing act that developed their skills at meeting the diverse needs of students, accreditors, and healthcare consumers. These nurses may be chief academic officers, provosts, or college presidents.

Nurses in Business

Many nurses work for companies that provide healthcare products and services, among them are EHR vendors, medical device manufacturers, and simulation product manufacturers. The for-profit nature of these companies can pose challenges because the Nursing Code of Ethics (American Nurses Association, 2015) requires nurses to place their patients first, ahead of corporate concerns about revenue and profit: "Nursing is about caring while business [is] about making money" (Elango et al., 2007, p. 201). Still, all businesses, including nonprofit healthcare providers and nonprofit colleges, require revenue to keep their doors open. Nonprofit businesses funnel all their revenue after expenses back into the business, whereas for-profit businesses must grow the business while generating income for owners and stock holders. While for-profit companies exist to generate profit, most of them have vision and value statements that make their work compatible with nursing's ethical requirements. For example, a for-profit medical device company would go out of business if it failed to offer its customers safe, reliable products. Nurses work at for-profit companies as trainers, product developers, subject-matter experts, and even in direct sales roles. Some become corporate CNOs. Nurses who work for healthcare vendors can significantly impact the way products are developed and delivered and help influence the way companies run their businesses. They are highly sought-after employees because of their broad understanding of healthcare, their trustworthiness, and their problem-solving abilities (Porter-O'Grady, 2001).

Nurses in Military and Government

Nurses have become an integral part of the U.S. military and the Veterans Administration. They also hold important positions in federal, state, and local government. Nurses lead public health agencies and serve in other governmental departments that value their patient care expertise. Three nurses were sworn into the 155th Congress of the United States of America in 2017: Karen Bass, an APRN from California; Diane Black, an RN from Tennessee; and Eddie Bernice Johnson, an RN from Texas (Wood, 2018). Nurses serve in state and local legislatures as well. During the Obama administration, Marilyn Tavenner, MHA, BSN, RN, served as the administrator for the Centers for Medicare and Medicaid Services, while Mary Wakefield, PhD, RN, served the Health Resources and Services Administration as that agency's leader (Mayer, 2014).

Questions to Ask Yourself

1. What am I passionate about?
2. Where would I go to learn more about business to help me decide if I wanted to be an entrepreneur?
3. How much am I willing to risk for the sake of an idea?
4. What barriers exist to following through with my idea?
5. Are these barriers external or internal?

Role Preparation: Knowledge, Skills, and Attitudes

Nursing and healthcare are constantly changing, and their future is hard to predict. There will always be patients in need of care, but no one can foresee what that care will look like, who will provide it, or how and where patients will receive it. There is no way to prepare nurses for all the possibilities that will present themselves during a career in nursing (Porter-O'Grady, 2001). While it is true that many nurses are motivated by and find personal meaning and fulfillment in their careers through being able to make their own decisions, experience professional growth, and have an impact on others' lives (Vannucci & Weinstein, 2017), the path to embracing new challenges can be fraught with personal, professional, and financial obstacles and difficulties. Innovation and entrepreneurship seem to require a special skill set for which nurses are often ill-prepared (IOM, 2010).

Knowledge and Skills

One way to discover the knowledge and skills required to become an innovator, entrepreneur, or intrapreneur is to ask nurses in those roles to identify the gaps and deficits they have overcome in their own preparation. In a study of NPs' attitudes about entrepreneurship, respondents felt they lacked sufficient knowledge of legal and regulatory issues, reimbursement practices, office management, billing, and personnel management (Elango et al., 2007). In another study of 44 self-identified nurse entrepreneurs, researchers found that the participants identified as most critical to their business success such skills as marketing strategy, networking, and mentorship (Vannucci & Weinstein, 2017). In a review of studies on gaps in nurse entrepreneurs' preparation for business, researchers identified four major categories of skill deficits that nurse entrepreneurs believed they lacked (Arnaert et al., 2018). The knowledge and skills identified in this review are summarized in Table 16.2.

Nursing education has risen to the challenge of providing leadership education to nurses at all levels, but it may be time for leaders in nursing education to consider how to equip students with some of the skills nurse innovators, intrapreneurs, or entrepreneurs believe they lack to be successful in business.

Table 16.2. Skill Deficits Identified by Nurse Entrepreneurs

Cognitive	Interpersonal	Business	Strategic
Managing the uncertainties of business ownership	Sales	Legalities and regulations	Finding a niche
Business know-how	Networking and finding mentors	Risk management	Planning
Understanding the larger systems in which the business operates, e.g., economic, regulatory	Obtaining referrals	Regulation	Problem-solving
	Navigating the role change with colleagues and other professionals	Documentation	Knowing when to ask for help
	Communicating	Marketing	
		Finance	
		Operations	

Based on Arnaert, A., Mills, J., Bruno, F. S., & Ponzoni, N. (2018). The educational gaps of nurses in entrepreneurial roles: An integrative review. *Journal of Professional Nursing, 34*(6), 494–501.

Attitudes

Whether entrepreneurs, intrapreneurs, or social entrepreneurs are born or made, they all have qualities in common. They tend to be self-confident and passionate; to have integrity, self-discipline, and tremendous determination; to have the courage it takes to seize opportunities and be risk takers; and to be able to communicate their ideas and inspire others to work with them to achieve their vision (Wilson et al., 2012). Others have identified similar characteristics summarized in Figure 16.1, which also identifies key steps in developing an innovation.

Given technology's increasing ability to replace humans in the workforce, Samuel (2018) offers some advice for remaining relevant in an unknowable workplace future. Although the focus of these tips is on raising children who

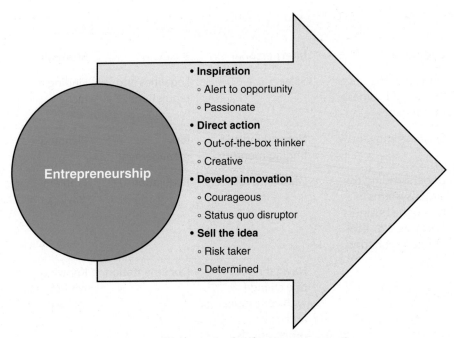

Figure 16.1. Key steps in developing an innovation.

will grow up to find meaningful work in a world full of robots that can do most human jobs, Samuel's advice, paraphrased below, is relevant for nurses seeking new roles:

- Gain an understanding of data, information, and knowledge so that you know the way information systems work.
- Nurture your creative side to stay flexible and be open to possibilities in the world around you.
- Computers cannot feel, so there will always be a need for emotional intelligence and interpersonal skills.
- Question rules.
- Learn constantly.
- Foster your inner entrepreneur.

Challenges

While nurses can lead innovative efforts to improve healthcare, barriers remain to their ability to effect widespread change (IOM, 2010), such as restrictive limits on APRN practice; payment and reimbursement issues; professional resistance from other healthcare providers; and the designation of nursing as a cost center, on a par with linen or housekeeping, rather than as a profit center. Innovative nurses and nurse entrepreneurs have been denied the kind of recognition afforded to other self-employed health professionals, and they often feel they work in isolation, without a safety net. They also encounter resistance or even hostility from colleagues (Wilson et al., 2012). In addition, nurses tend to feel they lack the expertise to express an opinion or take action, an inaccurate perception that inhibits their willingness to take risks. An important step on the road to a new career path is being "willing to take on opportunities that you are not completely sure-footed about" (Carlson, 2011).

Contemporary Nurse Entrepreneurs

Researchers in fields besides nursing can and do turn their findings and ideas into businesses, but most nurse researchers work in traditional ways to advance our understanding of topics that contribute to the body of knowledge in nursing. Sometimes, however, a researcher's work is so timely that it makes sense for the researcher to push the boundaries of conventional dissemination and make their work more widely available.

Cynthia Clark

Dr. Cynthia Clark's research on fostering civility and healthy work environments in nursing education and practice is an example of such timely and important work. Since beginning her doctoral studies in 2003, Clark has been a community-builder, researcher, educator, policymaker, and national and international expert on fostering civility. Her ground-breaking work has brought worldwide attention to the controversial issues of incivility in academic and practice environments, and her theory-driven interventions, empirical measurements, theoretical models, and reflective assessments provide best practices to prevent, measure, and address uncivil behavior and to create positive workplaces. She has developed several empirical instruments to measure incivility and civility, and revenue generated from the sale of her tools has provided funding for her continuing research. Clark has been a professional blogger for Sigma Theta Tau International for nearly a decade and the founder of Civility Matters in 2009, an online venue that provides practical resources, scientific research, and innovative ideas to foster civility and healthy work environments.

Clark began her nursing career working a job she loved, and "loving my work" has been a consistent theme throughout her illustrious career. One of her first nursing positions involved working with patients diagnosed with chronic illnesses and terminal conditions, and her predilection for engaging patients in conversation meant that at times she was not getting her work done. Her supervisor, noticing Clark's desire to spend more time in conversation with patients, suggested that her "true calling" might lie in the field of mental health. "Go back to school Cindy, you're clearly meant to be a psych nurse," the supervisor encouraged, and she did. Clark continued to advance her nursing education while earning additional degrees in substance abuse recovery, adolescent mental health counseling, and educational leadership. Clark found the special challenges of working with adolescents identified with violent behaviors and substance abuse issues particularly rewarding and managed inpatient, outpatient, and partial hospitalization programs for nearly 12 years before accepting a faculty position at a nearby university. Clark embraced her new role as an academician, and despite the significant reduction in salary, she began her tenure as a nursing professor in higher education—a role she enjoyed and cherished for nearly 20 years.

After several years as a successful nurse/therapist and clinical administrator, Clark came to academia as an outsider, not someone who had followed the usual path to a faculty role. Working with violent youth taught her many valuable and important lessons about managing the behavior of troubled youth. While not at the same level of intensity, observing nursing students respond to the difficulties they encountered in nursing school reminded her of the challenges many of her former patients experienced, including a lack of ability to engage in civil discourse and manage conflict in a constructive and respectful way. Her interest in this topic grew exponentially after the shooting deaths of three University of Arizona nursing faculty in Tucson in 2002. The resulting online discussion evidencing student disenfranchisement along with a growing sense that college student behavior was becoming more potentially threatening led Clark to see similarities between her prior work with troubled youth and college teaching. Many faculty-student interactions lack basic civility and have the potential for violence (Clark, 2017). Civility, "an authentic respect for others requiring time, presence, a willingness to engage in genuine discourse, and an intention to seek common ground" (Clark & Carnosso, 2008), became her passion, the subject of her doctoral work, and subsequent program of research and scholarship (Clark et al., 2015).

Conducting research for a dissertation is one thing; copyrighting the instruments you use and getting royalties from them is another. Then, turning that expertise into a successful speaking career is quite another. That is what Clark did, and that is what turned her from a nurse researcher to a social entrepreneur. She created something unique to fill a particular societal need and, despite obstacles, parlayed her research, her seven fully tested, valid, and reliable civility instruments, and her expertise in civility in nursing and healthcare into a vibrant career.

Clark credits a lot of people with her success, including her supportive spouse, dissertation advisor, and other amazing mentors along the way who helped fuel her passion to fulfill her life's mission, "leading the coalition for change: creating and sustaining communities of civility"(Clark, 2017, p. 118) (Clark, personal communication, June 4, 2018).

Diane Yeager

Diane Yeager took a circuitous route to starting her entrepreneurial business. She went to nursing school after starting her family and a short stint in business school. Determined to get a job right out of school in the specialty area of labor and delivery, where new graduates did not typically begin practice at the time, she moved her family to another state to a hospital that would allow her to start right in the specialty area without experience. That determination and willingness to take risks is a theme in Yeager's story. Even as a staff nurse, her entrepreneurial spirit and business abilities emerged as she helped a friend start a private business as a birthing coach.

In her first teaching job, she found a niche as the only faculty member who knew how to use a computer. Like Clark, Yeager came to the position as an outsider, without any teaching experience, which may have allowed them both to see possibilities that elude those who come to academia via more traditional routes. After an encounter with a state auditor, she rewrote the program's curriculum, an experience that would prove valuable later when she was developing her product. Around 2005, while teaching full-time and raising her family, Yeager began a website that gave open access to anyone wanting electronic games and activities for teaching and learning nursing. Although no longer supported or updated, the resource saw much use by nursing students and nursing faculty across the United States.

She was recruited by a large EHR company to become a curriculum developer for training nurses and left her teaching position at the college. She found the work interesting but unsatisfying and missed teaching. Then it came to her—talking with nursing instructors and hearing their struggles to teach documentation to students who are often unable to access a hospital's EHR system, she realized there was an opportunity. Her son was grown and had become a computer programmer, and in 4 months, they developed the framework for what would become EHR Tutor. Yeager left her job; her daughter left her job as a trainer and came onboard to do marketing; and Yeager's husband provided support and business advice. Even though there were large companies providing a similar product, the company took off.

Yeager has said she feels blessed; she credits a lot of her success to being in the right place at the right time. But her story reflects many of the attributes of the entrepreneur: she was alert to opportunity, listening to nurse educators concerns about students and EHRs; she had courage to risk leaving her secure job behind to pursue the vision she created with her son using out-of-the-box thinking (she admits she did not know other companies were selling products similar to EHR Tutor when she started); and she had determination to achieve her vision, recruiting her family to market and sell EHR Tutor to nursing schools. She remains active in the company training others and marketing the product (Yeager, personal communication, June 12, 2018).

Sharon Weinstein

Sharon Weinstein, a nurse entrepreneur, author, and CEO of SMW Group and the Global Education Development Institute, educates and trains employees and executives in healthcare and other high-stress industries internationally. She not only sought certification as a Certified Speaking Professional (CSP) but became president of the Washington, DC area National Speakers Association (NSA), is the Vice-Chair of the Certification Committee (NSA National), and has held such offices in other organizations. A fellow of the American Academy of Nursing (FAAN), she has become a recognized and sought-after expert in work-life balance and stress management (see In Their Own Words by Sharon Weinstein on p. 561).

In Their Own Words

Sharon M. Weinstein, MS, RN, CRNI-R, FACW, FAAN, CSP

Chief Executive Officer of SMW Group and the Global Education Development Institute and Past President, NSA-DC

The key points in understanding my role are... that I am not alone; I am following in the footsteps of nurse icons, like Florence Nightingale, and nurse colleagues, each of whom has embraced entrepreneurship, made mistakes along the journey, learned from those mistakes, and forged a future that has enhanced healthcare outcomes and services.

What keeps me coming back every day is... the joy that I derive from knowing that I have changed lives and created a sustainable future for others. As an entrepreneur, I have started an LLC and two not-for-profits. The LLC is the cornerstone of my business model and allows me to coach, consult, and speak. Clients have offered positive reviews, referred me to others, and scheduled follow-up work. This affirms that I am filling an unmet need and doing it well. My not-for-profits address global healthcare and environmental safety. They, too, keep me focused, expand my reach, and empower me to act on behalf of those who cannot act for themselves.

My greatest challenge is... working solo. It is difficult to structure one's day so that the focus is on business; it is important to work on the business and not in it. I am my company's brand, and as the brand, I need to be out in the communities I serve to maintain presence and make the right connections. Working from home means setting specific hours, remaining at one's desk or in meetings during those hours, and avoiding the temptations of a visit to the gym, the salon, or something else. Self-care is critical, especially for nurse entrepreneurs, but everything should be done in moderation.

I wish someone had told me... that I would benefit from a peer advisory board that could help me to solve issues, resolve questions, reach decisions, and grow my business. I now know how important that is, and I strive to help others to make great decisions that benefit their companies, families, and communities.

I need to be a lifelong learner because... I was told as a teenager that I should learn to type because I would never amount to a thing. At the time, I believed

(Continued)

my parents and learned to type (150 wpm). My nursing school scholarship provided roots for me, and I soon learned that I was capable of success in anything I set my mind to do. For me, lifelong learning is twofold: (1) it proves my parents are wrong, and (2) it sustains my personal and professional growth. My nursing platform is consistently used as the basis for all my endeavors, and I treasure my career and experiences. I returned to school for a baccalaureate, master's, and postgraduate education.

Another point to understand is... prior to entrepreneurship, I worked 100 hours per week, three countries per week in Central and Eastern Europe. I was tired, stressed, and when I missed a family event, I switched gears and "got a life." My new career was based on work-life balance. I wrote about it, spoke about it, and lived it. Stress and burnout can accompany self-employment, and these experiences may be related to factors such as balancing family and business demands, lack of social support, and financial uncertainty. Life is a balancing act, and nurses in all settings, especially entrepreneurial roles, can enhance well-being and productivity with effective self-care strategies.

These are just a few examples of nurses working outside traditional roles in education, administration, informatics, and research. They all exhibit many of the tendencies of entrepreneurs including passion, courage, determination, out-of-the-box thinking, and more.

Summary

Gaps in the way nurses are educated and socialized impede their ability to even consider alternatives to traditional forms of employment such as hospital, clinic, or agency-based roles. But the needs of the healthcare system for high-quality, widely available, and cost-effective patient care are opening opportunities for nurses with advanced education and skills who have the willingness to recognize and take advantage of those opportunities. Help is available, often without charge (see Web Resources), but forging a new path is not without risk—personal, professional, and financial. Role models and mentors exist, but innovation and entrepreneurship require courage, passion, and creativity. When the burdens and constraints of an oppressive history and practice restrictions are lifted, nurses can and will be vital change agents for the patient care of tomorrow.

Chapter Highlights

- The U.S. healthcare system has not embraced or encouraged the unique and innovative contributions nurses have made to patient care over the past century and a half. As a result, innovation that might emerge from nurses, who make up the largest percentage of the healthcare workforce, is discouraged and often lost.

- Because nurses touch every aspect of people's lives and because of advanced education in specialty areas and progressive state legislation expanding autonomy for advanced practice registered nurses, fewer boundaries exist today for nurses who have entrepreneurial, intrapreneurial, and social entrepreneurial ideas for improving the lives of the people they serve.

- Opportunities within the healthcare system abound for nurses with advanced education and skills and have the willingness to recognize and take advantage of those opportunities.

- Whether entrepreneurs, intrapreneurs, or social entrepreneurs are born or made, they all have qualities in common. They tend to be self-confident and passionate; to have integrity, self-discipline, and tremendous determination; to have the courage it takes to seize opportunities and be risk takers; and to be able to communicate their ideas and inspire others to work with them to achieve their vision.

- Entrepreneurial nurses are able to consider alternatives to traditional forms of employment.

- Entrepreneurial role models and mentors exist, but innovation and entrepreneurship require courage, passion, and creativity.

- When the burdens and constraints of an oppressive history and practice restrictions are lifted, nurses can and will be vital change agents for the patient care of tomorrow.

Certification and Professional Organizations

American Academy of Nurse Entrepreneurs: https://aane.us/
Edward Lowe Foundation: https://edwardlowe.org/
Entrepreneurs' Organization: https://www.eonetwork.org/
National Nurses in Business Association: https://nnbanow.com/

Startup Grind: https://www.startupgrind.com/
United States Association for Small Business and Entrepreneurship: https://www.usasbe.org/
Vistage: https://www.vistage.com/
Young Entrepreneur Council: https://yec.co/
Young President's Organization: https://www.ypo.org/

Web Resources

- The National Nurses in Business Association provides updates, information, and a place to network on their website. The organization also hosts conferences, workshops, and seminars: https://nnbanow.com
- The American Association of Birth Centers "promotes and supports birth centers as a means to uphold the rights of healthy women and their families, in all communities, to birth their children in an environment which is safe, sensitive, and cost effective with minimal intervention": https://www.birthcenters.org
- This site is "committed to accelerating the growth of sustainable nurse-led start-ups": https://www.nnpen.org/
- "SCORE is the nation's largest network of volunteer, expert business mentors, with more than 10,000 volunteers in 300 chapters. As a resource partner of the U.S. Small Business Administration (SBA), SCORE has helped more than 10 million entrepreneurs through mentoring, workshops, and educational resources since 1964": https://www.score.org/
- The Small Business Development Center (SBDC), part of the Small Business Administration (SBA) of the federal government, assists small businesses and entrepreneurs with business plans, manufacturing, financing, market research, and more: https://www.sba.gov/tools/local-assistance/sbdc
- This commercial site called Clinicians Business Institute (and NPBO) offers business training and services to help clinicians start and succeed in any kind of business: www.NursePractitionerBusinessOwner.com
- National Nurse-Led Care Consortium "is a nonprofit organization supporting and advocating for nurse-led care": https://nurseledcare.org/

References

American Association of Birth Centers. (2016). *An historical timeline*. https://www.birthcenters.org/page/history

American Association of Colleges of Nursing. (2019). *Nursing fact sheet*. www.aacnnursing.org/News-Information/Fact-Sheets/Nursing-Fact-Sheet#:~:text=Nursing%20i%20the%20nation's%20largest,84.5%25%20are%20employed%20in%20nursing

American Nurses Association. (2015). *Code of ethics for nurses with interpretive statements.* https://www.nursingworld.org/practice-policy/nursing-excellence/ethics/code-of-ethics-for-nurses/

American Nurses Association. (n.d.). *Isabel Adams Hampton Robb.* https://www.nursingworld.org/ana/about-ana/history/hall-of-fame/inductees-listed-alphabetically/

Arnaert, A., Mills, J., Bruno, F. S., & Ponzoni, N. (2018). The educational gaps of nurses in entrepreneurial roles: An integrative review. *Journal of Professional Nursing, 34*(6), 494–501.

Buhler-Wilkinson, K. (1993). Bringing care to the people: Lillian Wald's legacy to public health nursing. *The American Journal of Public Health, 83*(12), 1778–1786.

Bunger, J. D. (2008). Nurse entrepreneurs. *Nebraska Nursing News, 25*(4), 14–17.

Campaign for Action. (2018). *Percentage of U.S. nurse-led clinics in medically underserved areas.* https://campaignforaction.org/resource/percentage-u-s-nurse-led-clinics-located-medically-underserved-areas-mua/

Carlson, J. (2011). *For more hospitals and health systems, a clinical background has become the preferred track to the top jobs, including CEO.* Modern Healthcare. http://www.modernhealthcare.com/article/20110411/MAGAZINE/110409984

Clark, C. M. (2017). *Creating and sustaining civility in nursing education* (2nd ed.). Sigma Theta Tau International Publishing.

Clark, C. M., Barbosa-Leiker, C., Gill, L., & Nguyen, D. T. (2015). Revision and psychometric testing of the incivility in nursing education (INE) survey: Introducing the INE-R. *Journal of Nursing Education, 54*(6), 306–315. http://doi.org/10.3928/01484834-20150515-01

Clark, C. M., & Carnosso, J. (2008). Civility: A concept analysis. *Journal of Theory Construction and Testing, 12*(1), 11–15.

Dees, G. (2001). *The meaning of social entrepreneurship.* https://community-wealth.org/sites/clone.community-wealth.org/files/downloads/paper-dees.pdf

Elango, B., Hunter, G. L., & Winchell, M. (2007). Barriers to nurse entrepreneurship: A study of the process model of entrepreneurship. *Journal of the American Academy of Nurse Practitioners, 19*(4), 198–204.

Electronic Health Reporter. (2016). *How nurses are using health informatics to improve patient care.* https://electronichealthreporter.com/nurses-using-health-informatics-improve-patient-care/

Ely, L. (2015). Nurse-managed clinics: Barriers and benefits toward financial sustainability when integrating primary care and mental health. *Nursing Economic, 33*(4), 193–202.

Ernst, K., & Bauer, K. (2012). *Birth centers in the United States.* American Association of Birth Centers. http://docplayer.net/53044467-Birth-centers-in-the-united-states-kitty-ernst-cnm-mph-dsc-hon-and-kate-bauer-mba-american-association-of-birth-centers.html

Garofalo, M. E., & Fee, E. (2015). Lavinia Dock (1858–1956): Picketing, parading, and protesting. *American Journal of Public Health, 105*(2), 276–277. http://doi.org/10.2105/AJPH.2014.302021

Hahn, J., & Cook, W. (2018). Lessons learned from nurse practitioner independent practice: A conversation with a nurse practitioner entrepreneur. *Nursing Economics, 36*(1), 18.

Hayden, J. K., Smiley, R. A., Alexander, M., Kardong-Edgren, S., & Jeffries, P. R. (2014). The NCSBN national simulation study: A longitudinal, randomized, controlled study replacing clinical hours with simulation in prelicensure nursing education. *Journal of Nursing Regulation, 5*(2 suppl), S3–S40. http://doi.org/10.1016/S2155-8256(15)30062-4

Institute of Medicine. (2010). *The future of nursing: Leading change, advancing health.* http://books.nap.edu/openbook.php?record_id=12956&page=R1

International Council of Nurses. (2004). *Guidelines on the nurse entre/intrapreneur providing nursing service.* http://www.ipnig.ca/education/Guidelines-NurseEntre-ICN.pdf

Mayer, J. (2014). *Celebrating nurse leaders in government*. American Nurse. https://www.myamer-icannurse.com/celebrating-nurse-leaders-in-government/

Michals, D. (2015). *Clara Barton*. www.womenshistory.org/education-resources/biographies/clara-barton

National Association of Clinical Nurse Specialists. (n.d.). *Scope of practice*. http://nacns.org/advocacy-policy/policies-affecting-cnss/scope-of-practice/

Parry, M. S. (2006). Dorothea Dix (1802–1887). *American Journal of Public Health, 96*(4), 624–625. http://doi.org/10.2105/AJPH.2005.079152

Pollitt, P. (2015). Charlotte Rhone: Nurse, welfare worker, and entrepreneur. *American Journal of Nursing, 115*(2), 66–70. http://doi.org/10.1097/01.NAJ.0000460699.55628.4d

Porter-O'Grady, T. (2001). Beyond the walls: Nursing in the entrepreneurial world. *Nursing Administration Quarterly, 25*(2), 61–68.

Reverby, S. M. (1987). *Ordered to care: The dilemma of American nursing, 1850-1945*. Cambridge University Press.

Robert Wood Johnson Foundation. (2015). *New study explores impact of ACA on nurse practitioners*. https://www.rwjf.org/en/library/articles-and-news/2015/07/new-study-explores-impact-of-ACA-on-nurse-practitioners.html

Samuels, A. (2018). How you raise robot-proof children. *The Wall Street Journal*. https://www.wsj.com/articles/how-you-can-raise-robot-proof-children-1524756310

Vannucci, M. J., & Weinstein, S. M. (2017). The nurse entrepreneur: Empowerment needs, challenges, and self-care practices. *Dove Press, 2017*(7), 57–66. https://www.dovepress.com/the-nurse-entrepreneur-empowerment-needs-challenges-and-self-care-prac-peer-reviewed-fulltext-article-NRR#ref2

Whelan, J. C. (2012). When the business of nursing was the nursing business: The private duty registry system, 1900–1940. *Online Journal of Issues in Nursing, 17*(2), 6. http://doi.org/10.3912/OJIN.Vol17No02Man06

Wilson, A., Whitaker, N., & Whitford, D. (2012). Rising to the challenge of healthcare reform with entrepreneurial and intrapreneurial nursing initiatives. *The Online Journal of Issues in Nursing, 17*(2), 5. http://doi.org/10.3912/OJIN.Vol17No02Man05 and. http://ojin.nursingworld.org/MainMenuCategories/ANAMarketplace/ANAPeriodicals/OJIN/TableofContents/Vol-17-2012/No2-May-2012/Rising-to-the-Challenge-of-Reform.html

Wood, M. (2018). *115th Congress includes 3 nurses*. Becker's Hospital Review. https://www.becker-shospitalreview.com/payer-issues.html

17

Transitioning to APN/APRN Roles

Pegge L. Bell · Carolyn Hart

LEARNING OBJECTIVES

After completing this chapter, you will be able to:

1. Compare annual salaries of the advanced practice nurse (APN) and advanced practice registered nurse (APRN) roles.

2. Consider strategies for adding value to professional practice.

3. Develop a professional resume.

4. Prepare for an interview with a prospective employer.

5. Describe the process of contract negotiation.

6. Discuss the mentor's role with advanced practice nurses.

7. Discuss the preceptor's role with advanced nursing education.

KEY TERMS

Base compensation: The initial rate of pay for services provided, usually calculated as an hourly, weekly, monthly, or yearly salary that does not include benefits, housing, or other forms of pay for the employer.

Business plan: A document that describes what services will be provided by a business, how it will operate (including leadership, staffing, and finances), and all details needed to achieve success by outlining goals and the specific means of reaching those goals over a 3- to 5-year period.

Contract negotiation: A give-and-take process between two parties culminating in a final agreement, in this case, related to compensation and benefits.

Cover letter: A tool used during the job application process to help introduce a prospective employee to a potential employer in a memorable way.

Curriculum vitae (CV): A detailed document that outlines one's academic and professional history, usually used for positions at a college, university, or research institution.

Outcomes research: A broad term used to describe research that is focused on the effectiveness of healthcare interventions.

Professional development: A wide variety of specialized training or education that is intended to improve one's professional knowledge, competence, skill, or effectiveness in a particular role.

Profit sharing: A plan in which a designated percentage of annual profits are shared with employees only when the institution experiences a profit.

Resume: A one- to two-page document that summarizes one's work experience, education, and skills.

Translational science: The application of knowledge to address critical medical needs in a way that specifically improves health outcomes.

Triple Aim: The Institute for Healthcare Improvement's initiative to use integrated approaches to improve healthcare, improve population health, and reduce costs associated with healthcare, to which some clinicians have added the fourth dimension of finding satisfaction in providing healthcare serves (referred to as the Quadruple Aim).

Introduction

Professional considerations are important for future advanced practice nurses (APNs), as career choices are an investment of time and money. When considering future APN/advanced practice registered nurse (APRN) roles, nurses should give careful thought to why they are choosing a role and if they have a true passion for the role. Salaries will vary across the roles, but if compensation is the only consideration, the role could result in a higher cost—a career in a role that provides little joy. On the other hand, a role chosen early in one's career might have less appeal later in life. Fortunately, educational mobility is afforded through the post-master's and postdoctoral certificate programs. These allow APN/APRNs to build on previous educational preparation if, and when, they choose to add a second role or make a change to a new role.

This chapter provides an overview of professional considerations such as salary, finding and interviewing for a position, negotiating a position, developing a professional resume, and securing and serving as a mentor. Additionally, the chapter will introduce strategies for bringing value to the role and to the profession. Proving one's worth to an organization builds confidence for the role and allows employees to see the true value of securing an APN/APRN.

Compensation

Salary is certainly a consideration when seeking a position as an APN. Just as external factors such as type of facility (acute care vs. primary care, medical center campus vs. community hospital, for profit vs. not-for-profit, and geographic location) affect registered nurse (RN) salaries, they will also affect APN salaries. APNs face competition in the marketplace for positions advertised by healthcare facilities that could hire a physician, APN, or physician assistant (PA). Range and average salary are reported for each of the APN roles listed in Table 17.1. It should be noted that in some instances, APNs may receive additional monetary benefits and/or bonuses depending on partial ownership or stake in the business.

Within the salary ranges listed in Table 17.1, variation will occur based on geographical location, specialty, size of the institution, and practice setting. The years of experience held by the nurse can also influence pay. In addition to base compensation, some employers will offer bonuses or profit sharing. This means that if a practice setting does well and makes a profit, a certain percentage would be passed on to the individual employees who are instrumental in increasing the organization's bottom line.

Table 17.1. Comparison of APN Salaries

APN	Salary Range	Average Salary
CRNA[a]	$158,401 – $219,923	$187,382
CNM[a]	$94,072 – $139,438	$111,162
CNS[a]	$87,988 – $127,328	$107,705
CNP[a]	$95,275 – $128,715	$110,491
CNL[a]	$82,341 – $103,248	$90,489
Nurse Administrator[a]	$77,050 – $115,973	$95,280
Charge Nurse[a]	$76,687 – $107,749	$88,788
Nurse Manager[b]	$65,000 – $118,000	$86,000
Chief Nursing Officer[a]	$169,978 – $308,428	$235,220
Director of Nursing[a]	$114,483 – $194,280	$150,430
Director of Patient Services[b]	$51,000 – $140,000	$84,000
Assistant Professor[a]	$40,545 – $136,639	$66,988
Associate Professor[a]	$51,335 – $152,524	$79,753
Professor[a]	$60,613 – $182,546	$96,428

APN, advanced practice nurse; CNL, clinical nurse leader; CNM, certified nurse midwife; CNP, certified nurse practitioner; CNS, clinical nurse specialist; CRNA, certified registered nurse anesthetist.
[a]Salary.com, 2020.
[b]Payscale.com, 2020.

Considerations for First APN Position

When seeking an initial APN position, you should first use several strategies to identify vacant positions that best match career goals and professional skills. Introspection about where one sees themself in the next 5 years will help hone the search for the first position.

Questions to Ask Yourself

1. What do I want to accomplish in the next 5 years of my career?
2. What kind of populations do I want to serve?
3. What skills do I have that I want to maximize in my practice?
4. What skills would I want to minimize in my practice?
5. In what settings could I do the most good for myself?
6. In what settings could I do the most good for others?
7. What are my priority motivators for taking a position (salary, benefits, location, learning opportunities, work environment, type of patients)?

Each APN should weigh the match between the advertised position requirements and opportunities and their individual career goals. APRN clinicians should consider positions that build on their clinical and leadership strengths, as well as the competencies required for certification. For example, an APN who has experience with pain management or is proficient in epidemiology may want to consider a position that offers opportunities in these areas. APN educators should seek a position with opportunities to teach in the areas of their clinical experience. This would give them credibility with students and hospital staff when supervising students placed on specific clinical units. Clinical nurse specialists would need to match the population or disease focus of their educational and clinical experiences with those of an advertised position. They will have certification that matches a specific disease/population, so trying to stretch that into another disease/population would not be appropriate. APN administrators and clinical nurse leaders should consider the organizational aspects of a position to determine if it is a good match with their past leadership experiences or if it offers new opportunities that align with career goals. Aligning career goals with advertised vacant positions will foster a good match and minimize job frustrations.

Finding Your First Job

Career counselors suggest using several strategies to locate available positions. Suggestions include speaking with former professors and employers to inquire about available positions. Also, contacting former preceptors and fellow graduates may elicit opportunities either in your current state or elsewhere. Check the websites of professional organizations, professional employment agencies, and institutions where you might be interested in working. Government positions will be posted on state or federal websites such as the U.S. Department of Veterans' Affairs (VA) website or state agencies.

Posted positions found on professional nursing and job websites (Table 17.2) will include job descriptions and job requirements. It is important to review both aspects of the posting. While most job descriptions are a good match with the expected skills and competencies of each APN position, the job requirements will provide unique expectations. For example, at least 1 year of full-time experience may be required, or the APN may be required to speak a second language, depending on the geographic location. The details of the job requirement should be read carefully to increase the likelihood of a positive response on your application.

APN available positions can be found at several websites which provide posted job descriptions and requirements provided by individual prospective employers. A thorough review of these postings will provide applicants with the necessary information to determine not only what the job entails,

Table 17.2. Websites for Vacant APN Positions

Website	APN Role
advancedpractice.com	All roles
iHireNursing.com	All roles
iHireMidLevelPractitioners.com	CNM, NP, CNS, CRNA
Federalregister.gov/documents/ advanced-practice-registered-nurses	Government roles
https://job-openings.monster.com	All roles
https://www.glassdoor.com/index.htm	All roles
Indeed.com	All roles

APN, advanced practice nurse.

but also if there are any additional requirements of the job. Sample job postings are found below in Boxes 17.1 to 17.4.

As you review these sample job postings, consider the professional competencies provided by in the respective chapter of this text to compare what employers need and what you are being prepared to do upon graduation. These example job postings provide samples of what an APN can expect to see with job postings at various professional sites. Some postings provide

---

BOX 17.1

▶ NURSE PRACTITIONER JOB POSTING

Duties and Responsibilities

Prepare and maintain health records

Examine and treat patients

Collaborate with physicians on diagnosis and patient care

Write prescriptions and order for medical tests

Educate patients and families

Requirements

Active APRN Nursing license

Demonstrated knowledge and skill in customer service and conflict resolution

Experience working with collaborative team

Knowledge of electronic medical record

Ability to work flexible hours

Knowledge of Medicare, Medicaid, and other payer reimbursement and coding

BOX 17.2

▶ DIABETES CLINICAL NURSE SPECIALIST

Duties and Responsibilities

Clinical expertise in care and management of patients with diabetes.

Knowledge and skills of evidence-based practice and research, education, consultation, and leadership.

Knowledge and skills focused on three areas: patient/family, nurses and nursing practice, and organization/system.

Works collaboratively with other CNSs and specialists

Coordinates work across the clinical sites.

Requirements

At least 2 to 5 years of recent experience with diabetes

Active APRN license

Active CPR certification

Current national diabetes educator certification

Adapted from www.simplyhired.com

more information about what the job entails, what employers expect from the applicant, or the minimum educational or clinical requirements for the position. Many of these positions are posted on more than one professional site and may have more or less information provided at alternate sites depending on word limitations. Applicants should select the postings that best match individual career goals and then prioritize available positions based on those goals, future potential for growth, location and possible implications to family responsibilities.

BOX 17.3

▶ CERTIFIED REGISTERED NURSE ANESTHETIST POSITION

Duties and Responsibilities

- Interview patients preoperatively and assesses their status for anesthesia.

- Administers anesthesia and/or analgesia for surgical and/or obstetrical procedures.

- Reviews the patient's hospital record with the anesthesiologists regarding the anesthesia plan.

- Utilizes and prepares all essential equipment and supplies to enhance effective and safe anesthesia delivery.

- Monitors all necessary parameters to determine patient condition reaction to surgery and anesthesia.

- Advises and/or consults anesthesiologist regarding adverse reactions.

- Records the patient's status on the clinical anesthesia record prior to, during, and following anesthesia by anesthesiologists.

- Performs departmental duties as assigned.

- Performs 24-hour anesthesia coverage as required and/or directed.

- Provides emergency and resuscitative care for the entire Medical Center.

- Accomplishes required postoperative anesthetic visits using department forms or progress notes.

Requirements

Graduate of an approved nursing program.

Current RN license and CRNA license

Graduate of an approved anesthesia program.

Current certification with American Association of Nurse Anesthetists (or eligible).

Adapted from https://job-openings.monster.com

BOX 17.4

▶ NURSE FACULTY POSITION

Duties and Responsibilities

Evidence-Based Teaching/Learning and Master Instruction

- Implements the College's philosophy, curriculum and course objectives through classroom, online, clinical teaching, and service to College, community, health system, and profession.

- Develops curricular/teaching innovations in the annual preparation and revision of all assigned course(s).

- Monitors selected clinical agencies for appropriateness for student clinical experiences and ability to meet clinical course outcomes.

- Plans clinical experiences for and provides direct/indirect supervision and evaluation of nursing students delivering nursing care to an individual or group of individuals.

- Provides oversight for clinical preceptors/mentors for student clinical experiences and coordinates and evaluates those preceptors/mentors.

- Provides documented feedback to students on level of performance based on course outcomes.

- Serves as professional role model for students

- Advises students

- Serves on college committees

- Demonstrates scholarship through the Scholarship of Teaching, Discovery, Application, or Integration congruent with expectations of assigned rank.

Requirements

- Master's Degree in Nursing required

- Doctorate preferred

- Professional nurse licensure required

- A minimum of 2 years' nursing experience working in a clinical setting

- Experientially prepared for assigned courses

- Previous teaching experience preferred

- Excellent communication skills

Adapted from https://www.careerbuilder.com

In Their Own Words

Victor Ospina, DNP, APRN, ACNP-BC, CCRN
Corporate Director, Nursing and Health Sciences Research
Academic Affairs Department
Baptist Health System

Preparing for a Job Interview
How should applicants prepare for an interview?

- Applicants interviewing for the position of nurse in an advanced role should have a fair understanding of the institution's mission and vision. If possible, try to find information about the strategic plan or core commitments. The applicant would also want to have some a good understanding of the awards, accolades, and accreditations that the institution has received. What are they best known for? Finally, have an understanding of the communities that the institution serves; what are the various patient populations and service lines within the organizations. How would your goals and skills align with the strategic goals of the company?

What do you look for in a prospective applicant?

- This is a complex mix that includes level of experience, expertise, and level of commitment. We would also want to look at the applicant's history of employment and longevity in their role. "Job hopping" can be a drawback. In addition to these objective measures, we would also want to hear about

(Continued)

examples of caring and compassion; the applicant can also expect questions that relate to the institution's vision and goals.

- While answering questions, we also assess appearance and professionalism. We look more favorably upon someone who can clearly articulate responses and show signs of flexibility.

How can an applicant stand out from others?

- These things can be divided into two areas. The first are objective things such as any accolades or awards that the nurse has earned along with professional achievements. Community service can also help someone stand out from others along with excellent references, especially references from within the organizations.
- Just as important is the applicant's ability to engage the interview team and creating a sense of trust, truthfulness, and genuineness.

What are a few things applicants should try to avoid?

- Things that do not look good are applying for a job with minimal experience and job hopping. Applications and cover letters with poor grammar and spelling errors usually are filtered out and do not even make it to the review process.

Is negotiation an expected part of the process?

- Organizations that know their salaries are not the most competitive will usually expect some amount of negotiation. Things to consider when negotiating can include a cell phone allowance, delineation of privileges (depending on supervising physician/s), schedule, vacation time, loan payoff (for example, school loans), or special courses and training.

What things or factors do applicants often overlook?

- Applicants frequently forget that they need to remain flexible; the interview process is a give and take where, ideally, both parties believe they benefit. They also need to be willing to stretch themselves as these may be the assignments that result in professional growth.
- Other factors that are often overlooked are the mechanics of working for a particular institution and the expectations of being an employee. Consider things like the travel time, expected workload, and the culture of health system which will vary from entity to entity.

Questions to Ask Yourself

1. How will I be adequately prepared for my chosen role?
2. Do I have any educational gaps that will need to be addressed or will I have any educational opportunities while in the program?
3. How will this encourage me to be a more active participant with my learning?
4. What considerations should I give to selecting a preceptor and clinical site in order to seek a position upon graduation?

Applying for the Job

When a good match is found between educational and professional credentials and a posted position, the next step is to submit the documents required to apply for the job, either by mail or online. These may include a cover letter and resume or curriculum vitae (CV). It is very important to comply with any special instructions about the submission of these materials, such as word or page limits. If selected for consideration, the candidate will then participate in the interview and contract negotiation processes.

Interviewing

Preparing for your job interview is a critical step in landing your dream job. As the first step in preparing for a job interview, research the organization. Familiarize yourself with the mission and vision along with any strategic goals. Be sure to frame your responses keeping these values in mind. You may decide to articulate your skills in terms of the organization's mission. This information can also provide an opportunity for you to ask a pointed question during the interview (for example, "I was intrigued with your commitment to [X]; how would this influence expectations of performance in my role should I be hired?"). You should also be prepared to talk about how your professional values match those of the organization.

Resume

The resume is a brief summary of personal, educational, and professional experiences, usually captured on one page. When a good match is found between educational and professional credentials and a posted position, the next step is to submit a resume and cover letter (if requested) either by mail or online. The applicant should review the website of the hiring agency to determine if their organizational mission and goals are a good match with the APNs. If so, the match should be reflected in the applicant's career goals and details about their past work experiences and community involvement activities. An example of a resume found at: www.bing.com and is provided in Figure 17.1. A fictitious name has been provided to protect the identity of the author.

Lori Smith, MSN RN CNN CFNP

111 Diamond St • Sedona, Colorado 88888 • (555) 555-5555

Qualifications

Dedicated Family Nurse Practitioner with more than 20 years nursing experience.
Background in emergency, intensive care, internal medicine, critical care, neonatal and in-flight nursing.
Flexible, quick learner who adapts easily to new situations and enjoys a challenge.
Self-motivated professional with a commitment in providing quality nursing care.
Strong organizational and communication skills.

Credentials

	Basic Life Support
Registered Nurse (License #51436)	Advanced Cardiac Life Support
Nationally Certified Family Nurse Practitioner	Pediatric Advanced Life Support
Nationally Certified Neonatal Nurse Practitioner	Neonatal Resuscitation Program Regional Instructor

Certifications

Education

BSN, MSN, FNP, University of Colorado at Colorado Springs, May 1998
Neonatal Nurse Practitioner Certificate, Beth-El College of Nursing, Colorado Sprints, Colorado 1986
Associate Degree in Nursing, Mesa College, Grant Junction, Colorado, 1971 ~ 1973

Professional Experience

EMERGENCY DEPARTMENT STAFF NURSE, Memorial Hospital, Colorado Springs, CO	1999 – present
FAMILY NURSE PRACTITIONER, Dr. John Genrich, Colorado Springs, CO	1998 – present
NEONATAL NURSE PRACTITIONER, Memorial Hospital, Colorado Springs, CO	1986 – present

- Responsible for attending all deliveries and providing appropriate medical care, assessment, and case management in a LEVEL III regional medical center.
- Member of the neonatal transport team; selected as a clinical resource person for the institution.

FLIGHT NURSE/ER NURSE, St. Mary's Medical Center, Grand Junction, CO	1983 – 1985

- Provided nursing care during helicopter transfer of patients.

LEVEL II ICN NURSE, St. Mary's Medical Center, Grand Junction, CO	1982 – 1983

- Provided comprehensive nursing care to patients in LEVEL II ICN.

EMERGENCY DEPARTMENT STAFF NURSE, St. Anthony's Hospital, Denver, CO	1976 – 1982

- Served as a staff nurse in both the Emergency Room and Medical ICU.
- Hospital night supervisor.

Professional Affiliations, Research and Publications

- Chairperson of NNP quality improvement committee, Memorial Hospital NICU
- Member of the American Academy of Nurse Practitioners
- Co-investigator. (1992). Conventional versus high-frequency oscillatory ventilation following exosurf administration in infants with respiratory distress syndrome, Memorial Hospital
- Lemmons, M. P., Bruse C. E., Monaco, F. J. and Meredith, K. M. (1993). Conventional versus high-frequency oscillatory ventilation following exosurf administration in infants with respiratory distress syndrome: A preliminary retrospective review. Abstract published in *Pediatric Pulmonary*.

Figure 17.1. Sample Resume. (Please note: Information provided in sample resume is fictitious.)

The resume provides personal contact information and licensure and certification information. The applicant provides a brief overview of their qualifications which emphasizes their strengths and clinical experiences. Credentials and certifications are also provided. The educational background of the applicant is included starting with highest degree first. Professional experiences also start with most recent employment activities. Note that under each position a brief explanation is provided in one to two points to capture primary duties of the position. Lastly, the applicant provides scholarship and service activities starting with most recent first. Dates should be included for these activities to demonstrate a history of involvement. The Muse.com is an excellent source for information related to creating a resume. Table 17.3 is adapted from their *42 Resume Dos and Don'ts Every Job Seeker Should Know.*

Curriculum Vitae

A **Curriculum Vitae** (CV) is Latin for course of life. The information in a CV is more detailed and varied than the information in a resume. The primary differences between a CV and a **resume** are the length, what type of information is included, and the use of the CV. Academic settings require CVs of each faculty member—whether they are full-time with an academic appointment or part-time serving as clinical instructors—and many of these institutions have a template to provide uniformity. The CV usually requires personal information (name, address, contact information), as well as educational background. The CV contains a history of the activities in the three major missions of a university—teaching, research/scholarship, and service. Service can be to the university in the form of committees, while service to the external community can capture volunteer work and contributions to professional organizations. APA format is used to list publications, research projects, and presentations.

To demonstrate the difference in length and depth between a resume and a CV, an example of a faculty CV is provided below. The categories are standard for most colleges and universities; however, additions can be added. For example, a section for professional service could be added for faculty to track their committee involvement at the university level, department level, and in professional organizations. See Figure 17.2 for the CV components.

Applicants should note that this CV is an abbreviated sample of the faculty member's work. Faculty who have obtained higher ranks of associate or full professor will continue to add to their vitae, making it a very lengthy document.

Table 17.3. Insufficient Documentation Errors

Error	Example
Incomplete Progress Notes	Notes are unsigned, undated, missing details
Unauthenticated Medical Records	No provider signature, no supervising signature, illegible signature without a signature log or attestation to identify the signer, an electronic signature without the electronic record protocol or policy that documents the process for electronic signatures
No Documentation of Intent to Order Services and Procedures	Incomplete or missing signed order or progress note describing intent for services to be provided.
Physical Therapy Services	Documentation did not support the plan of care for physical therapy services; NPs signature and date of certification of the plan of care of progress note indicating the NP reviewed and approved the plan of care is required.
Evaluation and Management (E/M) Services (Office Visits Established)	Insufficient or no documentation, incorrect coding of E/M services to support medical necessity and accurate billing of E/M services.
Durable Medical Equipment (hospital bed, glucose monitors, manual wheelchairs)	Requires a valid detailed written order prior to delivery; NP must document a face-to-face encounter examination with a beneficiary in the 6 months prior to the written order for certain items.
Vertebral Augmentation Procedures (VAPs)	Missing signature and date on documentation that supports patients' symptoms, no evidentiary radiographs performed to support medical necessity, insufficient medical record documentation that supports the provider tried conservative medical management but it either failed or was contraindicated, no signed and dated attestation statement if the MD signature was missing or illegible.
CT Scans	Documentation must be sufficient to support medical necessity. Handwritten signature must be legible, include a signature, and if electronic, protocol should be submitted.

Adapted from Medicare Learning Network. (2017). *Complying with medical record documentation requirements*. https://www.cms.gov/Outreach-and-Education/Medicare-Learning-Network-MLN/MLNProducts/Downloads/CERTMedRecDoc-FactSheet-ICN909160Text-Only.pdf

As a novice faculty member, you may have a shorter version of this CV sample, but the categories are the same. The CV tracks the faculty member's development and progression in rank from instructor, assistant professor, and associate professor to professor and throughout the academic career. As more experience and engagement occurs in teaching, scholarship, and service, these will be reflected on the CV. It is also helpful to provide at least three professional references on the CV during the application period, or in the cover letter if one is required.

Title: John Adams, DNP, RN, FNPc
Address: 555 S. 10th Street
Livingston, IL 22222
Contact Information: Home Phone: (344) 524-2222
Cell: (344) 542-1111
Jadams@gmail.com

Educational Background: (Start with most recent educational experience)

University, College/School (date degree conferred), Degree earned (ex:)

Boston College, School of Nursing, June 2016, DNP

Emory University, College of Nursing, May 2010, MSN

University of Illinois, School of Nursing, December 2005, BSN

Licensure/certifications:

2010, APRN License #60655, Georgia

2010, APRN certification, Family Nurse Practitioner, American Association of Nurse

    Practitioners (June, 2010 – December, 2025)

2010, RN License #44407, Georgia (July, 2010 – July, 2022)

2005, RN License #52366, Illinois (2005 – 2010)

Professional memberships

2005 – present. American Association of Nurse Practitioners.

2005 – present. Sigma Theta Tau International Honor Society.

2005 – present. American Nurse Association.

Professional experience:

08/2018 to present. Clinical Coordinator, Davis Family Practice Clinical Services, Atlanta,

GA.

Figure 17.2. Components of Curriculum Vitae (CV). (Please note: Information provided in sample CV is fictitious.)

06/2010 – 08/2018. Family Nurse Practitioner, Advent Health, Atlanta, GA.

Honors & Awards

2017, Nurse of the Year, Georgia State Nurses Association

2005, Inducted into Sigma Theta Tau International, Phi Beta Chapter

Research projects (note funding source is applicable):

- Co-principle investigator: (with N. Jones, PhD), Cultural beliefs of Hispanic women regarding at home childbirth, April 2017 – December 2018, Funding source: Sigma Theta Tau, Gamma Alpha Chapter.

- Principle investigator: Assessing Culture: Pediatric Nurses' Beliefs and Self-reported Practices, December 2014 – June 2016, Doctoral dissertation, Funding source: ABC School of Nursing

Publications--peer-reviewed:

- Adams. J. (2019). Assessing Culture: Family Nurse Practitioners' Beliefs and Self-reported Practices, Journal of Public Health Nursing 14(4), 225-262.

Services proposals & grant

- Principle author: "Case Management in Community-based Clinic" submitted to: Helene Fuld Health Trust, New York, NY, March 2017 Funding requested: $100,000 Proposal request approved, no funded

Professional oral presentations

- Adams, J. Health Promotion Across the Lifespan, Emory University, Atlanta, Georgia, November 14–18, 2018.

- Adams, J. Childhood/Adolescent Obesity, Guest Lecturer, Theoretical Foundations of Family Practice, UCLA School of Nursing, March 7, 20018.

Figure 17.2. Cont'd

Cover Letter

Cover letters are usually requested to accompany a resume or CV. The cover letter introduces the applicant to the hiring agency and connects them to the specific posted position for which they are applying. The applicant should note the position title and number for which they are applying to avoid confusion. In the cover letter, the applicant can match their skills and experiences with those required by the position. The cover letter is an opportunity to stand out among other applicants; information should be well written with no spelling errors and articulate a clear intent to bring something of value to the organization. Cover letters should provide an explanation of why an applicant is interested in the position and what they have to offer to the organization. The letter can also serve to let prospective employers know the applicant is interested in getting to know more about their organization, mission, and goals and that they have something to offer the organization.

Helpful tips to have a cover letter that stands out include: (1) have a strong opening for the letter, give examples of why you would be the best person for the job; (2) provide compelling reasons for hiring you, give examples of how you contributed to your work environment in the past; and (3) keep it short and focused, employers receive multiple applications and will get bored with a lengthy letter. Other tips include: (1) watch the salutation and try to identify an individual rather than a generic "To Whom it may Concern"; (2) pay attention to details such as not addressing a female hiring agent as "Sir"; (3) ask someone else to proofread your document; and (4) follow the standard cover letter format.

Interview Process

Part of the screening process is identifying those candidates who should be interviewed. Some organization pare down the list of candidates to two to three and then schedule a phone interview, leaving the final "in person" interview for the top 1 to 2 candidates. Organizations put resources into developing all aspects of the hiring process including developing/refining the job description, posting the position, screening the applicants, interviewing the applicants, offering the position to the most qualified candidate, negotiating the terms of the contract, and finally hiring the individual.

The interview may be scheduled for 30 to 60 min, and in that time, the members of the search committee can determine who is the best candidate for their organization and the posted position. This puts much pressure on the applicant to determine if they are the best fit for the organization. The interview is where the organization will question applicants further about their cultural fit and work style (Glassdoor Team, 2019). It is important that you prepare for the interview by reviewing the organization's website to determine their goals and mission. Most companies ask similar questions to determine who would best represent them in the community and who would best work with their team.

This is a good time to analyze your nonverbal communication skills to make sure you do not fidget or avoid eye-to-eye contact. Verbal skills should also be in check. Practicing hypothetical answers to the typical questions provided in Box 17.5 can improve your ability to convey answers both grammatically correct and socially acceptable.

BOX 17.5

▶ PREPARING FOR AN INTERVIEW

1. **How to prepare:** Be sure to research the institution. What are their core values? What is the history of the institution? Do they have a publicly available strategic plan? What is their mission statement? What services do they provide? What populations do they serve? Based on this research, develop one or two questions that you might ask in the interview.

2. **What to wear:** Be conservative and neutral. It is always better to be too formal rather than too casual.

3. **What to say:** Plan on being asked to provide details about resume. You should also plan for standard questions such as: "Why are you a good fit?", "What are your strengths?", "What are your weaknesses?". You can also plan on being asked what questions you have, so be sure to have a minimum of one or two questions. Consider asking questions such as "Why is this a good place to work?", "Can you tell more about your organizational culture?", "How will I be evaluated?", or "What are the next steps in the hiring process?". Save questions related to the amount of sick or vacation time for your talk with HR.

4. **How to present yourself:** Interactions with others you meet prior to the interview can be vital. If you have waiting time with administrative staff, be polite and interested. Remember that your body language will speak volumes. Maintain good eye contact; sit straight but keep a calm appearance and smile.

> **BOX 17.6**

> ▶ **INTERVIEW RESOURCES**

> • 10 Best Interview Tips for Job Seekers: https://www.livecareer.com/career/advice/interview/job-interview-tips

> • How to Make a Great Impression: https://www.indeed.com/career-advice/interviewing/job-interview-tips-how-to-make-a-great-impression

> • Interview Tips: https://www.monster.com/career-advice/article/boost-your-interview-iq

> • The Ultimate Interview Guide: https://www.themuse.com/advice/the-ultimate-interview-guide-30-prep-tips-for-job-interview-success

Contract Negotiation

Once the organization decides the applicant they wish to hire, the prospective employee will be contacted and given an offer verbally and in writing. The terms of the employment will typically include the annual salary, title, job responsibilities, and benefits. It is essential to review all aspects of a contract to avoid future problems, and indeed, some will opt to hire an attorney to represent the APN in negotiating the contract. Brown and Dolan (2016) assert that a well-conceived contract offers protection to the employee, and thus, understanding the terms and conditions is essential. Although salary is an obvious point of discussion in contract negotiation, other elements that can be part of a compensation package include health insurance, employer-matched retirement plans, and vacation time. Elston (2017) blogs about less known benefits that are equally valuable:

• Administrative time—considered part of work hours, but ones in which a provider is not scheduled to see patients. While seeing patients is not applicable to educational and administrative APNs, the ability to perform a portion of administrative hours remotely can benefit all nurses.

• Consider asking to work four 10-hour days instead of the traditional 5-day work week for better work-life balance.

• Be sure to check on funds for professional development to defray costs of attending conferences. You will also want to make sure that education days do not require the use of vacation time.

• Make sure you understand the orientation process and what resources you will have as you adapt to your new role.

You should have an understanding of salary ranges that are appropriate to your geographic location. Do not expect to earn a New York City salary in a small, rural town. Checking with friends already working in a similar role can be one way to obtain this information, as can researching online salary websites such as payscale.com or salary.com. Remember that experience will also play a role in the salary that you can command. It also helps to consider the points of the contract from the employer's perspective. A good contract is one that is fair to both parties! Remember that in negotiating your contract, you are setting the stage for your relationship with your employer; collaboration and mutual respect will often yield the best outcome. APRNs who are expected to sign a collaborative practice agreement should review relevant information provided in Chapter 7.

Adding Value to Your Practice

You invested in yourself by continuing your education and advancing your career. Once you have the credentials, you need to consider how to add value to your practice. These are the things that you can do to ensure that you stay abreast of changes and remain marketable. Employers value innovative solutions to challenges that derail positive patient outcomes, staff retention, and high satisfaction rates among patients and staff.

In Their Own Words

Julia Burke, MSN, AWHONN, RNC C-EFM
Clinical Educator-Women's and Children's Department
Clinical Education & Professional Development
Jefferson Health

The key points in understanding my role are ... The healthcare needs of women and children are constantly evolving. As a staff nurse and then clinical nurse educator, my role has always revolved around elevating the care provided to women and children during some of their most joyful as well as their most

(Continued)

frightening times. Our population of laboring mothers, as a whole, has become older, and as a result of that coupled with other factors, there has been an increase in comorbidities which result in complications for them and their children. I was honored to partner with our Chief of Obstetrics to develop a severe hypertension in pregnancy bundle and a post-cesarean section infection prevention bundle to address some of the challenges faced during pregnancy. Our population has also experienced a dramatic increase in opioid use and abuse, which requires medical and psychosocial interventions that are new to many providers of care. In the quest to improve lives, I have spearheaded a project to provide an inclusive, patient-centered, evidenced-based care model for our infants at risk for neonatal abstinence syndrome. As a clinical nurse educator, I am afforded the opportunity to assist with development and implementation of programs to benefit women and children as well as the opportunity to educate other registered nurses as they continue their quest for excellence.

What keeps me coming back every day is … Assisting nurses in their personal quest for excellence, in addition to facilitating new parents in their quest to raise healthy, well-adjusted children through patient education resources, is my passion. By presenting education in an uncomplicated manner while providing encouragement and kindness, I receive the benefit of watching others grow and feel accomplished. Too often, information is presented in a judgmental fashion, causing the learner to miss the benefit of the education. By creating an appropriate learning environment, putting the learner at ease and providing positive reinforcement, I have been blessed with the gift of watching others flourish.

My greatest challenge is … Being patient has always been a challenge when there are so many projects and new ideas swirling in my head. I must do a better job to organize and prioritize ideas and future endeavors. Often, I receive feedback that I expect things to happen too quickly. I jokingly respond that "nurses only have one speed." However, I understand that there are financial and logistical restraints that must be overcome for ideas to come to fruition, irrespective of the excitement and anticipation of providing such benefit to our patient population.

I wish someone had told me … The role of healthcare IT becomes more intertwined with the role of the clinician every day. While clinical work is my passion, healthcare IT is unfortunately an area of weakness for me. It is something that I strive to improve and quickly find a resource who will assist with technical difficulties. Many years ago, when I was first a nurse, I never would have believed that there would be a technological component to almost every aspect of

(Continued)

nursing. While the benefits of the integration of technology in healthcare are numerous, sometimes I feel that we become focused on utilizing the technology at the expense of time at the bedside. I wish someone would have told me to major in nursing but minor in computer literacy.

I need to be a lifelong learner because … Practice changes based on evidenced-based practice are abundant in every specialty area including Women's and Children's nursing. It seems like every day we improve upon one process or another in obstetrics or pediatrics based upon verifiable research. Learning through professional journals, conferences, and literature searches provides an opportunity for me to practice with the benefit of current knowledge, but more importantly helps to fulfill my responsibility as a clinical nurse educator by ensuring that the information provided to staff and patients is current and clinically competent.

Another point to understand is … When I am asked about career choices and potential regrets, I truly cannot think of another profession that would be more fulfilling than nursing. Nursing provides so many unique opportunities that boredom is never an issue. Nurses can work at the bedside, healthcare IT, administration, education, healthcare policy, research, and many other areas once they complete their basic undergraduate degree. We earn an equitable wage, excellent benefits, respect, trust, and the honor of sharing many of life's most important moments with our patients. When it comes to my career choice, I genuinely have an "attitude of gratitude."

Business Plan

A business plan is an essential part of career mapping, and it provides a roadmap from where you are now to where you want to be in 1, 3, and 5 years. The first step is to determine where you want to be in 1, 3, and 5 years. Some nurses may find that shorter (3 months, 1 year, 2 years) or longer (3-, 5-, and 10-year) plans are better suited to their goals. What are the steps that must be achieved to reach these milestones? What are the costs that will be incurred along the way?

Healthcare organizations use business plans to create a new service/agency or add services to an existing agency. For example, nurse practitioners could find there is a service needed by all populations they serve such as mental health services. Teen suicides have become the top priority, and anxiety and depression are rampant across the adult and geriatric populations. A SWOT analysis would help delineate the problem and offer viable solutions. The SWOT analysis requires one to consider the strengths, weaknesses, threats, and opportunities that an individual or organization must face to grow and flourish. Figure 17.3 provides a sample SWOT analysis for a healthcare agency to consider when meeting the needs of their patients and community.

With a SWOT analysis completed, the next step would be to turn the analysis into a decision-making process by determining the overall strategic plan. The plan could be to create an after-hours mental health clinic. Stakeholders should be invited to help develop the plan, as they would provide referrals, possibly participate in treatment, and possibly serve as a referral from the clinic. Stakeholders may include hospital representatives, high school counselors, community outreach representatives, senior day care personnel, nursing home personnel, and family practice physicians and/or APRNs. Stakeholders can also help brainstorm other avenues for educating the community about mental health problems including public service announcements and social media. The use of social medical can help educate the community about common mental health conditions that require medical intervention.

Strengths	Weaknesses
Highly skilled APRN staff History of serving families across the life span High patient satisfaction rates with services Local community agencies are willing to participate	Only two APRNs on staff Office hours limited to 9a.m.–5p.m. Working families must go elsewhere for services after hours No flexibility within current schedule, as days are filled by patients with appointments No time to focus on mental health issues
Threats	**Opportunities**
Patient confidentiality could be risk Prime-Med is considering adding a psyche mental health APRN Insurance coverage for mental health services is limited	The local university has just graduated their first class of Psyche Mental Health NPs APRNs are open to flex time on selected week and weekend days Patients are very interested in extended office hours Local hospital is supportive of such a service, as their ER is inundated with patients with mental health needs Local hospital is allocating funds for a 20-bed mental health unit

Figure 17.3. Example of a SWOT analysis. (Adapted from Profitable Venture. (2019). *How to do SWOT analysis for a hospital or healthcare center*. https://www. profitableventure.com/do-swot-analysis-hospital-healthcare/)

Most importantly, you may want to consider what you do know, and what you do not know. It then becomes a matter of researching to find answers or contracting with someone who can fill in the gaps. Some state college extensions offer help to small businesses to provide their students with learning opportunities. You can also find excellent information at the U.S. Small Business Administration as well as tools for writing a business plan.

Professional Development

In stating, "Let us never consider ourselves finished nurses. We must be learning all of our lives," Florence Nightingale set the expectation that nurses would be engaged in professional development. Currently, professional development is seen as the means of ensuring that a nurse remain competent to practice which is a basic responsibility of our profession. Expectations for professional development can vary by state and may be required to renew one's nursing license. In addition to competency education, professional development can include learning new skills that can allow one to advance their career or to further specialize in an area. These additional skills can increase marketability, ability to transfer to new areas or locations, as well as to increase earning potential.

Learn a Second Language

Given the diversity of the United States, communities across the country are encountering challenges with providing care to non-English-speaking residents. The largest and growing non-White group includes Hispanics. In 2016, the Hispanic and Latinx population numbered 57.5 million, making it the nation's largest ethnic or racial minority (ACS, 2016). The number of Hispanics and Latinx in 2060 is projected to be 119 million, constituting 28.6% of the nation's population (Colby & Ortman, 2015). Over 40 million U.S. residents aged 5 years and older reported they spoke Spanish in 2016, a 133.4% increase since 1990, when Spanish-speaking Hispanics and Latinx numbered 17.3 million (U.S. Census Bureau, 2017).

APNs who speak a second language such as Spanish can help minimize the barriers to care for non-English-speaking patients. Language barriers prevent non-English-speaking patients from effectively communicating with their healthcare providers. Patient satisfaction and positive health outcomes have been linked to effective patient and provider communication and culturally sensitive and linguistically accessible services that are tailored to the unique needs of specific ethnic populations (DBP, 2016). Not only are these services improving patient satisfaction, but they have been proven to be more cost effective. Additionally, communication errors can be minimized when non-English-speaking patients are able to understand their healthcare provider. Communication errors impede the patient's ability to receive an accurate diagnosis, thereby contributing to additional health-related costs and poor health outcomes.

In a 2017 survey, the Centers for Medicare and Medicaid Services (CMS, 2017) found that 60% of the caregivers in their study estimated up to 20% of their patients spoke a language other than English at home, with an additional 9% estimating this number at 41% to 60%. The predominant non-English language spoken was Spanish (82%), followed by Chinese (46%), Arabic (22%), and Vietnamese (21%). Health provider participants were also asked the primary strategy they used to prepare for an encounter with a non-English-speaking patient. Twenty-four percent of participants reported they contract with interpreter services for in-person or telephonic services. Eight percent of providers reported hiring or training multilingual staff, and 16% reported they did not know how communication with non-English-speaking patients was expedited. Only 10% reported they track patient language preferences in medical records. Providers in private practice relied the least on interpretation services, using family members instead to facilitate communication with patients. More than 1,900 of the respondents (41%) reported they used bilingual staff to act as interpreters to meet their patients' language needs.

Learn a New Skill

Many options exist for APNs to enhance their clinical training that can add value to their practice. For example, some facilities offer nurse practitioner residency training programs—sometimes called fellowships—that give nurse practitioners an opportunity to hone their skills. Residencies can be found at federally qualified health centers, Veterans Affairs medical centers, private practices, and hospital systems (Andrews, 2018). Unlike the 3-year residency programs for doctors, fellowships for nurse practitioners are completely voluntary; a residency program is not required for certification or licensure. There is some debate about these residencies; however, they have been found to be beneficial for some nurse practitioners.

Workshops are offered to expand both knowledge and psychomotor skills of APRNs. For example, Advanced Practice Prep (2018) offers workshops for nurse practitioners on a variety of topics such as coding and billing procedures, joint injections, inserting intrauterine devices (IUDs) and contraceptive implants, casting and splinting, suturing, incision and draining, basic biopsies, and cryotherapy. The American Association of Nurse Anesthetists offers pain management workshops and fellowships to advance the CRNA's career in the management of acute or chronic pain (AANA, 2018).

Documentation Requirements of APN/APRNs

Compliance with legal requirements is standard for all registered nurses and APNs. One of the most basic requirements is documentation—regardless of the advanced practice role, all APN/APRNs will need to document planning, actual services provided, and outcomes. All who access the patient's record will be able to see this information and track the patient's outcomes and evaluation of patient care. The medical record is a legal document that all members of the team access to communicate about the patient.

APRN Documentation

APRNs not only document on the patient's medical record their examination findings—what they see (examination), feel (palpation), and hear (interview, auscultation and percussion) during their examination of patients—but they must also provide accurate and supportive medical record documentation for the billing of services rendered. A fact sheet provided by the Medicare Learning Network (MLN) notes insufficient documentation errors that hinder payment for billed services (MLN, 2017). Numerous claims are denied because the reviewer could not determine that the services were provided or that they were medically necessary. These documentation errors are included in Table 17.3.

APN Clinician Documentation

Clinical nurse leaders (CNLs) must comply with legal requirements of documentation when providing direct or indirect patient care services. In leadership aspects of their position, they should document any formal meetings in minutes. This will provide a record of decisions, priorities, and accomplishments that will aid in their annual evaluation by administration. Their job description could be adjusted to better reflect the daily requirements of the CNL and help educate administration about the role. Documenting any changes in patient care outcomes before and after planned initiatives can also provide evidence that the role is an effective addition that adds value to nursing services.

Nurse Educator Documentation

Nurse educators must direct students to document patient care services provided during their clinical rotations. Hospitals may have constraints about allowing students to directly record nursing notes on the patient's electronic medical record (EMR). A member of the nursing staff may be required to personally make the EMR entry for the nursing student. However, nursing students should know the mechanics of patient care charting and relay that to the clinical preceptor.

Documentation of student performance—especially if there are problems—is extremely important for nurse educators. In the clinical setting, nurse educators should note any problems (example: medication errors) so that remediation can be recommended and provided so that further progress can be monitored. Students choose to appeal or grieve their clinical grade if they were never apprised of a problem until the end of the semester. They need time and resources to remediate their errors/mistakes. Documentation provides a track record of what behaviors were observed, what was done about it, and what has happened. Documentation that is shared with the student and signed by the student can be powerful evidence that proper steps were taken to address a student's weakness. However, patient safety is paramount and if the student must be constantly watched and they are unable to perform without the threat of harm to the patient, then more serious steps would need to be taken.

Faculty will also want to document their own performance. Most colleges and universities have a mechanism for promotion and/or tenure. To advance in the faculty role to a higher rank requires evidence that the faculty member is performing at the higher rank in teaching, service, and scholarship. Faculty should collect evidence (e.g., student evaluations, peer evaluations, administrator evaluations, published articles, conference programs with poster entries, CE documents, committee minutes of course review/revisions, letters of appreciation for community service, certificates of service, institutional review board [IRB] approvals) and update their CVs throughout the year to reflect achievements. These documents should be saved until the highest rank is achieved, as faculty share their professional story each time they apply for a promotion.

Nurse Administrator Documentation

Nurse administrators—clinical and educational—oversee their unit's documentation that supports compliance with accreditation standards and the organization's mission and vision. They keep the minutes of meetings; personnel documents; policies and procedures; and administrative staff, nursing staff, and faculty handbooks. They provide documentation to stakeholders, lawyers, and their administrators to verify that the unit complies with accreditation standards, policies, and procedures. Nurse administrators must also keep documentation on those they directly supervise to aid in the annual evaluation of subordinates' performance.

Nurse administrators do not typically provide direct patient care services, but should the situation require this, they too should provide documentation on the patient's EMR. Providing an orientation to new staff and faculty on documentation would be very helpful in assuring that appropriate information is recorded on the EMR and that patient confidentiality is protected.

Engage in Research

APNs can contribute to the improvement of patient-centered outcomes by conducting research that focuses on improving communication between patients and their caregivers to facilitate patients making informed decisions about their care. The National Center for Advancing Translational Sciences (NCATS) defines translational science as "the process of turning observations in the laboratory, clinic, and community into interventions that improve the health of individuals and populations—from diagnostics and therapeutics to medical procedures and behavioral interventions." Outcomes research, as viewed by the Agency for Healthcare Research and Quality (United States Census Bureau, 2017), provides "evidence about benefits, risks, and results of treatments so [clinicians] can make more informed decisions." In aligning practice to outcomes, outcomes research and translational science are key to improving the means to monitor and improve the quality of care.

In understanding the importance of translational science, it is perhaps necessary to first understand that, among all Western nations, the United States ranks 37th in health outcomes despite being the country that spends the greatest amount of money on healthcare (Melnyk & Fineout-Overholt, 2019). Longstanding evidence supports the concept that evidence-based practice improves not only the quality and safety of healthcare (McGinty & Anderson, 2008; Melnyk et al., 2012), but also lends itself to meeting the Triple Aim (Melnyk, 2016). The Triple Aim, first developed by the Institute for Healthcare Improvement, is designed to improve the health of populations, enhance the experience of care for individuals, and reduce the per capita cost of healthcare within the United

States. The Triple Aim serves as a framework for transitioning from a focus on healthcare in general to improving health for individuals and populations. Nursing research leads to better care for patients (Blake, 2016). Bedside nurses need to engage in research and use research to support practice decisions to ensure the adoption of best practices that will improve outcomes.

Patients are interested in knowing what to expect with a given treatment or condition, what options they are offered that will provide the most benefit and reduce harm, how they can improve outcomes that are most important to them, and how clinicians can help them make their best decisions about health and healthcare (PCORI, 2012). Woo and associates (2017) studied the impact APNs on patient outcomes and found that APNs positively influenced quality of care, clinical outcomes, patient satisfaction, and costs of services. Two examples of the impact of APNs on patient outcomes included reduced wait times in the emergency setting and reduced time to treatment (for example, receiving analgesia within 30 minutes). APNs engaging in translation research can track their effect on outcomes as well as mortality rates and length of stay to explore how they directly affect patient care in their unique setting.

In Their Own Words

Joan M. Vitello-Cicciu, PhD, RN, NEA-BC, FAHA, FAAN
Dean of the Graduate School of Nursing
UMASS Medical School
Worcester, MA

Discovering the Role of Scholar Practitioner
The role of the scholar practitioner in my opinion is one who can bridge the gap between academia and practice blending both scholarly pursuits while translating, integrating, and applying knowledge in the practice setting. I did this for 14 years as a critical care clinical nurse specialist, followed by the last 25 years as a nursing administrator/executive both in practice settings and now as a Dean. My vision was to give back to our nursing profession and to improve the health

(Continued)

and well-being of populations. I tried to accomplish this by discovering new knowledge through both my research as well as others, participating in performance improvement activities, and engaging in implementation science. As a Dean I am now participating in developing, evaluating, and improving nursing curricula, student learning, and teaching methodologies. My scholarly pursuits involve translating and applying knowledge through presentations and publications. In this role as a scholar practitioner, I am guided by the following three principles:

- First, share your knowledge and expertise through presentations and publications.
- Second, maintain a spirit of clinical inquiry and intellectual curiosity.
- Third, always explore opportunities to change or enhance practice through innovation.

Sharing Knowledge

As a second-career nurse and as a new graduate in critical care back over 40 years ago, I developed a passion for caring for cardiovascular patients. I joined the Greater Boston Chapter (GBC) of the American Association of Critical Care Nurses (AACN). This network led me to be invited to publish my first article on atherosclerosis obliterans in the *GBC Chronicle*—a monthly newsletter. I then started to accept invitations to speak, and even though it was nerve wracking at first, I continued to develop an expertise as a cardiovascular speaker. I took several continuing education courses on giving presentations to develop more confidence in sharing my knowledge. My continued passion for cardiovascular nursing led me from Massachusetts to Birmingham Alabama to pursue my master's degree in cardiovascular nursing at the University of Alabama in Birmingham (UAB) in the early 1980s. At UAB, my faculty mentor and thesis advisor was a well-known editor of a major nursing journal. She invited me to publish my master's thesis after my graduation in this journal. I can still remember how excited I was to see my name in print! That excitement has remained as I continue to share my knowledge and clinical wisdom.

From being widely published in the early 1980s, I was invited to be a coeditor of the *Journal of Cardiovascular Nursing* from 1985-1995. During this time, I had the opportunity to share other author's knowledge to enhance our discipline of nursing. As one would note, most of my publications and presentations were mostly invitations, and I took advantage and made the time to follow through on each and every one to really become what I envisioned as a scholar practitioner.

(Continued)

Spirit of Inquiry

I was always a curious person. As a clinical nurse and then as a critical care clinical specialist, I was constantly reflecting on my own practice and asking questions like: What am I doing to enhance this patient's outcome? What could I do better? What is the effect of this intervention? What is ritualistic practice? Is what I am doing for patients evidenced based? Basically it was the "so what" that has led me to explore and then publish research on the recalled perceptions of patients receiving pancuronium bromide, the profile of patients requiring epicardial pacing after cardiac surgery, the correlation between the leadership practices and emotional intelligence of nursing leaders, and most recently the key characteristics of nursing leaders of innovation in order to develop the competencies as well as the requisite knowledge, skills, and attitudes that could guide the development of future educational programs. As a Dean, I have now become very interested in innovation as I believe we need more innovation in our nursing practice.

Always Explore Opportunities to Change or Enhance Practice

Last but certainly not least is to always explore opportunities to change or enhance one's practice through innovation. Nursing has been slow to embrace innovation and has varied in the strategic adoption of it. It is imperative that innovation begin with all of us as leaders to cocreate environments that allow for innovative practice to flourish. Taking the reins to initiate and advance innovation is now what I consider my work by challenging the status quo, embracing opportunities and taking risks.

Another Point to Understand is …

My advice for any nurse who wishes to become a scholar practitioner is to:

- Develop a specialty, i.e., an expertise in a specialty practice, or in an intervention, or in a technological advancement.
- Join your professional and specialty organizations and start contributing your expertise through publications or presentations.
- Accept and follow through on any invitation to speak or publish.
- Develop the habit of making the time to write—carve out just a few hours.
- Always question what you are doing for your patients that you are serving and how you can enhance that care.
- Remember that as a scholar practitioner the true benefactor will be your patients and their loved ones!

Refine Leadership Skills and Competencies

This section serves as a reminder of the skills discussed in the text that help build leadership in the advanced practice role that will be assumed upon graduation. Not only must leaders continue to engage in educational activities that increase knowledge, but leadership skills should continue to be honed throughout one's career.

Translational Science to Improve Patient Outcomes

The competency of translational science is presented in Chapter 3. APNs can contribute to the improvement of patient centered outcomes by conducting research that focuses on improving communication between patients and their caregivers to facilitate patients making informed decisions about their care. The National Center for Advancing Translational Sciences (NCATS), defines **translational science** as "the process of turning observations in the laboratory, clinic, and community into interventions that improve the health of individuals and populations—from diagnostics and therapeutics to medical procedures and behavioral interventions." Outcomes research, as viewed by the Agency for Healthcare Research and Quality (AHRQ, 2016) provides "evidence about benefits, risks, and results of treatments so [clinicians] can make more informed decisions." In aligning practice to outcomes, outcomes research and translational science are key in improving the means to monitor and improve the quality of care.

In understanding the importance of translational science, it is perhaps necessary to first understand that, among all Western nations, the United States ranks 37th in health outcomes despite being the country that spends the greatest amount of money on healthcare (Melnyk, 2016). Long-standing evidence supports the concept that evidence-based practice improves not only the quality and safety of healthcare (McGinty & Anderson, 2008; Melnyk et al., 2012), but also lends itself to meeting the **Triple Aim** (Melnyk, 2016). The Triple Aim, first developed by the Institute for Healthcare Improvement, is designed to improve the health of populations, enhance the experience of care for individuals, and reduce the per capita cost of healthcare within the United States. The Triple Aim serves as a framework for transitioning from a focus on healthcare in general to improving health for individuals and populations. Nursing research leads to better care for patients (Blake, 2016). Bedside nurses need to engage in research and use research to support practice decisions to ensure the adoption of best practices that will improve outcomes.

Patients are interested in knowing what to expect with a given treatment or condition, what options they are offered that will provide the most benefit and reduce harm, how they can improve their outcomes that are of most importance to them, and how clinicians can help them make their best decisions about health and healthcare (PCORI, 2012). Woo and associates (2017) studied the impact of APNs on patient outcomes and found that APNs positively influenced quality of care, clinical outcomes, patient satisfaction, and costs of services. Two examples of the impact of APNs on patient outcomes included reduced wait times in the emergency setting and reduced time to treatment (for example, receiving analgesia within 30 min). APNs engaging in translation research can track their effect on outcomes as well as mortality rates and length of stay to explore how they directly affect patient care in their unique setting.

Improve Quality and Safety

Improving quality and safety competency, as presented in Chapter 3, demonstrates the strong link between improving patient outcomes and the application of translational science. Key to improving patient, staff, or student outcomes is the importance of measurement. To announce quality and safety have been improved in one's practice setting, measurements should be in place (patient's length of stay, patient satisfaction ratings, or staff/student performance on a pretest). The ability to measure the "before" of an intervention with the "after" allows for quantitative results that can be conveyed to others. This dissemination of findings creates evidence-based findings for the profession.

As an APN/APRN there will be opportunities to improve patient and student outcomes by translating data-based findings into one's daily practice. Many times, the solutions to measurements that fall below the acceptable level can be found by reviewing the literature to find similar situations where other organizations were able to make improvements by translating science. Additionally, there are numerous professional journals that provide examples in one's area of expertise. Professional conferences and workshops also provide updated findings and usually host poster sessions where attendees can gain ideas about resources and references from the researchers themselves. Professional organizations also provide CE offerings on specific topics that are challenging to manage in one's practice.

Key to improving outcomes is the ability to continually survey the landscape of the work environment to find where small disruptions or miscommunications prevent the achievement of desired outcomes. These small disruptions can lead to bigger problems if not addressed. With confidence, the bigger problems can be addressed—and with others in the work environment.

Embrace Innovation

The Agency for Healthcare Research and Quality (AHRQ) defined innovation as a new way of doing things to improve healthcare delivery (2008). Innovations can be new products or services or processes, systems, or business models. To determine the appropriateness of an innovation one should ask four key questions: (1) Does the innovation fit? (2) Should we do it here? (3) Can we do it here? And (4) How will we do it here? In many occasions, the innovations are meant to address the Triple Aim by improving patient experience of care, improving the health of populations, reducing the cost of healthcare (Institute for Healthcare Improvement, 2020). Several of the change scenarios in Chapter 13 provide examples of changes that addressed one or more aspects of the Triple Aim.

Just as necessity has been called the mother of invention, disruptions have been credited with prompting innovations. The disruptive innovation theory is credited with explaining the process by which complicated, expensive products and services are transformed into simple, affordable ones (Christensen et al., 2015). The challenge is to create sustaining innovations—not disruptive innovations that are limited and temporary. Consumers consider disruptive innovations as inferior products that are less expensive but also lack the desired quality. With sustained innovations, consumers wait until quality can be established and then adopt the new product. Disruptions in healthcare delivery services require healthcare providers to quickly respond with innovative practices that minimize the barriers to access and the rising costs of goods and services.

The recent COVID-19 virus disrupted almost every segment of life with the need for social distancing. Educational institutions had to quickly become innovative with technology to avoid disrupting the learning process for students at all stages of their educational journey. Healthcare providers also had to become innovative to maintain contact with their patients—particularly the chronic patients who needed weekly to monthly monitoring.

Telehealth

The recent coronavirus pandemic demonstrated just how important the use of technology can be in maintain patient safety and health. Telehealth provides patients access to care service through technological aids such as computers and cellphones. States that rely heavily on telehealth, such as California, tout its benefits that increase access to healthcare, improve health outcomes, reduce healthcare costs, assist with the maldistribution of healthcare providers, support clinical programs, and improve support to patients and families (CDC, 2020). Organizational productivity is also maintained as patients can avoid absences from work when they can remotely access health services. Home monitoring of chronic diseases in the California network has also been found to reduce hospital visits by as much as 50% with daily monitoring.

Telehealth is the "utilization of electronic information and telecommunications technologies to support and promote long-distance clinical healthcare, patient and professional health education, public health and health administration. Telehealth is not a service, but a way to improve patient care and physical education. Telehealth expands beyond telemedicine, to cover non-clinical events like appointment scheduling, continuing medical education, and physician training" (HealthIT.gov, 2017). Telehealth applications include live (asynchronous) videoconferencing, remote patient monitoring, and mobile health.

Of concern for some practices has been the adherence to Health Insurance Portability and Accountability Act (HIPAA) standards. The U.S. Department of Health and Human Services (2020) has addressed this with a notification that during the COVID-19 emergency, healthcare providers subject to HIPAA rules may seek to communicate with patients and provide telehealth during the COVID-19 nationwide public health emergency. During nonpandemic times, practices have relied on HIPAA-compliant companies to assist with an organization's compliance with HIPAA rules.

Considering the use of telehealth could be an innovative approach to capturing clients who are challenged to make 9 a.m. to 5 p.m. office appointments, and with chronic patients who have difficulties making frequent office visits. Telehealth is an innovative approach that should be considered in situations where patient outcomes could be improved if only patients could have frequent monitoring and access to providers.

Influence Change and Innovation

As leadership skills are developed consider the need to create a work environment that fosters innovation. A work environment that encourages innovation provides staff with opportunities to discuss possible innovations while weighing the risks and benefits (Boston-Fleischhauer, 2016). This provides intellectual stimulation to staff members and fosters creativity in a safe, accepting environment.

Consider the development of leadership traits that foster innovation. Resilience has been identified as a necessary component for the transformational leader to learn and guide change among their staff members (Tyckowski et al., 2015). This sense of resiliency keeps leaders from avoiding failure or seeing it as a negative event instead of an opportunity to learn.

Promoting change and innovation helps drive policies and processes that improve healthcare services and make them more affordable for consumers. Be inquisitive about the financial costs of goods and services in your practice. Explore if there are alternative methods for achieving positive patient outcomes while decreasing costs. If change is overwhelming, then consider how you can make small changes for a greater impact. Eventually change and innovation will solicit positive responses that will benefit your professional growth and contribute to improvements in healthcare services for your patient population.

Give Back

Giving back is the means of devoting some of your time to allow others to experience opportunities that you may have had as you began your career. By giving back to our profession, we contribute to maintaining our standards of care and we have an influence on attitudes toward patient care. While giving back can include serving on the board of a professional organization, it also includes serving as a mentor or preceptor for others learning or entering a nursing role.

Serve as a Mentor

The transition from RN to APN can be very stressful. Wendling (2015) reports that NPs found the shift from provider of care to prescriber of care to be a daunting challenge. Novice NPs reported a mental shift with their new role, as they learned new ways of problem-solving, learning new skills, while disconnecting from their former roles as RNs. Fenwick et al. (2015) also found the newly graduate nurse midwives reported their workloads were "diabolical and unmanageable." Social support provided by mentors can ease the stress of the transition process, especially if the new APN feels supported at work (Robeano et al., 2019). The social support of an experienced APN can help novice APNs gain confidence in their new roles and ease the transition from RN to APN.

One of the most important contributions nurses can make to the profession is serving as a mentor (Johnson, 2016). Those who are mentored were found to be more satisfied with their careers, experienced more promotions and higher income, expressed more commitment to the organization, and were more likely to serve as mentors themselves (Johnson, 2014). Many newly hired APNs will have an opportunity to work with a mentor as they hone their skill in their chosen role. Mentoring is seen as a beneficial endeavor by both mentors and mentees, as well as their clients (Raftery, 2015). There are some agencies/institutes that assign new APNs a mentor, providing a mentor who invests time and energy in the new hire as they adapt to their new role.

Reh (2017) asserts that learning to serve as a mentor is a personal and professional development experience. The experience as a mentor not only helps the mentee (the person being mentored), but also forces the mentor to evaluate and reflect on their own action and behaviors over time. Newly graduated APNs may have limited experience in their advanced role, but they may have much experience as an RN. These RN-related experiences could provide opportunities for the APN to serve as a mentor to other healthcare personnel in the agency/institution.

Serve as a Preceptor

As APNs gain experience in their advanced role they should consider serving as a clinical preceptor for APN students. Universities/colleges that offer advanced nursing degrees rely heavily on clinical preceptors to support students' educational requirements. The American Association of Nurse Practitioners (AANP) encourages their members to serve as clinical preceptors and provides a tool kit for clinical preceptors. The tool kit can be found at: https://www.aanp.org/images/documents/education/PreceptorToolkit.pdf.

Resources for Cover Letters

- https://exclusive-executive-resumes.com/cover-letters/wowfactorcoverletter/

www.macleans.ca/work/jobs/how-to-write-cover-letters-that-stand-out/

Job Postings

aacnnursing.org/Career-Center/Faculty-Vacancies
advancedpractice.com
chroniclevitae.com/jobs/position_types/1
Federalregister.gov/documents/advanced-practice-registered-nurses
Glassdoor.com/index.htm
iHireMidLevelPractitioners.com
iHireNursing.com
Indeed.com
Jobopenings.monster.com

Web Resources

Agency for Healthcare Research and Quality: https://www.ahrq.gov/
The Small Business Toolkit: https://www.bplans.com/business-tools/
U.S. Small Business Administration: https://www.sba.gov/
Top Five Essentials for Outcomes Improvement: https://www.healthcatalyst.com/
Outcomes-Improvement-Five-Essentials
The Muse: https://www.themuse.com/
2018 Core Set of Adult Health Care Quality Measures for Medicaid: https://www.medicaid.gov/
medicaid/quality-of-care/downloads/performance-measurement/2018-adult-core-set.pdf
42 Resume Dos and Don'ts Every Job Seeker Should Know: https://www.themuse.com/
advice/42-resume-dos-and-donts-every-job-seeker-should-know

Summary

Chapter 17 has a broad focus, covering diverse topics related to professionalism in your nursing role. At the start of your career, creating cover letters and a resume or curriculum vitae showcases your abilities, which will be expanded as additional skills are added or employment changes occur. The next step in securing a first position is adequate preparation for a job interview. Once you land a job offer, carefully approach contract negotiation. This requires a good understanding of local salary conditions and differences between base pay and benefits. APRN positions may include a collaborative practice agreement. Details about these agreements are included in Chapter 7.

Once you become acclimated to your new role, you will begin development from novice to expert. APN/APRNs must continue to engage in professional development. Professional development is important in ensuring that your practice standards remain current, reflecting best practice and evolving evidence. Professional development can also be used to add value to your practice through the addition of new clinical/educational/administrative skills and other factors that can increase your marketability. Additionally, you will want to engage in outcomes research, or in translating research into standards for best practices that improve the health of individuals and populations.

Finally, the importance of giving back to your profession is discussed. As you move toward becoming an expert in your area, consider serving as a mentor or preceptor. These roles are vital in developing the next generation of nurses.

Chapter Highlights

- Preparing for one's first advanced practice role requires much consideration in order to identify a good match with career goals, role responsibilities, level of autonomy, and desired salary.
- Seeking an APN or APRN position requires an impressive cover letter and resume or CV along with adequate preparation for the interview process.
- Contract negotiations can be helpful in securing desirable salary, schedule, learning opportunities, work environment, and orientation.
- APNs and APRNs can add value to their position including creating a business plan, learning a second language, or participating in research or evidence-based projects that improve patient care outcomes.
- Developing one's leadership skills can lead to innovation and change that improves healthcare services and reduces costs.
- Serving as a mentor to others or a preceptor to APN and APRN students are opportunities to give back to the profession.

References

AANA. (2018). *AANA pain management resources.* https://www.aana.com/practice/practice-management/pain-management

Advanced Practice Prep. (2018). *Skills workshops and procedures courses.* www.advancedpractice-prep.net

Agency for Healthcare Research and Quality (American Community Survey (ACS). (2016). *Facts for features: Hispanic heritage month 2017.* https://www.census.gov/newsroom/facts-for-features/2017/hispanic-heritage.html

Andrews, A. (2018). *More nurse practitioners are pursuing residency training to hone skills.* www.npr.org/sections/health-shots/2018/07/03/624721718/more-nurse-practitioners-are-pursuing-residency-training-to-hone-skills

Blake, N. T. (2016). *Yes, nurses do research, and it's improving patient care.* https://www.elsevier.com/connect/yes-nurses-do-research-and-it-is-improving-patient-care

Boston-Fleischhauer, C. (2016). Beyond making the case: Creating the space for innovation. *Journal of Nursing Administration, 46*(6), 295–296.

Brown, L. A., & Dolan, C. (2016). Employment contract basics for the nurse practitioner. *The Journal for Nurse Practitioners, 12*(2), e45–e51. https://doi.org/10.1016/j.nurpra.2015.11.026

Centers for Disease Control (CDC). (2020). *Using telehealth to expand access to essential health services during the COVID-19 pandemic.* https://www.cdc.gov/coronavirus/2019-ncov/hcp/telehealth.html

Centers for Medicare & Medicaid Services (CMS). (2017). *How healthcare providers meet patient language needs: Highlights of a Medscape provider survey.* https://www.cms.gov/About-CMS/Agency-Information/OMH/Downloads/Issue-Brief-How-Healthcare-Providers-Meet-Patient-Language-Needs.pdf

Colby, S. L., & Ortman, J. L. (2015). *Projections of the size and composition of the U.S. population: 2014 – 2060.* https://www.census.gov/content/dam/Census/library/publications/2015/demo/p25-1143.pdf

Christensen, C. M., Raynor, M. E., & McDonald, R. (2015). What is disruptive innovation? *Harvard Business Review, 93*(12), 44–53. https://hbr.org/2015/12/what-is-disruptive-innovation

Diversity Best Practices. (2016). *The state of diversity & inclusion in the healthcare industry part 1: Industry overview.* https://www.diversitybestpractices.com/sites/diversitybestpractices.com/files/attachments/2017/10/healthcare_industry_report_overview.pdf

Elston, M. (2017). *7 Benefits every nurse practitioner should negotiate for.* Medelita Blog site.

Fenwick, J., Hammond, A., Raymond, J., Smith, R., Gray, J., Foureur, M., Homer, C., & Symon, A. (2015). Surviving, not thriving: A qualitative study of newly qualified midwives' experience of their transition to practice. *Journal of Clinical Nursing, 21*(13–14), 2054–2063.

Glassdoor Team. (2019). *How to improve your interview process.* https://www.glassdoor.com/employers/blog/improve-interview-process/

HIPAA Journal. (2020). *HIPAA compliance and covid-19 coronavirus.* https://www.hipaajournal.com/hipaa-compliance-and-covid-19-coronavirus/

Institute for Healthcare Improvement. (2020). *Triple aim for populations.* http://www.ihi.org/Topics/TripleAim/Pages/Overview.aspx

Johnson, W. B. (2014). Mentoring in psychology education and training: A mentoring relationship continuum model. In W. B. Johnson & N. J. Kaslow (Eds.), *The Oxford handbook of education and training in professional psychology* (pp. 272–290). Oxford University Press.

Johnson, W. B. (2016). *On being a mentor: A guide for higher education faculty.* Taylor and Francis.

McGinty, J., & Anderson, G. (2008). Predictors of physician compliance with American Heart Association guidelines for acute myocardial infarction. *Critical Care Nursing Quarterly, 31*(2), 161–172. https://pubmed.ncbi.nlm.nih.gov/18360146/

Medical Learning Network (MLN). (2017). *Complying with medical record documentation requirements.* https://www.cms.gov/Outreach-and-Education/Medicare-Learning-Network-MLN/MLNProducts/Downloads/CERTMedRecDoc-FactSheet-ICN909160.pdf

Melnyk, B. M., & Fineout-Overholt, E. (2019). *Evidence-based practice in nursing & healthcare: A guide to best practice* (4th ed.). Wolters Kluwer.

Melnyk, B. M., Fineout-Overholt, E., Gallagher-Ford, L., & Kaplan, L. (2012). The state of evidence-based practice in US nurses: Critical implications for nurse leaders and educators. *Journal Nursing Administration, 24*(9), 410–417. https://pubmed.ncbi.nlm.nih.gov/22922750/

Patient Centered Outcomes Research Institute. (2012). *Patient-centered outcomes research.* https://www.pcori.org/research-results/patient-centered-outcomes-research

Raftery, C. (2015). Mentoring: Supporting NP transition to practice. *The Journal for Nurse Practitioners, 11*(5), 560. https://www.npjournal.org/article/S1555-4155(15)00374-8/fulltext

Reh, J. (2017). *Mentoring and coaching in the workplace.* www.thebalancecareers.com/developing-and-serving-as-a-mentor-in-today's-workplace-2275287

Robeano, K., Delong, D., & Taylor, H. A. (2019). Optimizing transitional support for novice nurse practitioners. *Nurse Leader, 17*(4), 303–307.

Tyckowski, B., Vandenhouten, C. L., Reilly, J. R., Bansal, G., Kubsch, S., & Jakkola, R. (2015). Emotional intelligence (EI) and nursing leadership styles among nurse managers. *Nursing Administration Quarterly, 39*, 172–180.

United States Census Bureau. (2017). *Facts for features: Hispanic heritage month 2017.* https://www.census.gov/newsroom/facts-for-features/2017/hispanic-heritage.html

U.S. Census Bureau. (2017). *American community survey.* https://factfinder.census.gov/faces/tableservices/jsf/pages/productview.xhtml?pid=ACS_17_1YR_S1601&prodType=table

Wendling, T. (2015). *Transitioning novice nurse practitioners into practice through a blended mentoring program.* Sigma 26th international nursing research congress, July 23-27, 2015 in San Juan, Puerto Rico. https://stti.confex.com/stti/congrs15/webprogram/Peper72433.html

Woo, B., Lee, J., & Tam, W. (2017). *The impact of the advanced practice nursing role on quality of care, clinical outcomes, patient satisfaction, and cost in the emergency and critical care settings: A systematic review.* https://human-resources-health.biomedcentral.com/articles/10.1186/s12960-017-0237-9

Overview of MSN/DNP Essentials and APRN Competencies

MSN Essentials (AACN, 2011)	DNP Essentials (AACN, 2006)	CRNA (COA, 2018)	CNM (ACNM, 2014)	CNS (NACNS, 2018)	NP (NONPF, 2017)
Background for practice from science and humanities	Scientific underpinnings for practice	Science, physiology, pharmacology, and chemistry curricular requirements	Midwifery fundamentals	Patient/direct care sphere	Scientific foundation competencies
Clinical prevention and population health for improving health	Clinical prevention and population health for improving health	Ethical and multicultural curricular requirements	Midwifery care of women and care of the newborn; hallmarks of midwifery	Nursing practice sphere	Independent practice competencies
Health policy and advocacy	Healthcare policy for advocacy in healthcare	Health policy and healthcare finance curricular requirements	Professional responsibilities	Organization/systems sphere	Policy competencies
Informatics and healthcare technologies	Information systems technology and patient care technology for the improvement and transformation of healthcare	Informatics curricular requirements	Knowledge of information systems and other technologies to improve the quality and safety of healthcare	Organization/systems sphere	Technology and information literacy competencies

MSN Essentials (AACN, 2011)	DNP Essentials (AACN, 2006)	CRNA (COA, 2018)	CNM (ACNM, 2014)	CNS (NACNS, 2018)	NP (NONPF, 2017)
Interprofessional collaboration for improving patient and population health outcomes	Interprofessional collaboration for improving patient and population health outcomes	Interpersonal communication and collaboration curricular requirements	Collaboration with other members of the interprofessional healthcare team (hallmarks of midwifery)	Nursing practice sphere	Health delivery system competencies
Organizational and systems leadership	Organizational and systems leadership for quality improvement and systems thinking	Leadership and management curricular requirements	Development of leadership skills; midwifery management process	Organization/ systems sphere	Leadership competencies
Quality improvement and safety		Analysis of strategies to improve patient outcomes and quality of care curricular requirements	Midwifery management process	Organization/ systems sphere	Quality competencies
Translating and integrating scholarship into practice	Clinical scholarship and analytical methods	Evidence-based principles and science-based theory curricular requirements	Ability to evaluate, apply, interpret, and collaborate in research	Organization/ systems sphere	Practice inquiry competencies
Master's level nursing practice	Advanced nursing practice	Standards I through XI	Professional standards of practice	Patient/direct care sphere	Independent practice competencies
		Accountability, ethical and multicultural curricular requirements	Advocacy for informed choice, shared decision-making, and the right to self-determination	Nursing practice sphere; organization/ systems sphere	Ethical competencies

APRN, advanced practice registered nurse; CNM, certified nurse midwife; CNS, clinical nurse specialist; CRNA, certified registered nurse anesthetist; DNP, Doctorate of Nursing Practice; MSN, Master of Science in Nursing; NP, nurse practitioner.

Appendix B

Overview of MSN/DNP Essentials and Advanced Practice Role Competencies

MSN Essentials (AACN, 2011)	DNP Essentials (AACN, 2006)	Administrator (AONL, 2015)	CNL (AACN, 2013)	Educator (NLN, 2018)
Background for practice from science and humanities	Scientific underpinnings for practice	Foundational thinking skills	Essential 1: Background for practice from science and humanities	
Clinical prevention and population health for improving health	Clinical prevention and population health for improving health	Patient safety; outcome measurement and research	Essential 8: Clinical prevention and population health for improving health	Participates in Curriculum design and evaluation of program outcomes
		Professionalism		Facilitates learner development and socialization
Health policy and advocacy	Healthcare policy for advocacy in healthcare	Healthcare economics and policy; advocacy	Essential 6: Health policy and advocacy	Functions as a change agent and leader; functions within the educational environment
Informatics and healthcare technologies	Information systems technology and patient care technology for the improvement and transformation of healthcare	Information management and technology	Essential 5: Informatics and healthcare technology	

MSN Essentials (AACN, 2011)	DNP Essentials (AACN, 2006)	Administrator (AONL, 2015)	CNL (AACN, 2013)	Educator (NLN, 2018)
Interprofessional collaboration for improving patient and population health outcomes	Interprofessional collaboration for improving patient and population health outcomes	Communication and relationship building; change management	Essential 7: Interprofessional collaboration for improving patient and population health outcomes	
Organizational and systems leadership	Organizational and systems leadership for quality improvement and systems thinking	Knowledge of the healthcare environment; leadership	Essential 2: Organizational and systems leadership	Functions within the educational environment
Quality improvement and safety		Performance improvement/ metrics; risk management	Essential 3: Quality improvement and safety	Pursue continuous quality improve- ments in the nurse educator role
Translating and integrating scholarship into practice	Clinical scholarship and analytical methods	Evidence-based practice/out- come mea- surement and research	Essential 4: Translating and integrating scholarship into practice	Engages in scholarship
Master's level nursing practice	Advanced nursing practice	Business skills and leadership	Essential 9: Master's- level nursing practice	Facilitates learning; participates in curriculum design and evaluation of program outcomes; uses assessment and evaluation strategies

CNL, clinical nurse leader; DNP, Doctorate of Nursing Practice; MSN, Master of Science in Nursing.

Index

Note: Page numbers followed by "f" indicate figures, "t" indicate tables, and "b" indicate boxes.

CCS0121